NEUROLOGY OF THE OCULAR MUSCLES

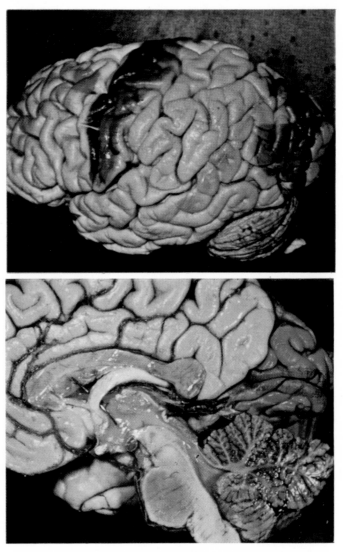

Formalin fixed brain which has been tinted to show pertinent structures on lateral surface of cerebrum (*upper picture*) and on medial surface of cerebrum, brain stem, and cerebellum (*lower picture*).

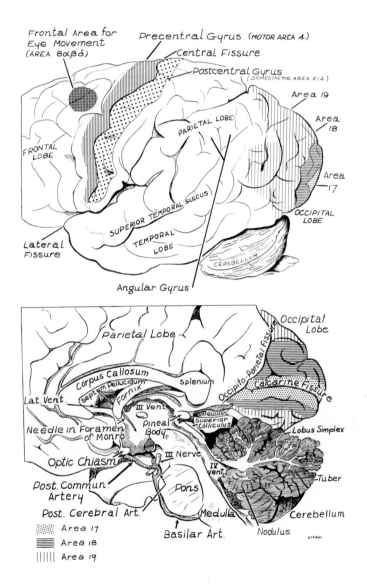

Frontal Area for Eye Movement (AREA 8αβδ)

Precentral Gyrus (MOTOR AREA 4)

Central Fissure

Postcentral Gyrus (SOMESTHETIC AREA 3,1,2)

Area 19

Area 18

Area 17

FRONTAL LOBE

PARIETAL LOBE

OCCIPITAL LOBE

SUPERIOR TEMPORAL SULCUS

TEMPORAL LOBE

CEREBELLUM

Lateral Fissure

Angular Gyrus

Parietal Lobe

Occipital Lobe

Corpus Callosum

Septum Pellucidum

Splenium

Occipito-Parietal Fissure

Calcarine Fissure

Lat. Vent.

Fornix

III Vent.

Needle in Foramen of Monro

Pineal Body

Superior Colliculus

Lobus Simplex

Optic Chiasm

III Nerve

IV Vent.

Tuber

Post. Commun. Artery

Pons

Post. Cerebral Art.

Medulla

Cerebellum

Nodulus

Basilar Art.

∷ Area 17

≡ Area 18

||||| Area 19

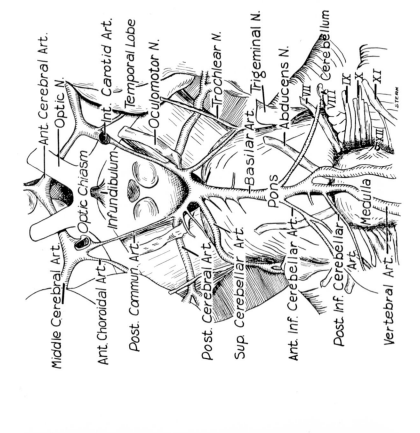

Base of brain illustrating arteries, nerves, and associated structures. The specimen was a normal brain removed at autopsy. It was not injected or otherwise treated.

Ant. Cerebral Art.

Optic N.

Int. Carotid Art.

Temporal Lobe

Oculomotor N.

Trochlear N.

Trigeminal N.

Cerebellum

VII

VIII

IX

X

XI

Basilar Art.

Abducens N.

STERN

XII

Pons

Middle Cerebral Art.

Optic Chiasm

Infundibulum

Post. Cerebral Art.

Sup. Cerebellar Art.

Ant. Inf. Cerebellar Art.

Medulla

Post. Inf. Cerebellar Art.

Vertebral Art.

Ant. Choroidal Art.

Post. Commun. Art.

Neurology

of the

Ocular Muscles

SECOND EDITION

By

DAVID G. COGAN, M.D.

Professor of Ophthalmology
Harvard Medical School
Director, Howe Laboratory of Ophthalmology
Boston, Massachusetts

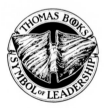

CHARLES C THOMAS · PUBLISHER
Springfield · Illinois · U.S.A.

CHARLES C THOMAS · PUBLISHER
BANNERSTONE HOUSE
301-327 East Lawrence Avenue, Springfield, Illinois, U.S.A.

Published simultaneously in the British Commonwealth of Nations by
BLACKWELL SCIENTIFIC PUBLICATIONS, LTD., OXFORD, ENGLAND

Published simultaneously in Canada by
THE RYERSON PRESS, TORONTO

Library of Congress Catalog Card Number: 56-9107

Printed in the United States of America

PREFACE TO SECOND EDITION

REVISION of a text is questionable practice, for the continuous and the orderly presentation is often lost with subsequent additions and graftings. Moreover, additions are so much easier to make than deletions that the original text must eventually lose its brevity. As anyone who has attempted to write must know, the problem is not what to include but what not to include; hence the increase in volume.

Thus, this second edition is presented with some misgiving. However, the recent upswing of interest in neuro-ophthalmology among students, the gracious insistence of the publisher, and valuable suggestions from numerous correspondents left little alternative. It is only hoped that an awareness of some of the pitfalls of revision may have mitigated their evils.

Aside from additions to the text compounded from the recent literature and from the author's experience, the organization has been considerably changed in places where this seemed expedient. Thus Chapter I of the first edition has been rewritten to emphasize the myopathies and re-set as Chapter III of the second edition. The section on the cerebellum has also been expanded to cover the recent advances in the recognition of anatomic and functional localization in this structure and the ocular motor counterparts of cerebellar disease. Internuclear ophthalmoplegia has been treated in considerably more detail in view of its importance as the major ocular motor manifestation of multiple sclerosis and in view of the recognition of a unilateral variety that is caused by vascular disease. A short section has been added on the enigmatic phenomenon of skew deviation.

An energetic attempt has been made to effect judicious deletions, but this was found difficult and only minor trimmings were accomplished. A section on the accommodative mechanism was again purposely omitted for, although accommodation has interesting physiologic implications and considerable ophthalmologic importance, it has only minor application in the neurologic field to which this little book is dedicated.

As in the original text the author has taken full liberty in the selection of subjects to be emphasized or to be omitted. In this there is inevitably a strong personal bias and lopsided reference to the author's interests and experiences. Only by this indulgence could the book escape being an uncritical and impersonal catalogue. Whenever pertinent, the work of others is cited so far as it is known to the author, and whenever controversial opinions are given, the source of information is presented by reference numbers.

PREFACE TO FIRST EDITION

THIS TEXT, an outgrowth of several years' postgraduate teaching in ophthalmology, attempts to correlate the clinical manifestations of disturbances of the ocular motor system with its neuroanatomic and neurophysiologic architecture. The familiar truism to the effect that clinical findings can be properly interpreted only with a knowledge of anatomic structures and physiologic principles is nowhere more cogent than in the case of the ocular muscles. The control of normal ocular movements is far from simple. Not only is each eye motivated by six extraocular muscles, each of which is acted upon by stimuli arising from numerous sources and traversing different pathways, but the two eyes are precisely coordinated in their movements. Furthermore, the action of the extraocular muscle is coordinated with the muscles within the eye, with those of the lids, and with those controlling head movements. Disease processes add a further host of variables all of which can add up to a confusing picture for the clinician who is expected to arrive at an adequate diagnosis after a relatively brief examination. This text aims to resolve this confusion, in some measure, by presenting the physiologic and anatomic bases for the ocular motor disturbances as indissociable from the clinical manifestation.

The data in this text are arranged according to objective signs rather than disease entities. More than most specialties, neuro-ophthalmology is concerned primarily with localization of disease and only secondarily with the nature of the underlying process. This placing of emphasis on the topographic analysis of signs and symptoms is contrary to the usual approach of the clinician. Charged with the responsibility of therapy, the latter customarily aims to arrive at an etiologic diagnosis as rapidly as possible. As a result, texts in medicine are arranged according to disease entities rather than signs and symptoms. But the clinical manifestations of disturbances of the ocular motor system vary more with the site of the lesion than with the nature of the lesion and the neuro-ophthalmologist is, more often than not, charged with the respon-

ix

sibility of localization only. The chapters in this text are therefore so arranged as to emphasize analysis of localizing signs and symptoms, and little or no space is give to treatment.

The extent to which a systematic presentation is possible on this basis must of course depend on the information available. In correlating the data one finds oneself in the ambiguous position of simplifying in the interests of lucidity and yet being critical of simplification in such a complex field as the ocular motor system. Accordingly, I have attempted to follow a course midway between dogmatism and nihilism, avoiding on the one hand a simplification that is unjustified by the data and on the other hand a skepticism that maintains that because some of our concepts will have to be altered in the future, all our present conclusions are therefore invalid. An effort has been made to set forth fairly the state of present knowledge of the clinical physiology of the ocular motor system and the conclusions that can be safely drawn from the facts available at the present time.

It is hoped that this text will be useful to ophthalmologists and neurologists and, above all, to those students of whatever branch or degree of training who are being inducted into this specialty within a specialty and who wish to have a comprehensive guide and outline at their command.

ACKNOWLEDGMENTS FOR SECOND EDITION

For the revision, as for the original text, my indebtedness is widespread and much of it indirect. Since the revision is largely based on the clinical material which I have had occasion to see and to study, my first indebtedness is to the patients who have tolerated examinations that often served the examiner's interests more than their own. I similarly have collective indebtedness to a group of loyal and thoughtful colleagues who have provided me with a wealth of "interesting cases" to study.

For more specific acts of service in the revision of this book, I have particular debts. Messrs. Charles C Thomas and Payne Thomas, as publishers, have facilitated my part in an exemplary manner; it has been a pleasure to work with them. Dr. David D. Donaldson provided the colored photographs for the Frontispiece and Dr. Sheldon D. Stern made the corresponding black and white drawings. The excellence of these preparations speak for themselves. For the bibliography, typing, proofreading, and endless details, I have had the assistance of Mr. Charles Snyder, Dr. Harvey A. Lincoff, Misses Therese Ecker, Sheila Gray, and Mary North.

D. G. C.

ACKNOWLEDGMENTS FOR
FIRST EDITION

THE INSPIRATION for writing this book is due in large measure to the students who patiently sat through the formative lectures. For their apparent interest and many helpful suggestions I am heavily indebted. The substance of the book has been taken from the available literature and compounded with the experience generously called the author's but in reality the experience of many persons, recognized and unrecognized, who have molded his opinion. The substance taken from the literature I have attempted to acknowledge by appropriate references throughout the text; the help of many who have made equivalent, albeit less tangible, contributions that cannot be directly referred to in the text, I can only acknowledge collectively but nonetheless with deep personal feeling.

For participating in the preparation of the monograph, I have certain specific obligations: to Dr. Mark Singer of the Department of Anatomy at the Harvard Medical School for several cross sections of the normal midbrain; to Dr. Charles Kubik of the Department of Neuropathology at the Massachusetts General Hospital for several neuropathologic specimens; to Dr. Frederick H. Verhoeff, my predecessor at the Howe Laboratory of Ophthalmology, for his criticisms of an earlier draft of the text; to Mrs. Irene M. Kinsey for proofreading; and to Miss Jeanette Loessl, librarian at the Howe Library of Ophthalmology, for her assistance in the compilation of the references.

D. G. C.

CONTENTS

NEUROLOGY OF THE OCULAR MUSCLES

Chapter I

GROSS ANATOMY AND ACTION OF THE EXTRAOCULAR MUSCLES

A. MUSCLE PLANES

THE MUSCLES controlling eye movements may be grouped in three pairs: the medial and lateral recti, the superior and inferior recti, and the superior and inferior oblique. Each pair may be represented by a plane, and each plane forms a characteristic angle with respect to the globe and to the walls of the orbit.

The medial and lateral recti form a plane that is approximately parallel to the floor of the orbit and coincides with the horizontal plane of the globe when the eye is in the primary position.

The superior and inferior recti form a plane that is vertical to the floor of the orbit and coincides with the central axis of the orbit. This plane makes an average angle of 23 degrees with the anteroposterior axis of the head (or with the medial wall of the orbit). It thus coincides with the vertical anteroposterior plane of the globe when, and only when, the eye is turned outward 23 degrees. If the eye could be turned inward 67 degrees, the plane of the superior and inferior recti would actually form a right angle with the anteroposterior plane of the globe (Fig. 1).

The superior and inferior oblique muscles form a plane that makes an average angle of 51 degrees with the anteroposterior axis of the head (or with the medial wall of the orbit). The muscle plane of the obliques thus coincides with the transverse or coronal meridian of the globe when the eye is rotated outward 39 degrees and with the vertical anteroposterior plane of the globe when the eye is rotated inward 51 degrees.

B. ORIGIN AND INSERTION OF THE EXTRAOCULAR MUSCLES

In the human being all the extraocular muscles except the inferior oblique arise at the apex of the orbit, i.e., the four recti muscles, the superior oblique, and the levator of the lid (Fig. 2). All these muscles arise from a membranous structure called the tendon of Zinn, made up of extensions of the periorbital fascia, the dura mater, and the tendons of the various muscles.[1055] The tendon of Zinn surrounds the optic foramen and part of the orbital foramina, forming the apex of the muscle cone. Various anomalies in the origin and insertion of the muscles occur frequently[335] but will not be considered here.

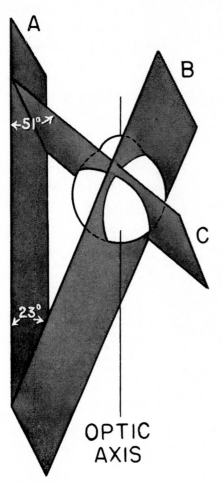

FIG. 1. *Planes of: (A) Medial orbital wall; (B) Vertical recti; and (C) Oblique muscles*

The four recti muscles fan out toward the globe to insert anterior to the equator at the following approximate distances from the limbus in the average adult eye:[181] medial rectus, 6.0mm.; inferior rectus, 7.3mm.; lateral rectus, 7.6mm.; and superior rectus 8.5mm.

The levator of the lid arises in close proximity to the superior rectus, on which it lies; it inserts by a broad, thin tendon into the subcutaneous tissue of the lid and, by means of a special band containing smooth muscle (Müller's muscle), into the superior margin of the tarsus.

The superior oblique muscle extends forward from the apex of the orbit to the upper portion of the anteromedial wall, where it is reflected, by means of a tendinous extension, over a pulley called the trochlea. Thus the superior oblique muscle, although arising from the apex of the orbit, actually approaches the eye from an anteromedial direction and, passing beneath the superior rectus, is inserted in the upper outer quadrant of the eye.

The inferior oblique muscle takes origin in the lower portion of the anteromedial wall of the orbit directly in line with the trochlea and, passing beneath the inferior rectus, is inserted in the lower outer quadrant of the eye. The insertion of the inferior oblique is a convenient landmark in surgery of the eye, since the macula lies approximately 2mm. above and 2mm. medial to the upper margin of the muscle's attachment.

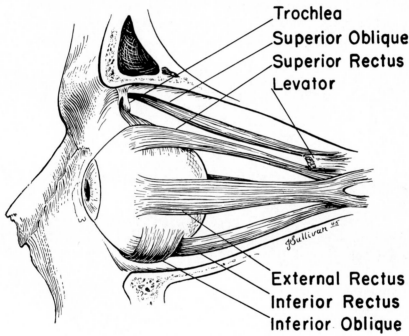

Trochlea
Superior Oblique
Superior Rectus
Levator

External Rectus
Inferior Rectus
Inferior Oblique

Fig. 2. *Origins and insertions of the extraocular muscles*

C. ACTION OF THE INDIVIDUAL MUSCLES

Although *all* the extraocular muscles probably actively participate in every movement of the eyes,[659, 286] particular muscles are especially effective in moving the eye in certain fields. The lateral rectus rotates the eye outward, and the medial rectus rotates it inward. There are no other important actions of these two muscles. The vertical recti and the obliques have functions that vary according to the position of the eye. This variable function is a common source of confusion for the student in first learning the functions of the muscles, but the changing action is nothing but what one would predict from the simple knowledge of the muscle planes. The actions should not be memorized categorically nor divided into "primary" and "secondary" functions.

From a consideration of Figure 3 it is obvious that when the eye is rotated outward 23 degrees (that is, when its optic axis coincides with the orbital axis) the superior rectus is a pure elevator and the inferior rectus is a pure depressor. On the other hand, if it were possible to rotate the eye inward 67 degrees so that the optic axis was at right angles to the orbital axis, the superior rectus would be a pure intorter of the eye, whereas the

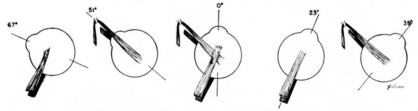

FIG. 3. *Diagram illustrating the positions and actions of the vertical recti and oblique muscles in different positions of gaze of the right eye*

inferior rectus would be a pure extorter. Similarly, the obliques have a variable function depending on whether the eye is turned inward or outward. Thus, again referring to Fig. 3 it is obvious that when the eye is rotated outward so that the plane of the oblique muscles is at right angles to the optic axis (which is the case when the eye is turned outward 39 degrees) the superior oblique is a pure intorter and the inferior oblique is a pure extorter. On the other hand, when the eye is rotated so that the optic axis coincides with the axis of the obliques (that is, when the eye is turned inward 51 degrees), the superior oblique is a pure depressor and the inferior oblique is a pure elevator. For all practical purposes it may be stated that the elevators and depressors of the eye are the superior and inferior recti when the eye is turned outward and the inferior and superior obliques when it is turned inward (Fig. 4). The torters, on the other hand, are the obliques when the eye is turned outward and the recti when it is turned inward. Obviously, vertical movements of the eye from the *primary position* are the combined functions of both muscle groups: vertical movements are chiefly, but not exclusively, executed by the vertical recti, whereas torsion is executed chiefly, but not exclusively, by the obliques.

The relative importance of the individual extraocular muscles varies in the different species, and the development of any one muscle can be correlated to a certain extent with the variations in function. In general, the higher the mammal is in the phylogenetic scale, the more highly developed are the extraocular muscles as a whole. This fact appears to be related to the progressively forward position of the eyes and to the development of foveal vision. As the eyes come to be placed forward in the head, the only way in which panoramic vision can be maintained is by acquiring greater ocular motility.

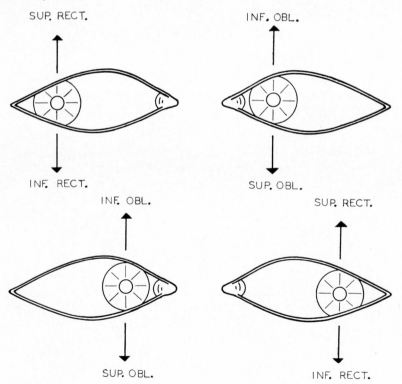

Fig. 4. *Diagram indicating the muscles chiefly responsible for vertical movements of the eyes in different positions of gaze*

Individual groups of muscles are selectively hypertrophied in certain species depending on functional requirements of these species. The obliques are hypertrophied in herbivora, in which the continual up and down movements of the head necessitate corresponding clockwise and counterclockwise rotation of the eyes. On the other hand, the medial and lateral recti are hypertrophied in carnivora, in which the predominant head movements are sidewise. The erect position in bipeds has led to a relatively greater development of the muscles turning the eyes downward (the inferior rectus and superior oblique) in comparison with the muscles turning the eyes upward (the superior rectus and inferior oblique). In consequence, the superior oblique muscle has been lengthened, and its effectivity in human beings has been increased by the development of a muscle inserting at the apex of the orbit, while the shorter inferior oblique muscle continues to insert at the margin of the orbit.

D. ACTIONS OF COMBINATIONS OF MUSCLES

Movements of the two eyes in the same direction are called *conjugate movements;* movements of the eyes in the opposite directions are called *disjunctive movements.*

It is obvious that conjugate movements are not executed by homologous muscles in the two eyes. Thus, in looking to the left, it is the lateral rectus of the left eye and the medial rectus of the right eye that are chiefly responsible for the conjugate movement. Similarly, on looking up, once the eyes are conjugately turned to the left, it is the superior rectus of the left eye and the inferior oblique of the right eye that act most effectively in the vertical plane (Fig. 4). These pairs of muscles, one in each eye, which act together in carrying out similar functions in the two eyes, are called *yoke muscles* (Fig. 4).

Disjunctive movements are movements of the two eyes in opposite directions. In the horizontal plane disjunctive movements are called convergence and divergence; in the vertical plane they are called sursumvergence. Disjunctive movements of a wheel-motion type in the clockwise or counterclockwise direction are called conclination and disclination, depending on whether the upper portions of the limbuses roll toward or away from each other.

The terminology for movements of the eyes and positions of the eyes is confusing. Whereas convergence and divergence are comprehensive terms designating movements of the eyes toward or away from each other in the horizontal plane, the same movements are termed adduction and abduction when brought about by use of prisms (see page 136). Similarly, sursumvergence is termed hyperduction when brought about by prisms; and analogous torsional movements, either conclination or disclination, induced by rotation of the field before one eye, are called cycloduction.[1046] Unfortunately, the terms adduction and abduction are also used to indicate medial or lateral movements of either eye alone and one must depend on the context to know whether the term refers to disjunctive movements of the two eyes or to medial or lateral movements of one eye.

Alternate terms have been recently proposed but have not received any wide use as yet. The suggestion[814] that exoduction and endoduction replace abduction and adduction for horizontal movements or that exorotation and endorotation replace exotorsion for wheel-like movements do not have any obvious advantage. But the suggestion[1053] that disjunctive movements be called contraocular movements would facilitate reference to the subtypes and at the same time distinguish them from conjugate movements. It is further suggested[1053] that contraocular movements be abbreviated to "cont" movements. Thus with the appropriate prefixes we would have exocont, esocont, right and left hypercont, and esocyclocont and exocyclocont.

A muscle that on contraction opposes the action of another muscle in the same eye is said to be the *antagonist* of that muscle. Thus, the medial rectus is the antagonist of the lateral rectus of the same eye, and the superior rectus is the antagonist of the inferior rectus. Contraction of one muscle is in practice accompanied by reciprocal relaxation of its antagonist, thus reducing any actual antagonism (Fig. 5). This relaxation is evident, for instance, with palsies of the lateral rectus; the paralyzed eye is turned toward the nose when the gaze is directed straight ahead, but may be brought to the midline by relaxation of the medial rectus when the gaze is directed toward the side of the paralyzed muscle.

Sherrington demonstrated reciprocal innervation experimentally on an animal in which all the nerves to the extraocular muscles were cut except that to the lateral rectus.[942] Although the

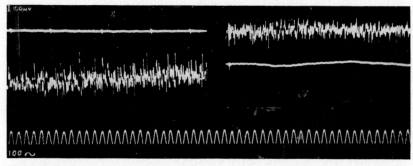

Fig. 5. *Electromyogram from the lateral recti (human) showing reciprocal activity on looking to either side*

The upper tracing records the activity from the right lateral rectus and the middle tracing from the left lateral rectus. The third tracing represents time recorded in 100 cycles/second. The left half of the graph shows the activity on extreme levoversion and the right half on extreme dextroversion. Thus, on levoversion there is complete inhibition of the right lateral rectus combined with marked activity of the left lateral rectus and vice versa on dextroversion. (Breinin and Moldaver, A.M.A. Arch. Ophth. 54:200-210, 1955)

eye was then turned outward, stimulation of the cerebrum resulted in a turning of the eyes toward the opposite side, and the eye with the paralyzed muscles reached the midline, a movement that could be brought about only by relaxation of the lateral rectus.

E. CLINICAL TESTING OF THE EXTRAOCULAR MUSCLES

A *muscle field* represents the limits within which the eye can be turned in all directions. With a little experience one learns to estimate, by direct observation, gross limitations of eye movements and for most practical purposes this is sufficient but for quantitative determinations the perimeter may be used. With his head fixed in the primary position and the eye that is to be tested in the center of the arc of the perimeter, the patient is required to follow the test object (for example, a flashlight) as it is moved along the arc of the perimeter. The muscle field determined by the extent to which the eye can follow the light is normally 45 degrees to either side of the primary position, 40 degrees above, and 60 degrees below. The muscle fields vary with the *effort* on the part of the patient, the *obstruction of vision* by the lids, nose, and brow, the *strength* of the extraocular muscles, and the *resistance* of the check ligaments.

With palsies of the extraocular muscles, the eye shows restricted movement *in the field of the paralyzed muscle*. Thus, movements outward are restricted with palsies of the lateral rectus; movements upward, once the eye is turned outward, are restricted with palsies of the superior rectus; and movements upward, once the eye is turned inward, are restricted with palsies of the inferior oblique.

Whereas gross limitations of movement offer no difficulty in interpretation, partial palsies in which there is little or no detectable restriction of movement are evaluated on the basis of diplopia (Fig. 6) or on the basis of the cover test.

The following rules for evaluating diplopia are offered for the beginner:

First, a colored glass (red is conventional) is placed before one eye, enabling the examiner to differentiate the images of the two eyes.

Secondly, the examiner determines whether the diplopia is horizontal, vertical, or both. The direction of gaze for this is unimportant. If the diplopia is purely horizontal, the examiner knows that the responsible muscle is either the medial or lateral rectus. If the diplopia is vertical, the responsible muscle may be either one of the oblique muscles or one of the vertical recti muscles. If the diplopia is *both* horizontal and vertical, the horizontal component should be entirely neglected at first, since a paresis of one of the vertical muscles may merely dissociate the eyes and thereby permit an esophoria or exophoria to become manifest.

Thirdly, the examiner finds that position of the eyes at which there is maximal separation of the images. Since maximal separation occurs in the field of action of the paralyzed muscle and one pair of yoke muscles acts predominately in one field, this procedure limits the search for the paralysis to one pair of yoke muscles. Thus, if the diplopia is purely a horizontal one and the maximal separation is present on looking to the left, the paretic muscle is either the left lateral rectus or the right medial rectus, since these two muscles turn the eyes to the left. Similarly, if there is maximal vertical separation of the images on looking down and to the right, the paretic muscle must be either the right inferior rectus or the left superior oblique, since the field of action of these two muscles is downward when the eyes are turned to the right.

Fourthly, and finally, the examiner determines which one of the yoke muscles is paretic by noting which eye is lagging. He now ascertains for the first time the relative position of the red and white images. The eye that is lagging of course projects the image farthest in the direction of gaze (that is, toward the side where its movement is limited), since the lagging of the eye causes the portion of the retina that is opposite to the direction of movement to be stimulated. In the example cited in the previous paragraph, in which the diplopia was horizontal and maximal on looking to the left, if the red glass were over the right eye and the white image were projected farther to the left than the red image, the paretic muscle would be the left lateral rectus. Similarly with the maximal diplopia on looking down and to the right, if the red glass were in front of the right eye and the white image were projected farther down than the red image, the paretic muscle would be the left superior oblique.

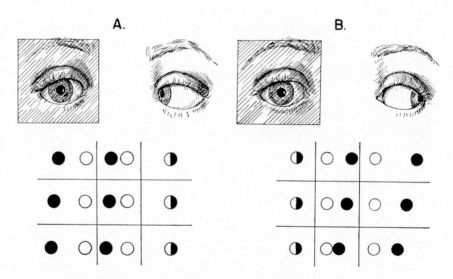

FIG. 6. *Diplopia fields with individual muscle paralyses*

The dark glass is in front of the right eye and the fields are projected as the patient sees the images.

A. Paralysis of right *lateral rectus*

Characteristic: right eye does not move to the right.

Field: horizontal homonymous diplopia increasing on looking to the right.

B. Paralysis of right *medial rectus*

Characteristic: right eye does not move to the left.

Field: horizontal crossed diplopia increasing on looking to the left.

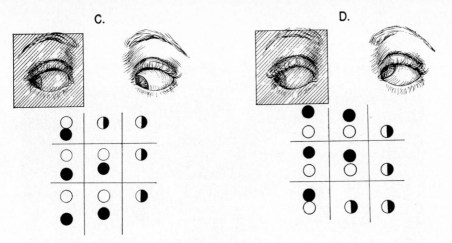

C. Paralysis of right *inferior rectus*
   Characteristic: right eye does not move downward when eyes are turned to the right.
   Field: vertical diplopia (image of right eye lowermost) increasing on looking to the right and down.
D. Paralysis of right *superior rectus*
   Characteristic: right eye does not move upward when eyes are turned to the right.
   Field: vertical diplopia (image of right eye uppermost) increasing on looking to the right and up.

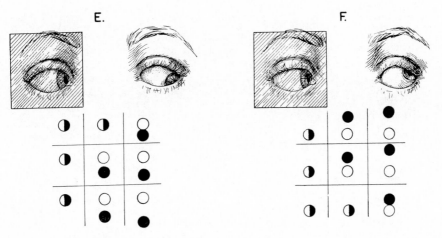

E. Paralysis of right *superior oblique*.
   Characteristic: right eye does not move downward when eyes are turned to the left.
   Field: vertical diplopia (image of right eye lowermost) increasing on looking to left and down.
F. Paralysis of right *inferior oblique*
   Characteristic: right eye does not move upward when eyes are turned to the left.
   Field: vertical diplopia (image of right eye uppermost) increasing on looking to left and up.

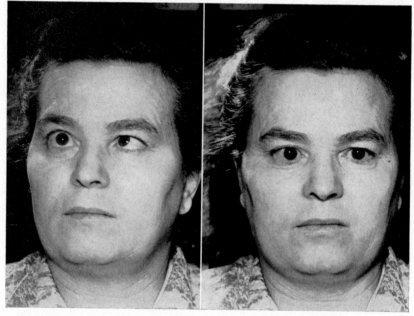

A   B

FIG. 7. *Right sixth nerve paralysis illustrating the gross difference between primary and secondary deviation*

In (A) the patient is fixating straight ahead with the paralyzed eye; in order to maintain this eye in the primary position she must put in a strong innervation for dextroversion with consequent overshoot of the non-fixing (left) eye. On the other hand, when she is asked to fixate with the left (non-paralyzed) eye, as indicated in (B), the only innervation required is that for the eyes to look straight ahead; there is then much less adduction of the non-fixing (right) eye.

The eye selected for fixation is determined more by acuity and refractive considerations than by the side of the paralysis. Failure to recognize that the deviating eye is not necessarily the paralyzed eye is a common source of error.

The cause of the opthalmoplegia in this patient was meningovascular lues. Aside from the predominant sixth nerve paralysis there was some third nerve involvement, as indicated by the larger pupil on the right and some weakness of elevation of this eye. The greater hypertropia of the left eye in (A) than the hypotropia of the right eye in (B) is a further illustration of the difference between primary and secondary deviation.

The separation of the images will be in the same direction irrespective of which eye is fixating the light, but the amount of separation will be greater when the eye with the paralyzed muscle is used for fixation (*secondary deviation*) than when the normal eye is used for fixation (*primary deviation*) (Fig. 7).

The cover test, made by alternately covering one eye and then the other eye in different directions of gaze, similarly determines the field in which there is maximal deviation of the eyes in respect to each other. The patient is required to look at some object, preferably at several meters distance, and, as his head is turned to produce various deviations of the eyes, that position is determined in which there is maximal movement of the eyes when they are alternately covered. The amount of movement may be measured by determining the strength of the prism necessary to neutralize the movement.

This position will tell us what is the field of action of the paralyzed muscle and the rest of interpretation is the same as in the diplopia test.

While the foregoing rules provide a systematic procedure for the interpretation of diplopia, there are occasionally other signs suggestive of muscle palsies that may be helpful diagnostic aids, especially in young children who cannot cooperate for the diplopia test. Most important is the presence of head turning on the one hand and head tilting on the other. *Head turning* occurs with paresis of one of the lateral rotators but is not pathognomonic of an individual muscle palsy. In order to maintain binocular vision, the eyes are turned away from the field of the paretic muscle; thus, in paresis of the left lateral rectus the eyes are turned toward the right side and in consequence the head is held turned to the left (Fig. 43). *Head tilting* occurs characteristically with paresis of the superior oblique or superior rectus, and rarely with paresis of the inferior rectus.[519] The tilting with palsies of the superior oblique or superior rectus muscle is toward the shoulder *opposite* the side of the paretic muscle. Since the eye with the superior oblique palsy is relatively extorted, the head is put in a position in which the opposite eye shows a corresponding degree of intorsion. (Fig. 8).

Since palsies of the superior oblique and of the superior rectus muscles induce head tilting to the opposite shoulder, their differentiation is often confusing; thus, as has been pointed out,[9] the literature records contradictory estimates of their relative frequencies. They may, however, be distinguished by the following three

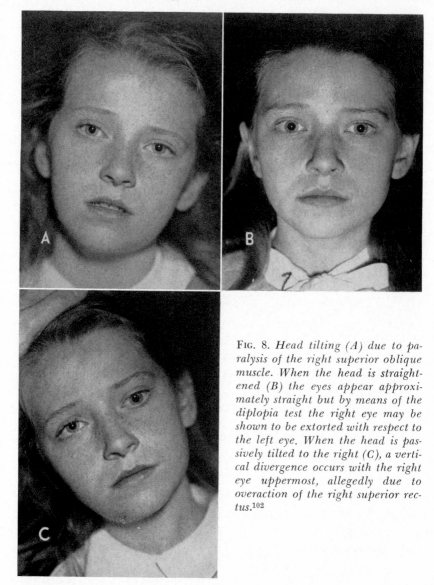

Fig. 8. *Head tilting (A) due to paralysis of the right superior oblique muscle. When the head is straightened (B) the eyes appear approximately straight but by means of the diplopia test the right eye may be shown to be extorted with respect to the left eye. When the head is passively tilted to the right (C), a vertical divergence occurs with the right eye uppermost, allegedly due to overaction of the right superior rectus.*[102]

criteria: (1) maximal separation of the eyes (and consequent maximal diplopia) occurs on attempted *downward* gaze with superior oblique palsies whereas maximal separation occurs on *upward* gaze with superior rectus palsies: (2) head tilting is never as marked with superior rectus palsies as with superior oblique palsies; and (3) the involved eye is relatively *elevated* with superior oblique palsies whereas it is *depressed* with superior rectus palsies. This latter has been explained as follows.[9] Although the superior oblique and superior rectus muscles are both intorters in the primary position of gaze, they have opposite and counterbalancing effects as regards vertical movements. Thus the superior oblique tends to *depress* the eye normally whereas the superior rectus tends to *elevate* it. When the *superior oblique* is paralyzed, the eye will be relatively elevated by the unopposed action of the superior rectus, and, conversely, when the *superior rectus* is paralyzed, the eye will be relatively depressed by the unopposed action of the superior oblique muscle.

The foregoing rules for the clinical testing of ocular motor function apply irrespective of which eye is fixating for they refer to the relative positions of the two eyes with respect to each other. The fixating eye is not necessarily the normal eye; that eye will be used for fixation which has the better visual acuity regardless of the motor paralysis. It is nevertheless a common error to assume that the deviating eye is the paralyzed eye.

Thus, when the right eye with a paralysis of its superior oblique muscle fixates, the right inferior oblique will require less innervation to turn the eye up than is usually the case. In consequence, the left eye which receives an equal innervation will be relatively depressed on levoversion and give the erroneous impression of a palsy of the left superior rectus. Application of the red glass test or of the prism test will, however, indicate the greatest vertical separation in the lower field and consequently indict correctly the superior oblique muscle.

Finally, it may be noted that partial paralysis of a muscle may be manifest not so much by the final positions of the eyes as by the lag in making a movement. This is particularly true of muscles acting in the horizontal plane. Thus, in weakness of a medial rectus function (as with internuclear ophthalmoplegia), the deficiency may be more evident in the relative lag in turning the involved eye to the opposite side then in a disparity of the final position of the two eyes.

SUMMARY

The muscles attached to each eye comprise three pairs, each pair forming a characteristic plane in respect to the orbit. The lateral and medial recti form a plane that is parallel to the floor of the orbit (or to the horizontal plane of the head); the lateral and medial recti always move the eye in the horizontal plane. The superior and inferior recti form a plane that makes an average angle of 23 degrees with the medial wall of the orbit (or with the sagittal plane of the head). The superior and inferior oblique muscles form a plane that makes an average angle of 51 degrees with the medial wall of the orbit (or with the sagittal plane of the head). The pull of these vertical and oblique muscles is always in a fixed plane, but the effect on the eye varies depending on whether it is turned inward or outward. The superior and inferior rectus muscles move the eye upward and downward when it is turned outward, and rotate it clockwise or counterclockwise when it is turned inward. On the other hand, the superior and inferior oblique muscles move the eye downward and upward when it is turned inward, and rotate it clockwise or counterclockwise when it is turned outward.

Simultaneous movement of the two eyes in the same direction is called conjugate movement, and the two muscles, one for each eye, that are primarily responsible for the movement are called yoke muscles. Movements of the two eyes in opposite directions are collectively called disjunctive movements. Disjunctive movements in the horizontal plane are called convergence or divergence; in the vertical plane, sursumvergence; and in the coronal plane, conclination and disclination.

Complete paralysis of one of the extraocular muscles is clinically manifested by a gross limitation of movements of the eye in the field of action of the paralyzed muscle. But interpretation of partial paralysis of the extraocular muscles usually requires the diplopia test. In this test the images of the two eyes are dissociated by a red glass, and the direction of gaze that produces maximal separation of the images is determined. In this position, the eye with the paralyzed muscle will be found to lag, and in consequence the image of this eye will be projected farther in the direction of the paralyzed muscle. Along with the diplopia, information may also be obtained from such associated signs as head turning and head tilting. Head turning occurs with partial paralysis of the lateral rectus and the turning is toward the side of the paralyzed muscle. Head tilting occurs with superior oblique or superior rectus paralysis and is directed to the shoulder opposite the paralyzed muscle but with superior oblique paralysis the eye on the paralyzed side tends to be elevated whereas with superior rectus paralysis the corresponding eye is depressed.

The eye with the better visual acuity is selected for fixation irrespective of the side of the ocular motor paralysis.

Chapter II

TONUS OF THE EXTRAOCULAR MUSCLES

Tonus represents the sum-total effect of the various neurochemical processes affecting the length of a muscle and, consequently, the position of an organ. In the case of the eyes, there is a continuous innervational tone acting on all the extraocular muscles and only when these are in equilibrium will the eyes be stationary. Movements of the eyes are brought about by increase in tone of one set of muscles or relaxation in tone of the antagonistic muscles, or, as is usually the case, by both.[945, 1020] It has been suggested that the tone of the ocular muscles, which is more persistently maintained than that of other skeletal muscles, stabilizes the movements of the eyes and counteracts overshooting and oscillations during fixation.[136]

The condition that most nearly approaches the atonic state—if, indeed, there is such a state—is one in which all innervation is removed, as in death or in complete ophthalmoplegia (for example, chronic progressive ophthalmoplegia externa). In these relatively atonic states, the eyes are directed straight ahead or are slightly divergent and are said to be in the *anatomic position of rest*. Contrary to common belief, the eyes do *not* assume the divergence of the orbital axes when all the muscles lose their tone.

Normally, no such state as atonic rest of the eyes exists. Even when the eyes are directed straight ahead and are immobile, the extraocular muscles are constantly receiving tonic impulses that may be detected and recorded as action potentials (see p. 33).[478, 586, 136] The position of the eyes induced by these tonic impulses, where all the stimuli but that for binocular vision are present, is called the *physiologic position of rest*. In man, this position is usually not far from the anatomic position of rest, and both usually approximate, within a few arc degrees, the primary position of the eyes (that is, with the gaze straight ahead).

The fact that a blind eye in the adult human being usually becomes divergent has given rise to the belief that the anatomic

20

position of rest is one of divergence; however, this is not in accord with the absence of any marked divergence when all innervation is removed or with the absence of divergence when *both* eyes are blind.[58] The divergence of a blind eye may be explained by assuming that when the stimuli for binocular vision are removed, there is a greater loss of convergence tonus than of divergence tonus. Convergence is more of a voluntary act than is divergence, being one of the first functions to be lost with progressive stupor.[737] It may be assumed to lose its tone with disuse more readily.[863] If both eyes are blind both convergence and divergence tonus decrease together and the eyes remain approximately straight as in death.

In childhood the situation is different. The hyperopia of childhood results in a greater convergence tonus, even in the absence of binocular vision, with the result that a blind eye in childhood usually becomes convergent.

Although the term tonus usually designates innervation of an involuntary nature only, the effect on the eyes is not basically different whether the innervation be involuntary or voluntary. Both will, therefore, be considered under the heading of tonus.

The extraocular muscles, like the skeletal muscles, receive impulses of tonic innervation arising from various centers in the central nervous system and reaching the muscles by different routes. In general, the source of tonic impulses and the pathways by which they reach the extraocular muscles, so far as they are known, are as follows:

A. LABYRINTH

According to the classic concept of labyrinthine control for the body musculature (including the extraocular muscles), *maintained postural deviations* are controlled by the otoliths in the inner ear, while *postural movements,* resulting from acceleration or deceleration of the body, are controlled by stimuli from the semicircular canals.[316, 681]

The parts played by the otolithic mechanism and the semicircular canals were studied separately by Magnus,[678] who used a technique devised by Wittmaack[1125] in which anesthetized guinea pigs were centrifuged at high speeds. The otolithic membranes were detached by the centrifugal force, whereas the canals, the ampullae, and the cristae remained intact. In such animals all labyrinthine reactions evoked by angular or rectilinear acceleration were present, but reflexes resulting from static posture were abolished.

The effect of the otoliths on the eyes is called *ophthalmostatic tonus;* the effect of the semicircular canals, *ophthalmokinetic*

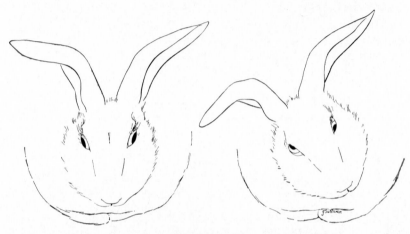

FIG. 9. *Compensatory position of the eyes with rotation of the head in rabbits*
    Labyrinthine control of eye movements are readily demonstrable in rabbits, which, having little or no voluntary movement of the eyes, show a fixed position of the eyes in the orbit for every position of the head in space. Thus, rotation of the head counterclockwise results in a compensatory vertical divergence of the eyes, tending to maintain the eyes in the primary position with respect to the ground.

tonus.[59] Ophthalmostatic and ophthalmokinetic tonus are universally present in all species having labyrinths and extraocular muscles, but are masked in the higher species, especially in man, by other types of eye movement. The lower the animal in the phylogenetic scale the more dependent is it on labyrinthine control.[677] The effect of the labyrinths is clearly demonstrable in rabbits, which possess little or no voluntary movements of the eyes (Fig. 9). In these animals *each position of the head* in space is accompanied by a corresponding deviation of the eyes. The eyes deviate with respect to the head as if attempting to maintain the primary position in reference to the ground. In *acceleration* the eyes deviate in the direction opposite the movement of the head.

In both cases it is as though the labyrinth provided the eye with inertia against change.[433] When the head is rotated backward, the eyes deviate downward; when it is rotated forward, they deviate upward. With rotation of the head about an anteroposterior axis, one eye rotates upward and the other rotates downward with respect to the head, the direction always being opposite to that of the head.

While most of the postural movements of rabbits' eyes have their counterpart in man, these animals, like all species with laterally placed eyes, have one movement not possible to anything like the same degree for species with frontally placed eyes. This is a vertical divergence whereby one eye is elevated and the other depressed as the head is rotated clockwise or counterclockwise about an anteroposterior axis.

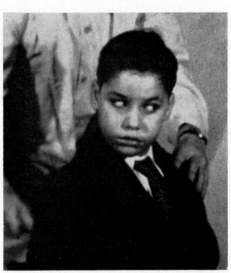

FIG. 10. *Patient with a paralysis of voluntary gaze to either side but intact vestibulo-ocular functions.*[217]

On rotation of the head to the right the eyes turn reflexly to the extreme left. This is variously called "doll's head" movement or Roth-Bielschowsky deviation; see pages 221-223.

In man labyrinthine control of ocular movements is best shown by the rolling or torsion movement, since for this there is no voluntary control. Javal[522] was one of the first to show that in man there is a partially compensatory rolling of the eyes on tilting the head. The cylinder that he was wearing in his glasses no longer corrected his astigmatism when his head was tilted. If the effect of the labyrinth is first abolished, this torsion does not occur.[570] The effect of the labyrinthine stimuli on vertical movements of the eyes can also be demonstrated in man under certain pathologic conditions in which volitional and fixational reflexes are abolished. Under these conditions in man, as in the rabbit, the eyes turn downward when the head is rotated backward and upward when it is rotated forward, an action that has been likened to that of a mechanical doll's eye (Fig. 60). Similar labyrinthinogenic movements may occur in the horizontal plane with paralysis of voluntary gaze (Fig. 10)

These maintained postural deviations disappear after labyrinthectomy or in deep narcosis. They are also absent in hereditary "waltzers" (guinea pigs[214] and rabbits[213]).

The ophthalmokinetic movements will be discussed under the heading of vestibular nystagmus (p. 201).

Each labyrinth exerts a continuous tonic innervation tending to turn and to tort the eyes to the opposite side. Removal of one labyrinth results, therefore, in a temporary turning of the eyes to the operated side[479] owing to the unopposed action of the intact labyrinth. The labyrinths exert a similar tonic effect on the contralateral skeletal musculature; this is seen most strikingly in rabbits which, on rotation of the body, assume a characteristic extensor reflex of the limbs opposing the rotation.

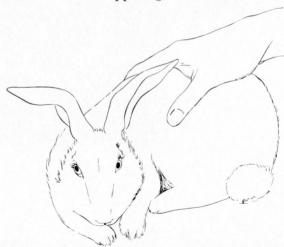

Fig. 11. *Deviation of the eyes in the rabbit resulting from proprioceptive impulses arising in the neck and trunk*
    Rotation of the body to one side results in a conjugate deviation of the eyes to the opposite side.

Just as one type of tonus may appear to be inhibited by superimposing on it another type, so the labyrinthine tonus may be inhibited or its effect may be masked by superimposing on it the tonus of voluntary or fixational movements.

While it is customary to consider the labyrinthine mechanism as having only gross effects on ocular movements, it probably influences ocular motor functions in much more delicate and precise ways than is generally believed. Thus abolition of labyrinthine control by 8th nerve lesions causes a measurable decrease in visual functions[691] and in visual acuity[212] during movement of the body.

B. PROPRIOCEPTION (kinesthetic sense)

The proprioceptive portion of the nervous system is concerned with the position of an organ or a part. The afferent arcs of proprioception arise on the one hand in the vestibular apparatus, and on the other hand in specialized nerve endings in the muscles themselves, which are generally believed to give rise to the so-called "stretch sense" or "muscle sense." These impulses arising in muscles are to be considered here, in so far as they affect the tonus of the extraocular muscles.

1. From Non-ocular Muscles

The extraocular muscles receive tonic impulses arising in various somatic muscles of the body; those from the neck muscles are especially effective and will, for instance, appreciably lessen the nystagmus induced by vestibular stimulation.[579] While this source (non-ocular muscles) of tonic innervation is present in practically all vertebrates, it may be masked in the higher animals by the voluntary eye movements. It is clearly demonstrable in animals having no voluntary eye movements, such as the rabbit (Fig. 11). Here a deviation of the eyes may be constantly produced by swinging the trunk on the neck or the rump on the trunk. The deviation of the eyes is always to the side opposite that toward which the trunk or rump is rotated.

The proprioceptive impulses arising in the neck and acting on the extraocular muscles have been studied by Bárány,[34] de Kleyn,[565] and others, special care being taken to eliminate the effects of the labyrinth. de Kleyn found that after removal of the labyrinths in rabbits there was a definite position of the eyes in the orbit for each position of the head in relation to the trunk; this deviation of the eyes from rotation of the head on the trunk did not occur after the first and second cervical nerves had been cut. The adjustments in the horizontal meridian were especially conspicuous.

This tonic innervation from proprioceptive impulses arising in the neck may have no great importance for man because of his highly developed voluntary eye movements. Indeed, these reflexes are difficult to demonstrate in man. They have, however, been shown in infants and premature babies,[39] in some central nervous system diseases of children,[568] in hydranencephaly,[212] and under special conditions in the adult (for example, once in postepileptic coma[958] and several times in persons with inexcitable labyrinths[415, 337, 367, 782]). They may also regulate to some extent the involuntary fixational movements of the eyes, for these movements, and consequent visual functions, are known to vary with different postures.[658, 199, 434, 212]

2. From Extraocular Muscles

To what extent there is an effective proprioceptive system arising in the extraocular muscles is a moot question. It was at one time thought that the extraocular muscles had a well developed proprioceptive system but this concept arose from the presumed need for such a system rather than from a critical evaluation of the characteristic features of position sense in the eyes. Moreover, it overlooked the possibility that coordination of the eyes might be more precisely served by afferent impulses from the two retinas than from the extraocular muscles. It is true that typical muscle spindles have been found in the extraocular muscles of some species, including man (see p. 37) and that afferent impulses have resulted from stretch of the muscles and have been recorded in the brain stem[232, 236, 233] but the spindles are lacking in other species[468, 1132] including the monkey,[278, 944] as are the afferent impulses resulting from muscle stretch.[240] Moreover, the psychophysiologic criteria which characterize position sense in other skeletal muscles appear to be lacking in the extraocular muscles.[510, 673, 667, 668] Thus, stretching of the individual muscles results in pain but produces no sense of turning of the eyes; passive turning of the eyes in the dark results in no sensation of movement of the eyes; nor can a vibration sense be detected in the extraocular muscles. All this makes it seem unlikely that there is a stretch sense in the extraocular muscles analogous to that which determines position sense in other organs or parts. One is aware of the position of one's eyes only by the knowledge that a certain amount of innervation has been supplied to turn the eyes and not by any stretch sense arising in the muscles themselves. When the eyes are moved passively by the hand or by the use of some reflex pathway at a sufficiently low level, as in Bell's phenomena, or in artificial stimulation of the semicircular canals, one is not aware of the actual position of one's eyes (see discussion on illusory movement of the environment, p. 185).

Conversely, when a muscle is paralyzed and one supplies an amount of innervation that is usually sufficient to turn the eyes, one believes that the eye is turned when it is actually stationary. Thus, it is the innervation furnished to turn the eyes that determines the position sense and not the stretch of the muscles themselves. Insofar as a patient has a conscious awareness of his limitation in eye movements, however this is accomplished, he will not have illusory movement of the environment (see p. 187).

Further evidence that there is no perceptual proprioceptive system in the extraocular muscles is seen in autokinetic eye movements in the dark. Weak, flickering light in an otherwise dark room after a time appears to move, owing to the spontaneous and involuntary eye movements. Indeed, while the observer may think that his eyes are fixed, the light may appear to wander 20 or more degrees excentrically owing to the involuntary eye movements. Lacking a proprioceptive sense, the subject is unaware of the fact that his eyes are moving.

Finally, the absence of proprioception in the extraocular muscles may be presumed from cases of alternating strabismus, in which the subject frequently does not know which eye is fixating and which eye is turned, and from congenitally blind persons in whom despite spontaneous movements of the eyes over wide arcs, the subject has no knowledge of the position of his eyes.

C. RETINA

1. Light

The tonic effect of light on ocular muscles is evident from a number of clinical observations. The following are two especially noteworthy and probably related instances: latent nystagmus, where darkening the field of one eye gives rise to a conjugate deviation of the eyes to the homolateral side (see p. 226); and the Bielschowsky phenomenon in persons with so-called alternating hypertropia (occlusion hypertropia[1050]) where darkening the field of the fixating eye results in a downward movement of the non-fixating eye.

The Bielschowsky phenomenon[123] may be elicited in persons with alternating hyperphoria or hypertropia by the following procedure. The patient's eyes are dissociated by holding a hand in front of one eye. A dark glass, preferably a graded photographic wedge, is placed in front of the fixating eye, and the nonfixating eye is observed behind the hand of the examiner. As the field of the fixating eye is progressively darkened, the hypertropic, non-fixating eye moves down toward or even below the level of the fixating eye.

The pathway by which these tonic light impulses reach the motor nuclei is obscure but it may be of significance that in lower animals there is a point-to-point representation of the retina in the superior colliculi overlying the ocular motor nuclei. These pathways have been thought to have some motor significance.[234]

The effect of light on the extraocular muscles is a special case of its effect on the general body musculature, which reaches its greatest development in the heliotropic reflexes in animals[59] but is also present in man. It can, for instance, be shown under suitable conditions that illumination of one eye or of homonymous halves of the retinas results in an increase in extensor tone of the contralateral limbs and a decrease in tone of the homolateral limbs.[724, 314, 735, 1091]

2. Disparateness of the Retinal Images

The retinal images are disparate when the images of an object do not fall on corresponding points in the two eyes. Muscle tone is concerned primarily with the disparateness arising from the maculas; only when there is no cause for disparateness in the center of one's field, will disparateness in the peripheral retinas be an important factor. When the object of attention is imaged on non-corresponding points in the two eyes, there is a redistribution of muscle innervation such that the images are brought on to corresponding points and maintained there. This phenomenon, commonly termed "fusion" but better termed "unification,"[1049] is the essential prerequisite for binocular vision.

The effect of image formation in stabilizing the eyes is seen with experimental blurring of the image. The blurring induces oscillations which have been likened to those of amblyopic nystagmus.[1015]

D. HIGHER CENTERS

The extraocular muscles receive a continuous tonic innervation from the cerebrum. Each hemisphere exerts a tonic discharge tending to turn the eyes conjugately to the opposite side. Normally, the tonic innervations to the two sides balance each other and the eyes are kept in the primary position, but if one hemisphere is removed or its activity is reduced on one side (as by cooling), there is a conjugate deviation of the eyes toward that side owing to the unopposed action of the opposite hemisphere.

Certain cerebral areas are especially noteworthy as being sources of tonic innervation for the eyes. These are the posterior end of the second frontal gyrus, most of the occipital lobe, and possibly the acoustic area in the temporal lobe. The frontal area has been considered the most important, since lesions occurring here produce more profound disturbances of the eye movements than do lesions elsewhere in the cerebrum.[65] But none of the higher centers are a potent source of tonic innervation; the cerebral tonic effects are normally masked by the effects of other stimuli. In certain abnormal states, however, the tonic effect of cerebral origin may become manifest. Thus, a lasting conjugate deviation of the eyes has been observed in a patient blind from infancy who developed an occipital lesion.[269] Similarly, in patients blind since early life, the aimless searching movements of the eyes tend to be more marked to one side or the other, depending on the cerebral dominance; for example, the eyes tend to turn to the right in right-handed blind persons.[59, 863]

Less is known of the higher centers for the tonic innervation of the disjunctive eye movements, convergence and divergence. It is nonetheless certain that these functions are tonically innervated, since removal of either results in an unopposed action of the other.

Further there is some evidence for localization of these disjunctive functions in the same areas of the frontal and occipital lobes as serve for the conjugate lateral movements.[858]

SUMMARY

Under the broad term "tonus" are included the manifold innervational complexes that determine the position of the eye. This term includes the impulses from the labyrinth, from the somatic muscles elsewhere in the body, from the retina, and from the higher centers in the cerebrum.

The labyrinthine impulses arising in the otolithic membranes determine the position of the eyes in response to maintained positions of the head, whereas those arising in the semicircular canals determine the movements of the eyes in response to acceleration. The tonic impulses arising in the somatic muscles produce the deviation of the eyes in response to changes of the head on the trunk and of the rump on the trunk. The effectivity of proprioceptive impulses arising in the extraocular muscles is open to question. The tonic impulses arising in the retina are of two types, those that are a function of light *per se* and those that result from disparateness of the retinal images in the two eyes. The former serves a phototropic function, which although demonstrable is nevertheless relatively unimportant in the higher species; the latter serves to coordinate the eyes and probably fulfills the same function for the eyes as the muscle sense does for *other* skeletal muscles. The impulses arising in the cerebrum, or at least mediated through it, are responsible for the ocular movements in the more highly integrated acts such as fixational and voluntary movements.

The impulses from all these so-called centers for ocular motor tonus arise symmetrically in the two halves of the body, and each half normally opposes the action of the other. With the eye at rest the innervation is equal from the two halves. Asymmetrical innervation from stimulation or depression of one half more than the other results in an eccentric position of the eyes.

Chapter III

CHARACTERISTICS OF THE EXTRAOCULAR MUSCLES

A. PHARMACOLOGIC

THE EXTRAOCULAR muscles differ from most skeletal muscles in being extraordinarily sensitive to drugs of the curare and choline group. Some ocular studies have been done with drugs of the former group (curare and quinine),[291, 448, 108, 165, 299, 953] which characteristically paralyze the extraocular muscles, but most interest attaches to drugs of the latter group (choline, acetylcholine, eserine, and nicotine),[291, 290, 327, 165] which stimulate directly or indirectly the extraocular muscles. These latter drugs act on the myoneural junction, causing a sharp muscle contraction, and also lower the threshold of the individual muscle fibers to direct electrical stimulation.[165] Their effect is demonstrable not only with intravenous administration of the drugs in the living animal but also with direct application to the muscle preparation *in vitro*. The reactivity is further enhanced by prior denervation.[95, 1077]

Normally acetylcholine is formed at the myoneural junction from some labile precursor[1] following stimulation of the nerve and is believed to mediate the impulse from the end-plate to the muscle fiber. It was Loewi in 1921 who advanced the proposal that the autonomic nerves caused an effector response through a chemical mediator, and it was Dale and his co-workers who established that stimulation of a motor nerve resulted in the liberation of an acetylcholine-like substance.[264] More recently Nachmansohn[758] calculated the number of molecules of acetylcholine that are formed. The chief difficulty in accepting the thesis of a chemical mediator for neuromuscular transmission is the rapidity of the muscular contractions and relaxations; recent evidence suggests that the process is not as simple as originally believed.[430] To the best of our current knowledge the motor end-plate acts like a leaky condenser where normally the potential

31

in the resting state is insufficient to bridge it, but impulses may be made to set it off either by increasing the potential (nerve stimulus) or by reducing the capacity of the condenser. Reduction in the capacitance is apparently brought about by either acetylcholine or potassium; these agents thus alter the end-plate membrane. Acetylcholine is accordingly interpreted as having a depolarising effect localized to the region of the nerve ending.[601]

Substances other than acetylcholine which are believed to have a direct stimulating effect on the myoneural junction of skeletal muscles are nicotine (in less than paralyzing concentrations) and potassium. It is true that potassium causes a liberation of acetylcholine,[164] but that potassium does not act simply through the liberation of acetylcholine is evident from the fact that potassium causes a contraction after curarization but acetylcholine does not.

The acetylcholine which is formed at the myoneural junction and which is responsible in large measure at least for the normal muscle contraction is rapidly hydrolyzed and inactivated by cholinesterase.* Thus any drugs such as physostigmine or neostigmine which inactivate the cholinesterase will prolong and potentiate the effect of the nerve stimulus. On the other hand there are drugs such as curare and quinine which abolish the effects of acetylcholine, not by impeding its formation but through blocking its utilization by the muscle. The action of curare appears to be one of depressing the myojunctional potential.† Thus as far as acetylcholine is concerned, curare and the cholinergic drugs are mutually antagonistic.[159]

Acetylcholine is to be found not only at the myoneural junction of skeletal muscles but also at the terminals of the parasympathetic nerves. In so far as these two effects differ pharmacologically they are spoken of as the "nicotine effect" referring to the action on the skeletal muscles and the "muscarinic effect" referring to the action on the parasympathetic end-organs.

The unusual sensitivity of the extraocular muscles to the choline group of drugs is shared to some extent with the facial muscles and possibly with the tongue muscles, but not with other striated muscles in mammals. This reaction is, however, comparable

---

* For a review of the acetylcholine-cholinesterase effect on neuromuscular transmission see Feldberg: *Physiol. Rev.,* 25:596, 1945.

† As shown for the lizard (Bucthal *et al.: Skandinav. Arch. Physiol.,* 77:224, 1937), and for the frog's isolated end-plate (Eccles: *Nature, 156:*680, 1945).

to that of skeletal muscles in birds[166] and in cold-blooded animals[263, 612, 868, 603, 327] and has been likened to the reaction both of mammalian skeletal muscle that has been sensitized by prior denervation[947, 362] and of fetal muscle that has not developed its nerve supply.[893]

The purpose served by this unusual sensitivity to the choline drugs is not apparent, but because of it the extraocular muscles are the ones most profoundly affected by systemic disturbances of the acetylcholine or cholinesterase mechanism, just as they are the ones most profoundly affected in curare poisoning. Thus, the first signs and symptoms of myasthenia gravis in the majority of patients with this disease are ptosis and diplopia.[710, 1072]

B. PHYSIOLOGIC

The fibers of the extraocular muscles are richly supplied with motor nerves;[148] for their size the extraocular muscles have the largest nerves in the body.[1105] The original estimate of one nerve fiber for every three muscle fibers[1016] does not make allowance for sensory fibers and may be unduly high. A conservative estimate is one nerve for every ten muscle fibers, as compared with one nerve for every one hundred and forty muscle fibers in other skeletal muscles.[378]

This abundant innervation of the extraocular muscles probably accounts for the fact that their contraction time, about 7 milliseconds, is the shortest of any muscle in the body.[235]

Along with the rich nerve supply, the ocular muscles yield action potentials of a uniquely high frequency and low voltage.[235] Thus, even at rest, frequencies of 50/sec. are common; these rise to 170/sec. with movements of the head.[867, 137] This compares with frequencies of 5-10/sec. for resting muscles elsewhere with a maximum of 80-90/sec. on contraction. No other muscles in the body have been found to have these small and brief motor unit action potentials whereas they are constant features of the ocular muscles.[940] They undoubtedly make possible the fine grading of ocular movements.

The extraocular muscles are also well supplied with blood vessels, and this probably accounts for the fact that they can continue actively contracting (as in nystagmus) for long periods of time without showing gross evidence of fatigue. It seems likely that, as in the case of the heart muscle, the better than average blood supply facilitates oxidation of lactic acid and removal of waste products from the local area, thereby prolonging the resistance to fatigue.

C. HISTOLOGIC

1. Muscle Fibers

Like skeletal muscles elsewhere, the extraocular muscles are composed of striated fibers. The fibers differ, however, from those of skeletal muscles in being smaller and more uniform and in running the whole length of the muscle.[165] The extraocular muscles have an unusual abundance of fibrous tissue[918] and elastic tissue;[918] this latter develops some time after birth.[542] Thick muscle fibers have been said to form a distinct entity within the extraocular muscles, clearly separable from the medium and from the thin fibers,[1132, 1126] but most investigators have found no such gradation of fibers on the basis of size.[388, 467] The thinner muscle fibers are, however, most numerous toward the margins of the muscle belly, especially in the distal portions of the muscle.

No convincing evidence has been adduced to account for this diversity in size of the ocular muscle fibers. It has been variously suggested: that the small fibers serve for the maintenance of muscle tone;[1129] that the small fibers are operative in the relatively slow pursuit movements whereas the large fibers are operative in the fast saccadic movements of gaze;[928] or that the small and large fibers account for the difference in contraction of convergent and conjugate movements.[1052] All of these hypotheses are admittedly speculative.

2. Nerve Fibers and Nerve Endings in the Extraocular Muscles

The nerves running to the eye muscles are made up of branches from the 3rd, 4th, and 6th (motor) nerves and from the 5th (sensory) nerve.[1122] The trunks consist of coarse medullated and fine non-medullated fibers, with a preponderance of the former. The nerves enter the recti muscles in the posterior portion of the middle third,[371] divide into numerous branches, and terminate on the muscle fibers in motor foot plates, in grapelike endings, and in bare terminal fibrils (Fig. 12). In approaching the muscle fibers, many of the terminal nerves form an encircling spiral that is not found in other muscles of the body.[266, 1130]

The *non-medullated* fibers are, in turn, divided into fine and thick fibers. The former consist of autonomic fibers to the blood vessels whereas the latter consist of autonomic fibers to both the skeletal muscle and to the blood vessels.[1131]

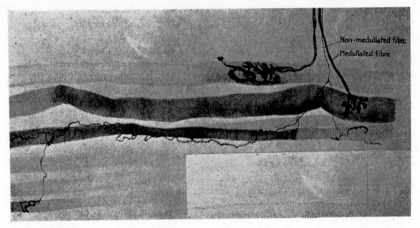

Fig. 12. *Types of nerve endings in the extraocular muscles (Woollard)*

The motor foot plates are especially prominent in the posterior two thirds of the muscle. There are 5 to 20 such plates for each nerve fiber.[469] They do not differ from the terminations of the motor nerves elsewhere in the body.

The grapelike endings and bare terminal fibrils, on the other hand, are not to be found in most skeletal muscles of mammals,[1114, 1132] and their presence in the extraocular muscles has given rise to considerable speculation. They are found chiefly in the insertional third of the muscle, innervating the thinner muscle fibers[1134] and terminating both on and beneath the muscle cell wall (epilemmal and hypolemmal endings respectively). While there is general agreement as to the morphologic characteristics of these endings in a wide variety of species, there is considerable divergence of opinion regarding their functions. Most investigators have thought them to be sensory.[157, 499, 250, 278, 1026, 944, 741] They are, however, unlike sensory endings elsewhere in muscle;[1132, 1133] they show no degeneration following destruction of either the trigeminal nerve or the trigeminal nucleus,[240]* and no action potentials can be recorded from the trigeminal nucleus or trigeminal nerve on stimulating the peripheral portions of the oculomotor nerve.[239]

The assumption that these grapelike endings belong to the sympathetic nervous system[142] is also not borne out, since removal of the cervical sympathetic ganglia is without effect on their histologic appearance.[468]

A number of investigators have felt constrained to assume that these peculiar endings belong to the kinesthetic system,[944, 1132, 239] since the typical muscle spindles that initiate the proprioceptive impulses are lacking in the extraocular muscles of many species. There is, however, no unequivocal evidence that the extraocular muscles have any proprioceptive system in the usual sense, and there is much functional evidence against such an assumption [510, 673, 667] (see p. 26).

Fairly conclusive evidence has recently been obtained with the Horsley-Clarke technique, which enables one to place an electrode with considerable precision, indicating that the cells giving rise to the atypical nerve endings, as well as those for the typical foot plates, are situated in the large-cell motor nuclei of the oculomotor nerves.[239, 240] Although this does not necessarily shed any new light on their function, it is strongly suggestive of a motor function for all the described endings.

Although not found in most other skeletal muscles, grapelike endings similar to those described above are present in skeletal muscles of cold-blooded animals,[603] a fact that leads one to believe that the endings may have something to do with the extraordinary sensitivity of both groups of muscle to cholinergic drugs. Why the extraocular muscles should retain this primitive type and

---

* It is true that removal of the orbital contents leads to retrograde chromatolysis in the mesencephalic root of the trigeminal nucleus (Freeman, 1925, Sheinin, 1933), but the weight of evidence is against origin of the lesions in the extraocular muscles (Kohnstamm and Quensel, 1908) or in the motor nerves running to the eye muscles (Corbin and Harrison, 1942; Tozer, 1912). It seems more likely that the changes in the trigeminal nucleus are due to lesions of the nerves running to the fascia and the ethmoid (Corbin and Oliver, 1942), which are known to arise in this portion of the nucleus.

reactivity of muscle while at the same time acquiring the ordinary motor foot plate is far from clear.

The presence of muscle spindles in the extraocular muscles has been a subject of moderate investigation and considerable speculation. Elsewhere in the body, muscle spindles are believed to be concerned with the perception of tension and consequent proprioception.[947] In some species, including man, muscle spindles have been found to be abundantly present in the extraocular muscles;[266, 231, 720] in other species they are lacking.[201, 1132, 468] The absence of any true proprioceptive sense arising in the ocular muscles (see p. 26) has given rise to the suggestion that the spindles here are concerned with some feed-back mechanism different from the usual kinesthetic sense.[668] On the other hand, the similarity to muscle spindles elsewhere (though the ocular spindles are more like fetal spindles[231]) is strong evidence of analogous functions. The matter must remain, for the present, inconclusive.

D. LESIONS WITHIN THE MUSCLES

1. Myasthenia Gravis

Myasthenia gravis is a disease characterized by paralysis of the skeletal muscles and is of particular interest to ophthalmologists because the initial symptoms in approximately half of the patients, and later symptoms in practically all the patients, are referable to the extraocular muscles. Since the ophthalmologist is often the first physician to be consulted, it behooves him to be familiar with the pathogenesis and symptoms of the disease and the means for its differential diagnosis.

Myasthenia gravis may occur at any age. Most of the patients are adults, but in the literature there are reports of 37 cases in children under 17 years[1028] and one case in an infant of 21 months. The ocular symptoms of which the patients complain are drooping of the lid and diplopia (Fig. 13). The ptosis is typically bilateral but usually asymmetric. The furrowing of the forehead, so characteristic of patients with bilateral ptosis, is less apt to be a conspicuous feature in patients with myasthenia gravis because of the associated weakness of the frontalis muscle. The diplopia is sometimes horizontal and sometimes vertical with a characteristic variation in amount from time to time. The ocular movements are limited in all directions. Despite this apparent weakness of the extraocular muscles, the intraocular musculature (pupillary and accommodative functions) is entirely normal.

The disease has spontaneous remissions lasting for days, weeks, or years. Its symptoms are related to fatigue and are characteristically worse in the evening than in the morning.

Both males and females have myasthenia gravis, but the disease is more apt to have an abrupt onset in men of middle age with rapidly progressive and severe manifestations occurring within a few months' time. In women of middle age the disease is more apt to be intermittent with relatively slight involvement over many years, often involving only one group of muscles.

While there is reported to be a type of "ocular myasthenia" in which the eyes only are involved,[1075, 655] most patients with myasthenia gravis ultimately show involvement of other skeletal muscles as well, manifest, for example, by easy fatigability of the legs on climbing stairs or of the arms on combing the hair.

The pathogenesis of myasthenia gravis is of general biologic interest since the disease is an example of an altered physiologic process. Specifically, it is referable to an alteration in the acetylcholine-cholinesterase mechanism whereby the chemical mediation of the nerve impulse appears to be lacking at the myoneural junction.

Although the muscle excitatory action of the cholinergic drugs and muscle depressing action of the curare-like drugs was well known, its relation to myasthenia gravis was not recognized until Walker[1065, 1066] reported the relief of myasthenic symptoms by physostigmine and neostigmine. This marked one of the dramatic episodes in the history of therapeutics. There are few reactions more striking than that of a myasthenic patient who unable to raise his eyelids, move his eyes, or contract his facial muscles will nevertheless have practically normal movements within a few minutes after a single injection of neostigmine (Fig. 13).

The test dose of neostigmine is 1.5 mgms. and to this is added 0.5 mgms. of atropine to minimize the muscarinic side-effects (intestinal cramps, sweating). Within 15-30 minutes after an intramuscular injection of the test dose there is considerable improvement in the ophthalmoplegia and ptosis. But it should be noted that neither is ordinarily made normal by the drug and often the eyes, while still paretic, develop a curious flutter on changes of

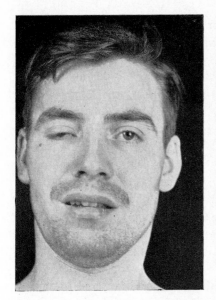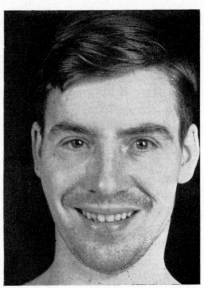

Fig. 13. *Myasthenia gravis before and after prostigmine*
This twenty-eight-year-old patient developed ptosis of the right lid as his first symptom two months previously; when the lid was passively raised, the patient saw double. The ptosis and diplopia were worse in the evening when the patient was fatigued, and shortly before the pictures were taken there developed dysphonia, dysphagia, and some weakness of the extremities.
The first picture was taken as the patient attempted to smile and shows the ptosis and profound weakness of the facial muscles. The second picture was taken fifteen minutes after receiving a diagnostic dose (1.5 mgms.) of neostigmine and shows the marked relief of symptoms.

fixation, suggesting a hyperexcitability, while under the influence of the drug.

Why the extraocular muscles are preferentially affected in myasthenia gravis is not clear, but they are known to be peculiarly excitable by acetylcholine and may, therefore, more than other skeletal muscles be unusually dependent on acetylcholine. By the same token any disturbance of the acetylcholine mechanism may be manifest first in these muscles.

The deficiency in transmission across the myoneural plate in myasthenia gravis may be thought to result from either a deficiency in acetylcholine itself, an abnormally rapid breakdown from excess of cholinesterase, or a curare-like substance which blocks the acetylcholine. That it is simply a deficiency of acetylcholine seems unlikely since the muscarinic or parasympathetic functions are normal. It also seems unlikely that it is simply an excess of cholinestrase for again this would affect the muscarinic as well as the nicotinic functions, and moreover the cholinesterase has been found to be normal in patients with myasthenia gravis.[531, 406, 1115] The pathologic presence of a curare-like substance is a possibility,[447] and there is some suggestive evidence of such a substance in the serum of patients with myasthenia gravis,[1116] and in the infants born of a mother with myasthenia gravis,[1005, 608, 719] although this evidence must be qualified by the fact that a curare-like substance is also found in the serum of normal patients after active or passive exercise.[1023] That this hypothetical substance may be especially deleterious in patients with myasthenia gravis is evident in the alleged worsening of a myasthenic ptosis by exercise of the hand muscles.[1067]

The finding of a tumor of the thymus in a significant percentile of patients with myasthenia gravis[716] and the relief of myasthenic symptoms following thymectomy[138, 446] suggest a role of this gland in the pathogenesis of the disease. Moreover extracts of the thymus have been reported to depress myoneural transmission[116, 229] and acetylcholine synthesis.[1022, 1021, 1027] Nevertheless, it must be admitted that no thymic abnormality has been demonstrated in the majority of patients with myasthenia gravis,[558] and thymic enlargement, when it does occur with myasthenia, may merely reflect a generalized endocrine disturbance in this disease rather than be causally related to it. Hyperactivity of thyroid function is similarly frequent with myasthenia gravis.[729]

Sections of the somatic muscles in myasthenia gravis usually reveal nothing abnormal but sections of the extraocular muscles are apt to show groups of lymphocytes (lymphorrhagia) and occasional degeneration of muscle fibers. The pathologic changes are neither striking nor characteristic.

Just as myasthenia gravis is a pharmacologic disease that simulates a deficiency of the acetylcholine mechanism at the myoneural junction, the reverse condition in which there appears to be an excess of this substance exists in the entity of myotonia (Thomsen's Disease). This is characterized by an increased tone of the skeletal muscles and impairment of relaxation of muscle contraction. Those drugs which benefit myasthenia gravis, physostigmine and neostigmine, make myotonia worse, while those drugs which are deleterious in myasthenia, curare and quinine, are symptomatically curative for myotonia. Nevertheless, the ocular motor signs in myotonia are of little significance. They are often absent altogether or consist merely of lid retraction (like the Graefe sign of hyperthyroidism) or of some slowness of ocular movements and occasionally ptosis. This contrasts with the preferential involvement of the ocular movements in the pharmacologic opposite, myasthenia gravis.

The differential diagnosis of myasthenia gravis will be discussed in the subsequent sections. It is one of the disturbances of eye movements with lid involvement but without pupillary involvement and in which the muscles involved do not accord with any one nerve pattern. It most clearly simulates abiotrophic ophthalmoplegia externa from which it can be distinguished only by the history of diurnal variation and by a definite response to the neostigmine test.

Its treatment is beyond the scope of ophthalmologic practice. Its necessitates determining the dose of an appropriate cholinergic drug—neostigmine is most widely used—which produces the maximal benefit and minimal side-effects.

2. Abiotrophic Ophthalmoplegia Externa

Although external ophthalmoplegia occurs with many disease processes, the condition which is often called chronic progressive ophthalmoplegia externa, and more accurately designated the abiotrophic form, is a definite entity. It is characterized by the gradual development of ophthalmoplegia and ptosis with sparing of the pupil and accommodation. Both eyes are involved but not necessarily to the same degree. Usually it goes on to total ophthalmoplegia but it may remain limited to the lids or to a combination of the lids and elevators of the eyes (Fig. 14).

The clinical picture is practically identical with that of myasthenia gravis. In somewhat less than half the cases, it is associated with weakness of the facial muscles (although selective involve-

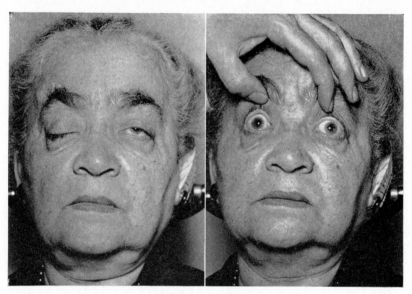

A   B

FIG. 14. *Chronic progressive ophthalmoplegia externa*

   The patient was a sixty-four-year-old woman who developed ocular symptoms consisting of ptosis and diplopia for the first time one year previously. Since onset the lids have become progressively drooped and ocular motility has gradually lessened. When unsupported the lids are seen to be asymmetrically drooped (A), and when they are passively raised (B), the eyes are found to be practically fixed in the primary position of gaze. The general appearance and findings are similar to those in myasthenia gravis, but unlike the latter there is no history of diurnal fluctuation and no response to the injection of neostigmine.

ment of the orbicularis oculi is the rule) and with the pharyngeal muscles. Rarely it is associated with other abiotrophic degenerations such as retinitis pigmentosa and spinocerebellar atrophy. Frequently it is familial but not as frequent as the literature would suggest.

Abiotrophic ophthalmoplegia externa involves both sexes and

may occur at any age. In general, the later in life it begins, the slower is its course and the better the chance it will never attain complete ophthalmoplegia.

Classifying a disease as an abiotrophy is, according to some, tantamount to saying the cause of the disease is unknown, but the implications of this are not altogether justified. Abiotrophies, as a class of diseases, are as well defined as are infections, neoplasias, and allergies.[226] The characteristic features of abiotrophies are the extraordinary specificity for one particular tissue or part of a tissue, the bilaterality and approximate symmetry, the apparently spontaneous occurrence in a tissue having previously normal function, the ultimately complete annihilation of this function, and the tendency to occur in families. Abiotrophies are presumably genetic in origin; in few instances has anything other than symptomatic therapy been found effective in their treatment.

Idiopathic chronic progressive ophthalmoplegia externa illustrates the characteristics of an abiotrophy in showing highly selective involvement of the voluntary motor functions of the eye, sparing of the pupillomotor functions and the functions of the structures between the ocular motor nuclei. Analogous abiotrophies elsewhere in the nervous system are Friedrich's ataxia affecting the posterior columns of the spinal cord, the Werdnig-Hoffman atrophy affecting the motor cells in the spinal cord, and retinitis pigmentosa affecting the outer layers of the retina.

Until recently abiotrophic ophthalmoplegia externa was thought to be due to a primary degeneration of the nuclei in the brain stem; indeed it is frequently called Nuclear Ophthalmoplegia. But, on the one hand, the changes in the brain stem have been disproportionately slight in view of the profoundness of the ophthalmoplegia[559] and, on the other hand, sections of the ocular muscles have shown degenerations interpreted as indicating a primarily local process within the muscles.[376, 904, 932] Why the extraocular muscles should be selectively, and often exclusively, involved is one of the paradoxical predilections common to all abiotrophies.

The chief problem of differentiation is myasthenia gravis; both diseases produce similar signs and symptoms. In favor of abiotrophic ophthalmoplegia is an absence of diurnal fluctuations, a lack of any relationship to fatigue, and the absence of involvement of the limbs; but conclusive differentiation is made only with test doses of neostigmine which produce little or no improvement with abiotrophic ophthalmoplegia but uniformly positive results with typical myasthenia gravis.

Less often, problems in differentiation occur with the other ocular myopathies (to be described) and occasionally with bilateral brain stem or basal ganglion disease (pseudo-ophthalmoplegia, see p. 223).With this latter, however, the lids are less apt to be affected, and there is preservation of the vestibulo-ocular reflexes (doll's head movements).

Treatment of abiotrophic ophthalmoplegia externa is symptomatic and consists of the use of ptosis crutches and occasionally of ptosis surgery. The latter must be done with caution, if at all, because of the coincident involvement of the orbicularis oculi and consequent danger of overcorrection with inability to close the eyes.

3. Dysthyroid Ophthalmoplegia

A curious ocular myopathy occurs occasionally in patients who have or have had hyperthyroidism and may lead to a clinical picture of ophthalmoplegia bearing some resemblance to ophthalmoplegia from other cause. The pathogenesis is obviously linked up with that of the exophthalmos to which the swelling of the muscles contributes a substantial part. It is incorrect to assume that the exophthalmos per se causes the ophthalmoplegia as the exophthalmos may be profound and the ophthalmoplegia slight, or vice versa; moreover, it is unlike the mechanical ophthalmoplegia simply from exophthalmos inasmuch as there is usually a selectivity in the muscles involved.

The pathogenesis of the exophthalmos in disturbances of the thyroid is far from clear. The concept that it is due simply to sympathetic stimulation as suggested by the lid retraction seems untenable for the following reasons: stimulation of the sympathetic nerve in human beings does not lead to exophthalmos;[755, 832] dysthyroid exophthalmos may occur in the presence of sympathetic paralysis; and pupillary dilatation which is the most sensitive index of sympathetic stimulation is absent in dysthyroid exophthalmos. The highly suggestive experimental evidence that some cases are due to excess secretion of the thyrotropic hormone by the pituitary gland have yet to be substantiated by the finding of excess of this hormone in patients with dysthyroid exophthalmos. To date no quantity of the hormone has been found in patients comparable to that in animals with the alleged counterpart of the disease. Nevertheless one must grant there is striking similarity between the histologic findings in the ocular muscles of patients with severe dysthyroid ophthalmoplegia and of the experimental animals.[960] We must conclude, therefore, that while there are many suggestive leads, the pathogenesis of the dysthyroid myopathy, as of the exophthalmos, is not definitely settled.

From the clinical point of view there are two types of dysthyroid exophthalmos (Fig. 15), the one occurring with hyperthyroidism and usually improving as the hyperthyroidism is controlled and the other type coming on more often following a state of hyperthyroidism, as after thyroidectomy, when the metabolism may be normal or subnormal. The chief objective sign distinguishing these two types is the absence of congestive signs in the former and its presence in the latter. Hence the former may be called the *noncongestive type* of exophthalmos with dysthyroidism and the latter the *congestive type*. The clinical criteria differentiating these two types are:

(a) *Orbital resiliency.* This is normal in the non-congestive type and reduced in the congestive type. It is a sign which was first reported by Basedow[71] but its usefulness has been largely ignored. The resiliency may be conveniently estimated by the ease with which the eye may be pushed back into the orbit. The normal eye or the eye with non-congestive exophthalmos may be replaced several millimeters while in congestive exophthalmos orbital resiliency is diminished. Pressure is made against the upper and lower lids with the eye open so that movements of the globe can be observed grossly. The amount of displacement may be measured with the exophthalmometer, although this is usually unnecessary since the reduction in orbital resiliency, when significant, is obvious simply by the gross manipulation. There are types of apparatus, the so-called piezometers or orbitonometers,[237] which quantitate the changes but simple manipulation is usually sufficient. A change in the orbital resiliency is probably the best index as to whether a patient is getting better or worse, for it precedes all other signs of congestion.

(b) ***Engorgement of veins over lateral recti.*** This is highly characteristic of the congestive type of dysthyroid exophthalmos. The vessel or vessels appear as large tortuous sinusoids beginning and ending in the muscle or tendon. They are not to be confused

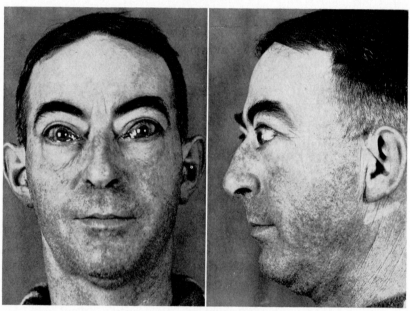

Fig. 15. *Congestive type of dysthyroid exophthalmos*
    Examination showed exophthalmos, finger-like edema of upper lids, congestion of eyes, marked reduction in orbital resiliency, and complete paralysis of upward gaze.

with the simple angular dilatation of vessels fading out toward the cornea. Such sinusoids as are seen in congestive exophthalmos are never seen in the non-congestive type.

(c) ***Evidence of myopathy.*** Although retraction of the lids is frequent there is no other characteristic of the non-congestive type referable to the extraocular muscles. With the congestive type, however, there is a characteristic paralysis of some of the muscles and diplopia is usually a presenting complaint. The elevators are much the most frequently affected; thus, the patients with congestive dysthyroid exophthalmos assume a characteristic head-back posture favoring the downward gaze position of their eyes. Next to the involvement of the elevators, the abductors are affected so that such patients are occasionally diagnosed as having a bilateral sixth nerve paralysis. Rarely all the extraocular muscles are involved, but the lids are characteristically spared in dysthyroid exophthalmos so that ptosis which is so characteristic of other ophthalmoplegias is absent usually in the dysthyroid type.

(d) *Edema of lids.* With congestive exophthalmos of dysthyroidism there is usually a finger-like swelling of the upper lids and puffiness of the lower lids. This is either absent or much less conspicuous in the non-congestive type.

(e) *Relation to hyperthyroidism.* The congestive type comes on most frequently following a thyroidectomy and becomes apparent usually about two weeks after the operation. The time of onset, however, is extremely variable, and it may not come on for many years after a thyroidectomy. It has also followed treatment of hyperthyroidism with thiouracil, roentgen radiation of the thyroid, and treatment with radioactive iodine. It also occurs following treatment of obesity with thyroid extract or ingestion of large amounts of thyroid extract by normal individuals. It may come on during the active stages of hyperthyroidism and may occur idiopathically without evident thyroid disease. Curiously it has not been reported with simple pituitary disease. The exophthalmos of the congestive type may remain stationary indefinitely, but usually it regresses eventually.

(f) *Retraction of the lids.* This is a relatively insignificant, but interesting, feature in the differentiation of the congestive from the non-congestive type of dysthyroid exophthalmos. In the non-congestive type the lid retraction is greatest on downward gaze, the typical Graefe sign, whereas in the congestive type the retraction, when present, is greatest on upward gaze. This latter is undoubtedly secondary to the weakness of upward gaze and not an irritative sign.

(g) *Visual disturbances.* The congestive type may be accompanied by irregular scotomata.[508] When these involve the central portion of the field they may produce an alarming reduction in vision. Their pathogenesis is obscure, but the prognosis for eventual recovery of vision is good. They do not occur with the non-congestive type.

The pathology in the extraocular muscles in the dysthyroid

myopathy has been studied in both clinical and experimental cases, but the findings are not germane to the present discussion except to state there are sufficient changes in the muscles to account for the paralyses simply on a local basis. There is considerable edema and round cell infiltration with varying amounts of degeneration of the muscle fibers. In view of the severity of the degeneration in some specimens it is surprising how much muscle function may be recovered clinically after prolonged paralysis.

The congestive type of dysthyroid exophthalmos is characteristically self-limited, and this is sufficient reason to avoid the names progressive or malignant exophthalmos which are so frequently applied to it. If the cornea is not threatened by exposure and one can temporize the exophthalmos and myopathy will ultimately get better. Marked improvement in the myopathy may occur after a latent period as long as several years, during which time the condition may be stationary. Because of its self-limited or self-curative nature it is easy to get the impression that various therapeutic measures are effective. Thus improvement has seemed to follow: treatment with thyroid, with iodine, with neostigmine, radiation to the pituitary, and radiation to the orbits. As none of these have resulted in dramatically rapid improvement, and as other cases have shown gradual improvement without treatment, it is difficult to assess the procedures. It seems reasonably certain, however, that elevation of the head at night results in symptomatic improvement. It is also certain that when the exophthalmos is so great as to endanger the corneas, removal of portions of the orbital wall will permit sufficient expansion of the orbital contents until there is a spontaneous remission. This may be done by removing the roof as in the Naffziger procedure[759] or the ethmoids as in Schall's procedure[915] or the lateral wall as in the Kroenlein procedure.

4. Myopathy of Pseudotumor

The so-called pseudotumor of the orbit is a clinicopathologic entity of obscure etiology characterized by infiltration of one orbit, including the extraocular muscles, with chronic inflammatory cells. It is a self-limited disease, occurring preferentially in young men, and owes its name to the fact that it simulates tumor of the orbit.

The reason for including it in the present section is that ophthalmoplegia is usually present and may often be marked. Moreover, the process may be limited to the region of one of the extraocular muscles[292] and thus simulate an isolated ocular motor palsy.

Differentiation from the foregoing ophthalmoplegias is usually not difficult in view of its unilaterality and its frequent association with inflammatory signs (including preauricular lymphadenopathy) and exophthalmos.

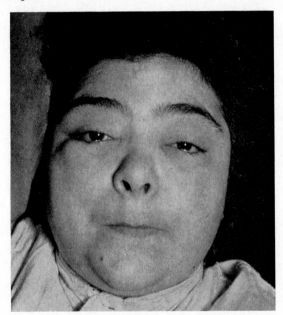

FIG. 16. *Swelling of lids and congestion of eyes with trichinosis.*
Three weeks previously the patient had eaten some pork which was said to have been inadequately cooked. She developed diarrhea, swelling of lids, "stiffness" of the eyes, chills and fever. Eosinophiles accounted for 25-45% of the white blood cells.

5. Miscellaneous Myopathies

Ophthalmoplegia due to direct involvement of the extraocular muscles may occur with diverse processes affecting skeletal muscles elsewhere. *Trichinosis* is not infrequently accompanied by a "painful stiffness" of the eyes due to trichinae in the muscles. The diagnosis is usually evident from the associated inflammation (with characteristic petechial hemorrhages of the conjunctiva) and the systemic signs of fever, eosinophilia, and gastrointestinal symptoms, (Figs. 16 and 17). Systemic *amyloidosis* may on occasion so infiltrate the ocular muscles as to produce a clinical picture similar to that of abiotrophic ophthalmoplegia externa.[105] (Fig. 18). Differentiation may be made only by recognition of the general disease. Finally, isolated ophthalmoplegias may occur with any of the group of *collagen diseases* due to foci of inflammation in the

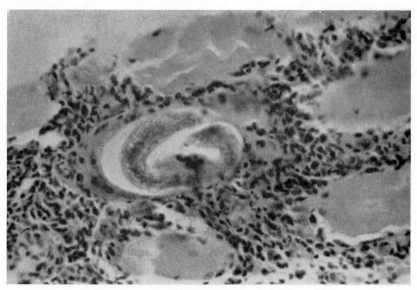

Fig. 17. *Biopsy from gastrocnemius muscle in the foregoing case. Specimen shows a typical trichinella spiralis*

muscles; thus reversible ophthalmoplegias occur occasionally with rheumatoid arthritis,[656] lupus erythematosus, etc.

SUMMARY

The extraocular muscles are striated muscles, but they differ pharmacologically from most skeletal muscles in being more sensitive to drugs of the curare (paralytic) and choline (excitatory) groups and in being more susceptible to such pathologic alterations of the acetylcholine mechanism as myasthenia gravis.

The extraocular muscles also differ from most skeletal muscles in having a greater ratio of nerve fibers to muscle fibers, and in having a richer blood supply, thus permitting more rapid and finer movements of the eyes and greater resistance to fatigue.

While some of the neural foot plates in the extraocular muscles are similar to those in other muscles, there are also grapelike endings that in the higher animals are peculiar to extraocular muscles. Various hypotheses have been advanced to account for their presence, but it seems most reasonable at the present time to consider them as motor in function and related in some way to the aforementioned pharmacologic peculiarities.

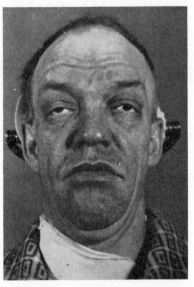

The ocular myopathies of clinical significance occur with myasthenia gravis, abiotrophic ophthalmoplegia externa, dysthyroid ophthalmoplegia, pseudotumor, and a miscellany of systemic diseases.

Myasthenia gravis is a disease referable to the cholinergic mechanism of neuromuscular transfer with a predilection for the ocular motor system. It is characterized by ptosis and intermittent ophthalmoplegia which are responsive to test doses of cholinergic drugs. Abiotrophic ophthalmoplegia produces similar ocular symptoms except that they are not intermittent and are not relieved by cholinergic

FIG. 18. *Ptosis and almost complete external ophthalmoplegia associated with amyloidosis*
The patient had generalized weakness of 3 years' duration with ptosis and diplopia of 10 months' duration. Prostigmine test was negative. Histologic studies showed diffuse infiltration of skeletal muscles with amyloid.

drugs. Dysthyroid ophthalmoplegia is a curious abnormality of the ocular muscles having some relation to the thyroid-pituitary axis and occurring most commonly after treatment of hyperthyroidism. It is associated with generalized orbital disease and consequent congestive exophthalmos. The entity known as pseudotumor produces a unilateral exophthalmos and frequently ophthalmoplegia. Its etiology is totally obscure. Ophthalmoplegia occurs less commonly with other inflammatory processes (trichinosis and collagen diseases) and infiltrative (amyloid) processes.

Chapter IV

NERVES TO THE EXTRAOCULAR MUSCLES

A. GENERAL ARRANGEMENT

THE BRAIN STEM has lost much of the segmental arrangement that it is presumed to have had originally. It has been widely held that the 3rd, 4th, and 6th cranial nerves, comprising the nerve supply to the extraocular muscles, represent the motor components of the first three metameres, while their sensory counterparts have been fused into the trigeminal nerve,[1107] but there is also phylogenetic evidence that all the ocular muscles arose from one metamere.[305] The evolutionary changes through which the original myotomes have come to serve exclusively ocular movements are lost in antiquity. In contemporary vertebrates, however, the pattern is relatively fixed. The 4th nerve supplies the superior oblique muscle, the 6th nerve supplies the lateral rectus (and, when present, the rectractor bulbi), and the 3rd nerve supplies all the other

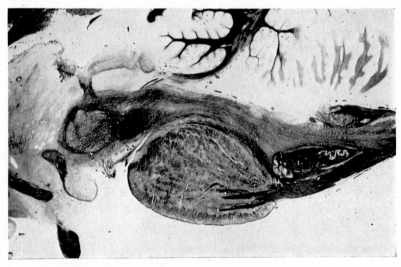

FIG. 19. *Longitudinal section of the brain stem (unretouched)*

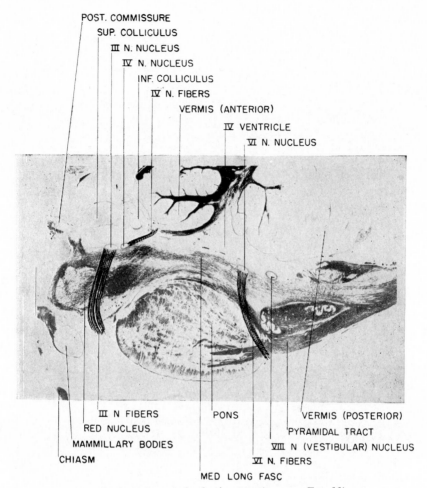

POST. COMMISSURE
SUP. COLLICULUS
III N. NUCLEUS
IV N. NUCLEUS
INF. COLLICULUS
IV N. FIBERS
VERMIS (ANTERIOR)
IV VENTRICLE
VI N. NUCLEUS

III N FIBERS   PONS   VERMIS (POSTERIOR)
RED NUCLEUS   PYRAMIDAL TRACT
MAMMILLARY BODIES   VIII N (VESTIBULAR) NUCLEUS
CHIASM   VI N. FIBERS
MED LONG FASC

FIG. 20. *Longitudinal section of the brain stem* (*same as* FIG. 11)
The photograph has been underdeveloped and retouched to show the ocular motor nerves and nuclei.

extraocular muscles including the superior rectus, medial rectus, inferior oblique, inferior rectus, and levator palpebrae (Figs. 19 and 20).

Aside from the purely motor fibers, the 3rd, 4th, and 6th cranial nerves also contain the parasympathetic and some of the sympathetic fibers. The parasympathetic fibers accompany chiefly that branch of the 3rd nerve to the inferior rectus and inferior oblique muscles; branches of the sympathetic fibers accompany all the motor nerves as well as the trigeminal branches. Whether or not the motor nerves relay sensory fibers is a controversial question. In the embryo there are clearly sensory cells along the fibers (presumably distal representatives of the gasserian ganglion), but in the adult, section of the motor nerves causes no retrograde degeneration in the trigeminal nucleus.[239] There is therefore no certain evidence that sensory fibers exist in the adult ocular motor nerves.

All three motor nerves to the extraocular muscles enter the orbit and the muscle cone by way of the superior orbital fissure. They enter the sheaths in the posterior third of their respective muscle bellies.

B. INDIVIDUAL NERVE SUPPLY

1. Oculomotor or 3rd Cranial Nerve

(a) *Anatomy and physiology.* The 3rd nerves arise from a paired group of motor cells extending approximately 5 mm. in length just beneath the central gray substance of the mesencephalon at the cross-section level of the superior colliculi (Figs. 19 and 20). As seen in a cross-section of the midbrain, the nuclei are arranged in the form of a V, with the medial longitudinal fasciculi forming the lateral and ventral boundaries (Figs. 21 and 22).

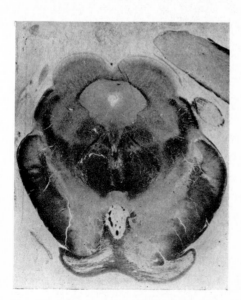

FIG. 21. *Cross section of the brain stem through the third nuclei (unretouched)*

The main mass of cell bodies in the oculomotor nuclei is situated along the arms of the V. These cells are for the most part typical large multipolar cells similar to those in the anterior horns of the spinal cord. There are, however, numerous smaller cells, about one-third the size of the others, scattered throughout the nuclei.[1033, 605] At different levels in the crotch of the V are various cell masses. In the midzone there is an unpaired group of larger motor cells similar to and not clearly demarcated from the lateral cell nuclei,[107] called Perlia's nuclei.[824] In the extreme anterior portion of the oculomotor nucleus is a paired group of characteristically small cells called the Edinger-Westphal

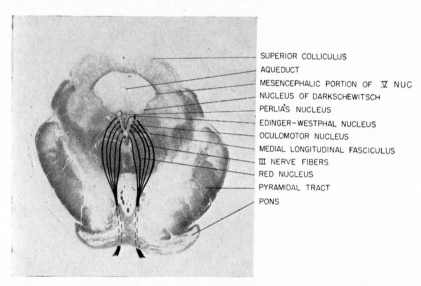

SUPERIOR COLLICULUS
AQUEDUCT
MESENCEPHALIC PORTION OF Ⅴ NUC
NUCLEUS OF DARKSCHEWITSCH
PERLIA'S NUCLEUS
EDINGER–WESTPHAL NUCLEUS
OCULOMOTOR NUCLEUS
MEDIAL LONGITUDINAL FASCICULUS
Ⅲ NERVE FIBERS
RED NUCLEUS
PYRAMIDAL TRACT
PONS

Fig. 22. *Cross section of the brain stem through the third nerve nuclei (same as* Fig. 21)
The photograph has been underdeveloped and retouched to show the third nerves and nuclei.

nuclei.[306, 1103] These cells are situated on either side of the midline anterior to Perlia's nucleus and between the upper ends of the arms of the V, so that they lie just beneath the central gray substance. They are similar to the small cells that, as previously mentioned, are scattered throughout the lateral or main nuclei.

The *functions* of the various portions of these cell complexes are a matter of dispute. There is little doubt that the main bulk of the oculomotor nerve comes from the large cells in the arms of the V. It has long been known[112] and amply confirmed that section of the oculomotor nerve causes retrograde degeneration in these

cells. The dispute revolves about the localization of function
within the lateral nuclei and about the significance of the nuclei
of Perlia and Edinger-Westphal.

The representation of the individual extraocular muscles in the
oculomotor nucleus has been recently reinvestigated. Bernheimer's
scheme,[111] based on retrograde degeneration studies in the monkey,
has been most widely accepted. According to this there is a front-
to-back representation arranged in the following order: levator
palpebrae, superior rectus, medial rectus, inferior oblique, and
inferior rectus. The rostral portions of the nucleus are believed
to innervate the muscles of the homolateral eye; the intermediate
portions (representing both medial recti) innervate both eyes; and
the caudal portions innervate the contralateral eye. There is some
experimental[1084] and clinical[268, 162] evidence in support of this
arrangement as well as clinical evidence against it.[1068] It must be
realized, however, that such clinical evidence is obtained almost
exclusively from chronic palsies and the histologic evidence in
these cases is not satisfactory.[361]

Until recently, techniques for stimulating separately the various
portions of the nuclei have been too coarse to permit accurate
localization but the recent application of the Horsley-Clarke stereotaxic electrode with minimal excitatory currents has indicated
an arrangement within the third nerve nucleus quite different
from that inferred from retrograde chromatolysis. These experiments in the cat[1010, 267] and in the monkey[106] have indicated a strictly
homolateral representation of function in the nuclei. Successive
stimulation in a rostral to caudal direction causes the eye to turn
successively downward, downward and inward, inward, inward and
upward, and finally it causes an elevation of the lid; thus, downward movements of the eye are represented rostrally and upward
movements, together with elevation of the lid, are represented
caudally. Conclusions based on these electrophysiologic experiments are not only more reliable than those based on retrograde
degeneration but accord more with the general architecture of
functional representation in the nervous system elsewhere.

It may be argued, of course, that there is no fixed localization
of function within the oculomotor nuclei. As evidence for this

may be cited the experiments on transposition of various extra-ocular muscles, with an alleged subsequent rearrangement such that muscles carry on functions different from their original ones.[702, 805, 626] These experiments must, however, be interpreted cautiously, since it has not been proved that the original functions are not still being effectively carried out through pull on Tenon's capsule[1048] or through the original muscles,[54] and especially since a comparable condition in human beings, the pseudo-Graefe phenomenon, in which nerve fibers innervate muscles other than those for which they were originally intended, never do develop any readjustment of function (see p. 71f). Until, therefore, there is more convincing evidence to the contrary, it seems most reasonable to assume that the oculomotor nucleus, like other motor nuclei in the central nervous system, does have a discrete and immutable localization of muscle function.

Perlia's nucleus is obviously a motor nucleus, since it consists of typical motor cells. Moreover, it is undoubtedly concerned with the oculomotor mechanism, since its cells are indissociable from the rest of the 3rd nerve complex and since it shows retrograde degeneration with lesions of this nerve.[162] But its particular function can only be inferred. Since it does not develop until relatively late in embryonic growth,[693, 820] and since it is highly developed only in the human species,[19] it is generally assumed to serve the function of convergence, which is well developed only in the higher species. Occasional cases of medial rectus palsy have been reported with degeneration in Perlia's nucleus.[162]

The *Edinger-Westphal nucleus* is not so obviously motor in function, nor indeed is it necessarily associated with the 3rd nerve nucleus. Bernheimer[112] originally reported that retrograde degeneration occurred in this nucleus after removal of the intraocular structures, whence these cells were assumed to be associated with pupillary and accommodative functions. His experiments were not confirmed[701, 28]; nevertheless his thesis has persisted. Removal of the ciliary ganglion has, however, resulted in retrograde degeneration in the Edinger-Westphal nucleus[632, 635, 605] indicating that the thesis may have been correct even though the experiments were in error. Stimulation experiments by the relatively crude methods previously available,[459, 114] as well as by the modern Horsley-Clarke apparatus,[107, 106] are consistent with a pupillomotor function of the Edinger-Westphal complex.[1010] Most disturbing to this thesis at the present time are the facts that no fibers have been traced from the Edinger-Westphal nucleus into the oculomotor group; that section of the oculomotor nerve has not resulted in retrograde degeneration in the Edinger-Westphal nucleus;[761] and that its destruction has not resulted in loss of pupillary function.

There is no unequivocal evidence for the representation of accommodation in the oculomotor complex, but the location may be presumed to be in close proximity to the centers for miosis and convergence, since accommodation is associated with these functions in the near reflex. Accommodation may be represented in the Edinger-Westphal nucleus.

Finally, there is another paired group of cells, the nuclei of Darkschewitsch, which may be mentioned in passing. These cells are situated anterior and lateral to the oculomotor complex. They consist of small cells similar to those in the Edinger-Westphal nuclei. They were originally assumed to be concerned with the ocular motor mechanism, and are now occasionally reported to be associated with vertical movements of the eyes,[1121, 390, 392] but it seems more likely that they serve some nonocular function, probably connected with the origin of the commissural fibers.

The fibers of the 3rd cranial nerve, arising in the oculomotor nuclei, pass ventrally through the brain stem and in their intramedullary course traverse successively the medial longitudinal fasciculus, the red nucleus, the substantia nigra, and the anterior margin of the pons (Fig. 22). The trunks of the 3rd nerve emerge from the central nervous system in the interpenduncular fossa at the angles formed by the peduncle and the pons.

Thence the nerves course forward and somewhat laterally, covered by pia, through the subarachnoid space to penetrate the dura mater and enter the cavernous sinus just lateral to the posterior clinoid process. The 3rd nerves extend forward in the cavernous sinuses with the other ocular motor nerves and emerge at its anterior part, passing lateral to the carotid artery in close proximity to the uncus of the temporal lobe and enter the orbit through the superior orbital fissure. As the oculomotor nerve enters the orbit, it divides into a superior branch destined for the su-

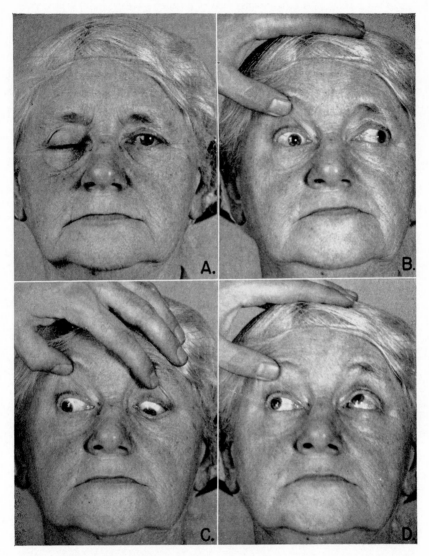

FIG. 23. *Third nerve paralysis*

Right-sided paralysis of (A) levator palpebrae (ptosis); (B) medial rectus; (C) inferior rectus; and (D) superior rectus.

The patient was a seventy-three-year-old woman who had hypertension. The paralysis developed spontaneously two weeks previously, gradually lessened, and completely resolved in eight weeks from onset.

perior rectus and levator palpebrae muscles and an inferior branch destined for the medial rectus, inferior rectus, inferior oblique, and a short branch of the latter to the ciliary ganglion. The pupillo-constrictor fibers are believed to be concentrated in the superior portion of the third nerve in the region of its exit from the mid-

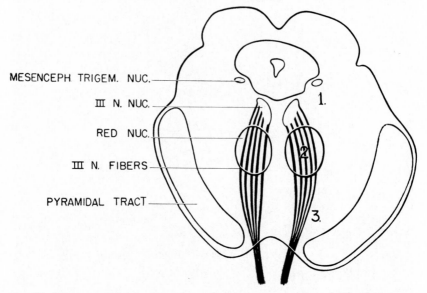

MESENCEPH. TRIGEM. NUC.

III N. NUC.

RED NUC.

III N. FIBERS

PYRAMIDAL TRACT

1.

2.

3.

FIG. 24. *Diagram of brain stem through third nerve nucleus indicating structures involved by lesions at different levels*
     Lesions at level 1 result in homolateral third nerve paralysis and homolateral anesthesia of the cornea. Lesions at level 2 result in homolateral third nerve paralysis and contralateral tremor (Benedikt's syndrome). Lesions at level 3 result in homolateral third nerve paralysis and crossed pyramidal tract signs (Weber's syndrome).

brain; in consequence, preferential involvement of the pupil is especially characteristic of lesions in this region.[1007]

(b) *Clinical disturbances.* Total paralysis of the 3rd nerve produces ptosis,* inability to rotate the eye upward, downward or inward, a dilated nonreactive pupil (iridoplegia), and paralysis of accommodation (cycloplegia) (Fig. 23). When the nonparalyzed eye is fixating straight ahead, the paralyzed eye is held in a posi-

---

  * The ptosis is due to the tone of the orbicularis, which is unopposed when the levator is paralyzed. If the orbicularis is paralyzed (7th nerve) as well as the levator (3rd nerve), the ptosis is much less than when only the 3rd nerve is paralyzed.

tion of divergence but can be brought to the midline by directing the gaze to the side opposite the paralysis. Incomplete palsies of the 3rd nerve produce various combinations of the foregoing signs. When only the intraocular structures are paralyzed (dilated pupil, paralysis of accommodation), the condition is spoken of as *internal ophthalmoplegia.*

The site of the lesion producing 3rd nerve paralyses determines to some degree the extent of the involvement and, of course, to a large degree the association of other signs and symptoms with it. Lesions of the 3rd nerve fibers *within the central nervous system* are accompanied by other neurologic signs and symptoms (Fig. 24). Involvement of the 3rd nerve fibers in the red nucleus gives rise to *Benedikt's syndrome* characterized by homolateral oculomotor paralysis with contralateral intention tremor (Figs. 25 and 26). Involvement of these nerve fibers in the cerebral peduncle produces *Weber's syndrome* characterized by homolateral oculomotor paralysis and crossed hemiplegia. Involvement of the 3rd nerve fibers in the

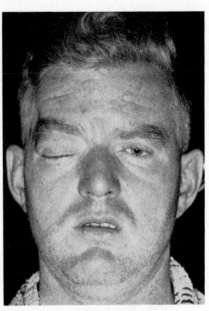

Fig. 25. *Right third nerve paralysis due to a vascular anomaly in the brain stem*
With the right sided ophthalmoplegia, the patient had a gross tremor of the left arm. (Benedikt's syndrome) and a hemiparesis on the left (Weber's syndrome).

cavernous sinus and at the *superior orbital* fissure is almost invariably accompanied by involvement of the other ocular motor nerves as well. With lesions of the cavernous sinus, the extraocular muscles are affected earlier than are the intraocular muscles whereas the reverse is true with lesions between the cavernous sinus and the brain stem (see p. 176). Lesions in the region of the superior orbital fissure or of the cavernous sinus produce only a moderate dilatation of the pupil owing to the simultaneous involvement of

the sympathetic nerves, in contrast to the full dilatation characteristic of other peripheral lesions where the sympathetic nerves are
not involved. Not infrequently the pupillary functions may be
entirely normal with lesions of the superior orbital fissure despite
total external ophthalmoplegia.

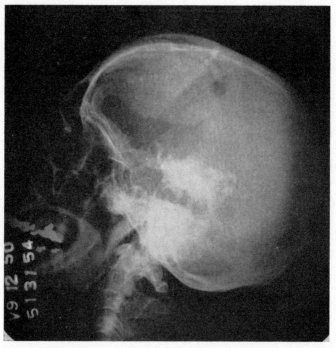

Fig. 26. *The vascular anomaly in the foregoing patient, visualized by arteri-
ography, is indicated by a diffuse plexus of vessels in the brain stem. This
contrasts with the discrete lobulation seen with aneurisms (compare with*
Fig. 33)

The lesion responsible for the clinical signs presumably involved the right
midbrain area in the region of the red nucleus and pyramid. The X-rays
also show a bony defect corresponding to a previous operative site.

The lesions responsible for 3rd nerve palsies are of various
types. Rarely do *congenital lesions* involve the entire 3rd nerve,
although selective paresis of the levator and superior rectus muscles, either singly or together, is fairly common (Figs. 27 and 28).
Inferior rectus, inferior oblique, or medial rectus palsies rarely
occur as isolated congenital phenomena[1001, 197, 519, 1104, 1140, 187] and still
more rarely as sequelae of trauma.[688]

Conditions simulating isolated ocular muscle palsies may result from anomalous adhesions of the muscle sheaths.[335] These result in mechanical limitations of the eye movements and may be detected, and differentiated, only by forced passive movements of the eye with forceps.[527, 167]

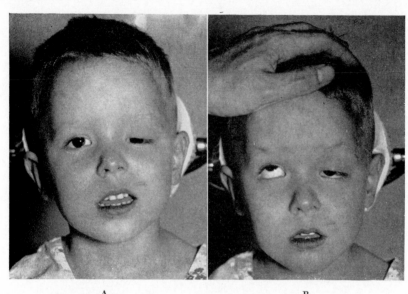

A   B

FIG. 27. *Congenital paralysis of left levator palpebrae muscle and left superior rectus muscle*
(A) Patient looking straight ahead; (B) patient looking up.

Third nerve palsies occur with a variety of inflammatory conditions, vascular lesions, tumors, and degenerative diseases (Figs. 29 and 30). Some of these are especially noteworthy. Among the inflammatory processes it should be noted that *syphilitic and tuberculous meningitis* are especially apt to produce 3rd nerve paralysis because of the tendency of these inflammatory processes to localize between the chiasm, pons, and temporal lobes, where the 3rd nerves emerge from the central nervous system. The paralysis is usually bilateral. *Purulent* meningitis is more likely to produce 6th nerve paralysis, and even when the 3rd nerves are found at autopsy to be bathed with pus, there may have been no evidence of functional impairment during life. *Poliomyelitis* may rarely cause oculomotor ophthalmoplegia.[1137, 560] *Polyneuritis* from a variety of toxins (al-

cohol, lead, arsenic, carbon monoxide, and the toxins of diabetes)
may involve the 3rd nerve as it does any peripheral nerve. *Herpes
zoster* is especially apt to affect the 3rd nerve, a paralysis developing five to seven days after the appearance of the skin eruption. The
medial rectus, levator, and sphincter pupillae are said to be espe-

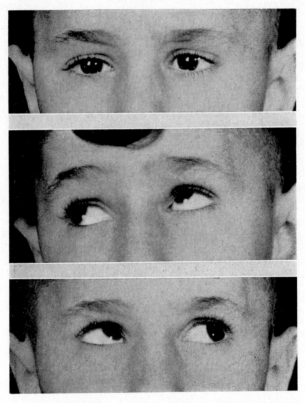

Fig. 28. *Congenital paralysis of both superior recti muscles with secondary
"overaction of inferior oblique muscles.*

cially prone to involvement,[360] but the entire 3rd nerve may be
affected. *Mumps* also occasionally causes 3rd nerve paralysis.[188]
Cavernous sinus thrombosis produces 3rd nerve paralysis, but
here other ocular motor nerves are also involved, which, together
with the exophthalmos, venous stasis, and obvious sepsis, leaves
little doubt about the diagnosis. With cavernous sinus thrombosis[1073] and other lesions in the sphenoidal region,[846] the involve-

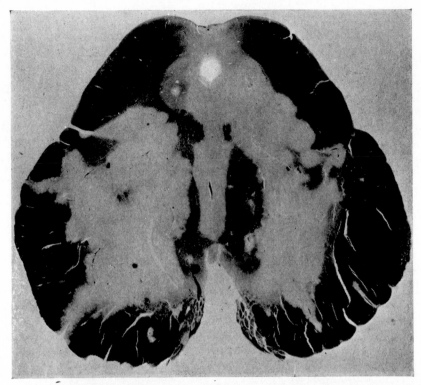

Fig. 29. *Extensive demyelination and gliosis (encephalomyelitis) of the brain stem in the region of the intramedullary portion of the third nerve*
 The patient was a twenty-eight-year-old man who first developed drooping of the left lid and then a complete bilateral third nerve paralysis, spasticity of gait, stupor, and death within five weeks after the onset of symptoms.

ment of the extraocular muscles is apt to precede that of the intraocular muscles. Unilateral paralysis of the 3rd nerve with a relatively miotic pupil[89] along with involvement of the other ocular motor nerves, and frequently of the optic nerve as well, comprises an entity variously known as the *syndrome of the superior orbital fissure,* sphenoidal syndrome, or syndrome of the lateral wall of the cavernous sinus.[350] It may result from suppuration of the sphenoidol sinus, from other focal inflammation, from skull fracture, hemorrhage, or from tumor. The common tumors are sphenoidal ridge meningioma, nasopharyngeal tumors, and metastatic carcinomas.

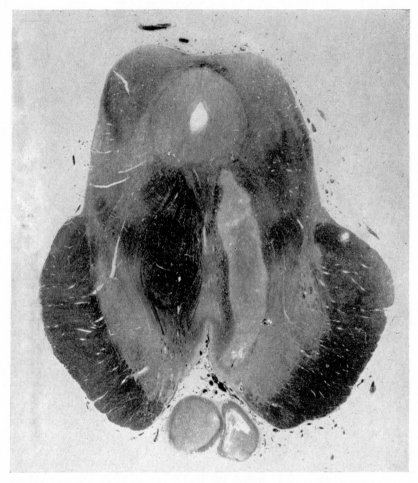

Fig. 30. *Localized area of softening along the course of one of the third nerves due to an embolic infarct*

The patient was a fifty-eight-year-old man with acute vegetative endocarditis who one month prior to death, suddenly developed a third nerve paralysis on the left side and a hemiplegia on the right side (Weber's syndrome).

Oculomotor paralysis with diabetes merits special consideration because of its frequency. It comes on suddenly with, often, severe pain on the same side of the head. In consequence, it is generally believed to be of vascular origin; in favor of this is its predominant occurrence in persons with hemorrhagic retinopathy and other evidence of vascular disease.[1088, 298] The only pathohistologic observation that has been made in a case of recent diabetic oculomotor palsy indicated a gross swelling of the intraorbital portion of the nerve with extensive destruction of medullated fibers in the central portions of the nerve.[3]

Isolated internal ophthalmoplegia from inflammatory lesions may occur with botulism and following grippe. *Paralysis of accommodation* without coexistent involvement of the pupil may occur with diphtheria,[1079, 1080] but it also occurs without obvious cause.[92]

The one vascular lesion that characteristically produces 3rd nerve

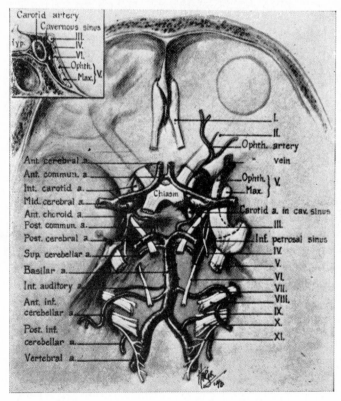

Fig. 31. *Drawing of the base of the skull showing the relative positions of the arteries and cranial nerves (Walsh and King)*

Especially noteworthy in connection with intracranial aneurisms is the proximity of the internal carotid artery with its bifurcations to the third and fifth cranial nerves.

paralysis is rupture of an *aneurism* at the base of the brain[524, 1075] (Figs. 32, 33, and 34). This nerve is especially vulnerable by reason of its proximity to the branching of the internal carotid artery, where these aneurisms are prone to be situated[669] (Fig. 31). The characteristic signs of rupture of these aneurisms are 3rd nerve paralysis, pain about the eyes and face (5th nerve involvement)[1077] and generalized headache.[514] These symptoms do not necessarily occur concomitantly. The 3rd nerve paralysis is due to hemorrhagic infiltation of the nerve and not to pressure alone; in its intracranial course the nerve is covered by pia only and hence relatively easily infiltrated by blood. Occasionally aneurisms of the arteries (congenital, arteriosclerotic, or traumatic) rupture into the cavernous sinus, producing pulsating exophthalmos and other signs of congestion about the eye.[523, 892] Despite the 3rd nerve paralysis in these cases, the pupil may not be dilated, owing to the simultaneous involvement of the sympathetic fibers. Also often presumed to be vascular in origin are the *recurrent 3rd nerve paralyses* that occur as manifestations of migraine.[151,1018]

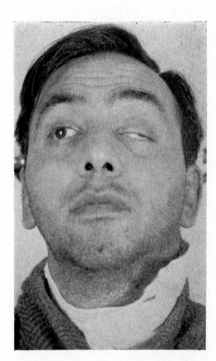

FIG. 32. *Left third nerve paralysis due to intracranial aneurism.*

The patient was a twenty-year-old man who, six weeks previously, developed a severe left-sided headache lasting several days. Three weeks later the headache recurred and was accompanied by a left third nerve paralysis. Lumbar puncture showed xanthochromic spinal fluid.

Third nerve paralyses occur occasionally with occlusions of the basilar artery, especially with *emboli* (whereas 6th nerve paralyses are more frequent with *thromboses* of the basilar artery).[597]

The herniation of the temporal lobe through the tentorium that occurs with supratentorial expanding lesions may so press on the 3rd nerve as to result in an oculomotor paralysis. Autopsy of such cases shows the 3rd nerve impaled with the temporal lobe in the tentorial foramen. The pupillary fibers appear to be the most vulnerable[1007] and mydriasis may be the only sign of such a lesion.

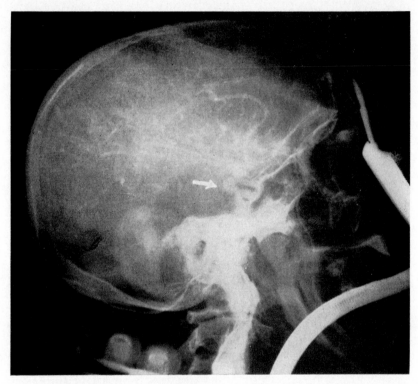

FIG. 33. *Arteriogram of same patient*
The left carotid artery is apparent and the aneurism can be seen as a diverticular mass measuring 1 cm. in diameter arising from the first knee of the internal carotid artery just above the posterior clinoid processes.

A similar herniation consequent to cerebral edema has been proposed to account for the cyclic ophthalmoplegia of migraine.[443]

Tumors of the base of the skull frequently involve the 3rd nerve, sometimes alone but usually in association with other ocular motor nerves and the trigeminal nerve. These tumors may arise in the nasopharynx, the sella turcica (pituitary adenomas[47] and chordomas), from the meninges (especially of the sphenoidal ridge), from

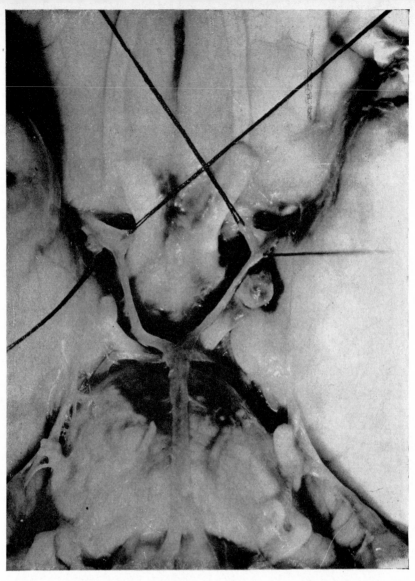

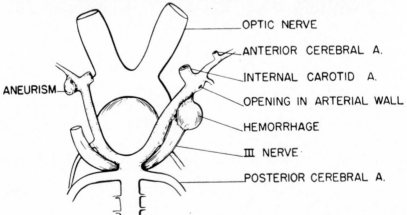

OPTIC NERVE

ANTERIOR CEREBRAL A.

INTERNAL CAROTID A.

ANEURISM

OPENING IN ARTERIAL WALL

HEMORRHAGE

III NERVE

POSTERIOR CEREBRAL A.

the brain itself (especially frontal and temporal lobe gliomas) and by metastasis from distant foci.

Aberrant regeneration occasionally follows lesions of the 3rd nerve when the stumps of the nerve have not been properly re-aligned[127] or when there is a delay in restoration of function. It

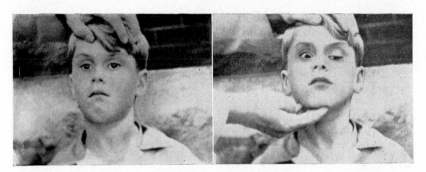

FIG. 35. *Retraction of the lid (right) on downward gaze due to aberrant regeneration of the third nerve fibers*
The patient was an eight-year-old boy who had a third nerve paralysis at birth. The lid was observed to show the anomalous retraction at five months of age. Examination at the present time shows, aside from the retraction of the lid on downward gaze, a paresis of the right inferior rectus and right medial rectus.

does not occur if the nerve recovers function within 6 weeks but is relatively common when recovery does not take place for several months. Frequently the nerve fibers that were originally connected with the inferior rectus grow down into the sheaths of the levator, and sometimes the fibers originally connected with the medial rectus grow into the distal sheaths of the pupillary pathways (and even into the ciliary muscle pathways[98]). Thus,

←◀◀◀

FIG. 34. *Inferior brain surface and diagram showing multiple aneurisms (presumably congenital) of internal carotid arteries*
The patient was a twenty-year-old girl who, three weeks prior to death, suddenly lost consciousness for eighteen hours, but recovered with only mild headache and drowsiness; ten days before death she developed a complete third nerve paralysis on the left side and a stiff neck. The photograph shows one recently erupted aneurism coming from the left internal carotid artery and adherent to the left third nerve. Another aneurism, unerupted, may be seen coming from the right internal carotid artery in the angle formed by this vessel with the anterior choroidal artery.

when an attempt is made to look downward, the affected eye moves little or not at all, but the lid rises (Fig. 35); when an attempt is made to look to the opposite side, the eye moves little or not at all, but the pupil constricts. The miosis is all the more striking since the pupil is otherwise semidilated and nonreactive to light. The retraction of the lid on downward movement of the eye gives it the name "pseudo-Graefe phenomenon" because of the superficial resemblance to lid lag (Graefe's sign) in thyrotoxicosis. Since this name does not include various other bizarre movements that do not have lid retraction and yet result from the same process, a better name is *"aberrant regeneration of the 3rd nerve."** Thus, the pupil alone may constrict when an attempt is made to use the medial rectus (a pseudo-Argyll-Robertson pupil[353]); or, if the medial rectus receives fibers from the proximal stump of the superior rectus nerve fibers, the eye may turn in when an attempt is made to look upward (Fig. 36). A particularly curious anomaly occurs when the elevator mus-

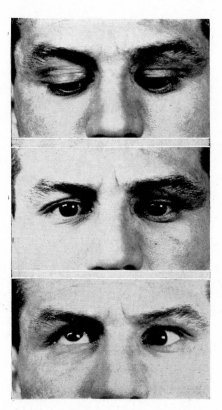

FIG. 36. *Anomalous adduction of the left eye on upward gaze due to aberrant regeneration of the third nerve fibers*

The patient was an eighteen-year-old boy who had had a third nerve paralysis at birth. Examination at the present time shows (Top) a slight retraction of the left lid on looking down but (Center and Bottom) a conspicuous adduction of the left eye on looking up and a constriction of the pupil. When tested monocularly, the left eye showed a complete paralysis of the superior rectus and inferior oblique muscles.

* This name would presumably not be acceptable to those few who do not accept the implied pathogenesis.[1083]

cle receives fibers originally connected with the superior rectus muscle. The lid then elevates not only with the normal voluntary upward movements of the eyes but also with involuntary upward movements (Bell's phenomenon) on attempted closure of the lids.[395] At other times the lid is ptotic. In other words, the lid opens widely when an attempt is made to close it!

Aberrant regeneration of the 3rd nerve is a permanent condition, not unlike the aberrant regeneration that sometimes follows 7th nerve lesions and that results in bizarre facial movements[653] (see p. 146f). The lesions responsible for the 3rd nerve paralysis are nonspecific; for example, syphilis,[377] fractured skull,[127] saccular aneurism,[1077] tumor,[97] and birth injuries.[212] It has been produced experimentally in the chimpanzee[101] and in the monkey.[98]

2. Trochlear or 4th Cranial Nerve

(a) *Anatomy and physiology.* The 4th nerves arise from a paired group of motor cells situated just beneath the central gray sub-stance in the mesencephalon at the cross-section level of the posterior colliculi (Figs. 19 and 20). The cell bodies are continuous anteriorly with the nuclei that make up the 3rd nerve complex and are separated from them only by a thinning out of the cells. Like the cells of the 3rd nerve, those representing the 4th nerves are bounded laterally and ventrally by the medial longitudinal fasciculi (Figs. 37 and 38). The cells are mostly typical motor cells but contain a few smaller cells. [821]

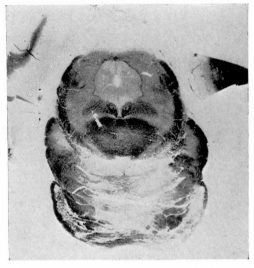

Fig. 37. *Cross section of the brain stem through the fourth nerve nuclei (unretouched)*

Although there is no anatomic separation of the cell bodies of the 4th nerves from those of the 3rd nerve, their ocalization offers no difficulty, since the 4th nerve fibers may be traced directly into the nuclear complex. Also, stimulation of the nuclei by means of the Horsley-Clarke apparatus has located a trochlear reaction (intorsion of the contralateral eye) when the electrode has been placed deep at the posterior end of the 3rd nerve nucleus.[106]

The fibers arising from the 4th nerve nucleus course dorsally and laterally about the central gray substance, to decussate completely in the roof of the mesencephalon and emerge just behind the posterior colliculi. Of all the motor nerves the 4th cranial nerves are unique in emerging from the central nervous system dorsally and in decussating practically completely. The reason for this anoma-

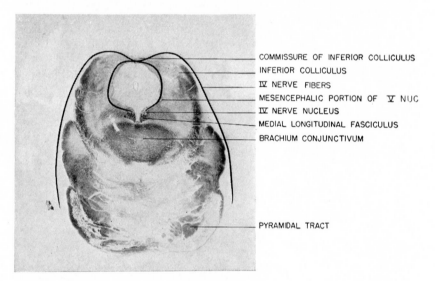

COMMISSURE OF INFERIOR COLLICULUS
INFERIOR COLLICULUS
IV NERVE FIBERS
MESENCEPHALIC PORTION OF V NUC
IV NERVE NUCLEUS
MEDIAL LONGITUDINAL FASCICULUS
BRACHIUM CONJUNCTIVUM

PYRAMIDAL TRACT

FIG. 38. *Cross section of the brain stem through the fourth nerve nuclei (same as* FIG. 37)
The photograph has been retouched to show the course of the fourth nerve fibers.

lous behavior is not known, but it is a pattern that was set in early phylogeny, for it is universally present.[817]

After emergence from the central nervous system, the 4th nerves pass anteriorly and ventrally about the superior margins of the cerebral peduncles. Thus, passing in the subarachnoid space to the base of the brain stem, they pierce the dura mater to enter the cavernous sinus just behind the level of the posterior clinoid processes. In the cavernous sinus the 4th nerves are closely associated with the 3rd and 6th nerves, and the three nerves emerge from the anterior end of this sinus together to enter the superior orbital fissure. Thence the 4th nerves are directed to the superior oblique muscles.

(b) *Clinical disturbances.* Paralysis of the 4th nerve results in an extorsion of the eye and a weakness of downward gaze. The extorsion is more marked as the gaze is directed outward, and the weakness of downward gaze is more marked as the gaze is directed to the opposite side. Because of the limitation in downward gaze, it

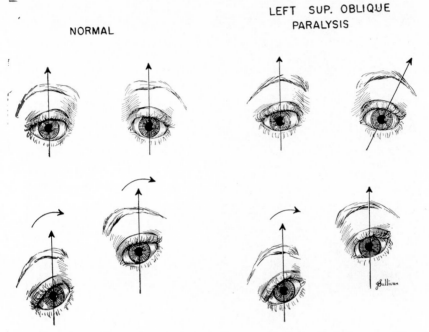

NORMAL

LEFT SUP. OBLIQUE
PARALYSIS

Fig. 39. *Sketch illustrating torsion of the normal eye and of the eye with a paralysis of the superior oblique muscle on tilting of the head*
The pairs of eyes on the left represent the normal condition; those on the right represent the condition of a left superior oblique paralysis.
Since the eye with the paralysis of the superior oblique muscle is extorted and since extorsion of one eye and intorsion of the other eye is a normal ophthalmostatic reflex on tilting the head, a patient may obtain binocular alignment of his eyes by tilting his head to the opposite shoulder.

is not surprising that patients with 4th nerve paralyses complain of special difficulty in going downstairs.

Head tilting is especially characteristic of 4th nerve palsies (Fig. 8), and may even result in a scoliosis.[49] By tilting the head to the opposite shoulder, patients with such paralysis may obtain binocular vision, for in this position extorsion of the upper eye and

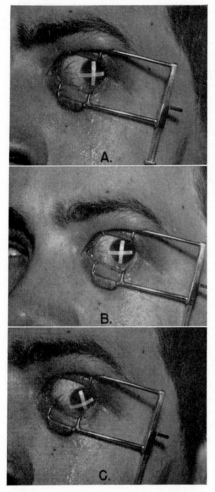

FIG. 40. *Intorsion of the eye due to the action of the superior oblique muscle in the presence of a third nerve paralysis*

Strips of filter paper were placed on the anesthetized cornea. The patient was fixing with the right eye in (A) the primary position, (B) looking up, and (C) looking down. There is a slight extorsion on looking up and a conspicuous intorsion on looking down. The presence of torsion indicates that although the third nerve is paralyzed, the fourth nerve is functioning.

intorsion of the lower eye constitute a normal ophthalmostatic reflex (Fig. 39). In congenital palsies of the 4th nerve the head tilt may so well compensate for the ocular motor paralysis that the cause of the torticollis may not be recognized. Indeed, some of these patients are reported to have had tenotomies of their sternocleidomastoid muscles under the impression that the fault lay in the neck muscles!

The testing of superior oblique function in the presence of a 3rd nerve paralysis offers a special problem since the eye cannot be turned inward where the vertical actions of the oblique muscles can be tested. If, however, the patient *attempts* to look to the opposite side and then directs his gaze up and down, the action of the superior oblique will be evident by a distinct intorsion of the eye on attempted downward gaze (Fig 40). The blood vessels are ordinarily the best landmarks for observing the intorsion of the globe.

Paralysis of the 4th nerve occurs with many of the conditions that cause paralysis of the 3rd nerve (polyneuritis, meningitis, herpes zoster, diabetes, lesions of the cavernous sinus and superior orbital fissure) but it is also produced by lesions which are peculiar to it. It is not infrequent following trauma with fracture of the superior orbital rim. Some of the operations on the frontal sinus, such as Killian's operation, in which the trochlea is displaced are accompanied temporarily by an effective paralysis of the superior oblique muscle. Although this is, no doubt, a mechanical effect and not a true paralysis, the clinical result is the same and hence may be included here. The palsies that occur with *Paget's disease* and with *hypertrophic arthritis*[1053] may also be due to mechanical disturbances of the trochlear process. It is surprising that the superior oblique function is only rarely involved with ethmoiditis.

Fourth nerve paralysis occurs not infrequently with *arteriosclerosis* owing either to hemorrhage in the roof of the midbrain or to direct involvement of the nerve by the adjacent posterior cerebral and superior cerebellar arteries.

3. Abducens or 6th Cranial Nerve

(a) *Anatomy and physiology.* The 6th nerves arise from a paired group of motor cells situated in the floor of the 4th ventricle on either side of the midline (Figs. 41 and 42). The situation of these nuclei are demarcated in the gross specimens by eminences, the facial colliculi, produced by fibers from the facial nerve. These latter nerve fibers, making a peculiarly circuitous course in the brain stem, surround the 6th nerve nuclei and thereby form an appreciable elevation in the floor of the 4th ventricle.

The 6th nerve nuclei lie just anterior to the rambling complex of cells that make up the vestibular nuclei, and probably lie in close proximity to the pontine centers for conjugate lateral gaze. Medial to the

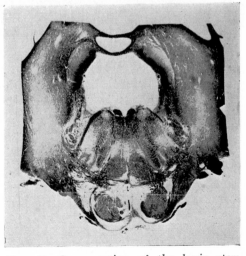

Fig. 41. *Cross section of the brain stem through the sixth nerve nuclei (unretouched)*

6th nerve nuclei and separating them from each other are the *medial longitudinal fasciculi.* The fibers from the 6th nerve nuclei course ventrally, without decussating, through the tegmentum and pons, to emerge from the brain stem on either side of the midline at the posterior border of the pons.

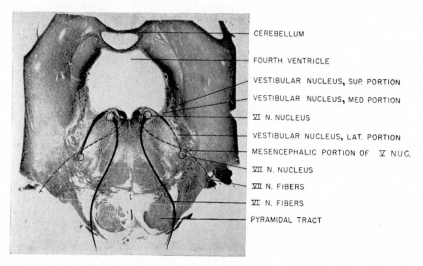

CEREBELLUM

FOURTH VENTRICLE

VESTIBULAR NUCLEUS, SUP. PORTION

VESTIBULAR NUCLEUS, MED PORTION

VI N. NUCLEUS

VESTIBULAR NUCLEUS, LAT. PORTION

MESENCEPHALIC PORTION OF V NUC.

VII N. NUCLEUS

VII N. FIBERS

VI N. FIBERS

PYRAMIDAL TRACT

FIG. 42. *Gross section of the brain stem through the sixth nerve nuclei (same as* FIG. 41)

The photograph has been retouched to show the nuclei and course of the sixth and seventh nerves.

After emerging from the central nervous system, the 6th nerves pass forward and laterally over the *petrous tip of the temporal bone,* to which they are bound by the overlying petrosphenoidal ligament (Dorello's canal), and pierce the dura mater alongside the dorsum sellae to enter the cavernous sinus. Here they come in contact with the lateral wall of the carotid artery. Thence they pass forward with the 3rd and 4th cranial nerves out of the cavernous sinus, and together the three nerves enter the orbit through the superior orbital fissure.

(b) *Clinical disturbances.* Paralysis of the 6th nerves results in a convergent strabismus, with inability to turn the eye lateralward beyond the midline (Fig. 43). With *complete* paralysis, diplopia is the rule, but with *incomplete* paralysis, binocular vision may be maintained by turning the *head* toward the side of the paralyzed muscle. The eyes are then conjugately turned toward the non-paralyzed side. Unlike the compensatory positions of the head previously mentioned with superior oblique and superior rectus palsy, that with external rectus palsy is a *turning of the head and not a tilting.*

With *fresh* palsies of one external rectus, the strabismus is *greater* when the paralyzed eye is used for fixation *(secondary deviation)* than when the nonparalyzed eye is used *(primary devia-*

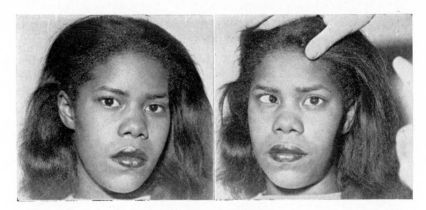

FIG. 43. *Paralysis of the left lateral rectus muscle showing (A) compensatory head turning to the left and (B) inability to turn the left eye to the left*
The patient was a twelve-year-old girl who developed pain in the left face and paralysis of the left lateral rectus following a left middle-ear infection and mastoiditis (Gradenigo's syndrome).

tion). With fresh palsies the phenomenon of *past-pointing* is also demonstrable; that is, when a patient is asked to fixate with the paralyzed eye on an object placed to the side of the paralyzed muscle, he believes that his eye is turned more than is actually the case. Hence, if he is asked to close his eyes and point to the object he has been attempting to look at, he overshoots the mark.

Old 6th nerve paralyses are apt to be accompanied by progressive *contractures* of the medial recti so that the convergence increases with time. This is not true, curiously, with congenital palsies.

Paralyses of the 6th nerves occur with many of the conditions that cause 3rd and 4th nerve paralyses, such as diabetes, herpes zoster,[385] poliomyelitis,[560] poisoning with lead, arsenic, etc. Rarely the 6th nerves are involved in interstitial hypertrophic neuritis[212] and chronic adhesive arachnoiditis. With cavernous sinus thrombosis all the ocular motor nerves, at least on one side, are usually affected. The 6th nerves are more apt to be affected than are the other ocular motor nerves with *purulent* meningitis, skull fractures, and especially with increased intracranial pressure. The predisposition for the 6th nerves in these conditions is no doubt due to their *longer* intracranial course, to the fact that they are *sharply angulated* over the crest of the temporal bones, or possibly to strangulation by the transverse branches of the basilar artery.[262] Sixth nerve involvement occurs occasionally with tuberculous meningitis.[1039, 375] Owing to the proximity of the 6th nerves to the arteries at the point of emergence from the central nervous system (the antero-inferior cerebellar artery behind and the internal auditory artery in front) and to the internal carotid artery in the cavernous sinus, the 6th nerves are occasionally involved with intracranial aneurisms. Wheras emboli of the basilar artery, lodging high up at its bifurcation, produce 3rd nerve paralyses, it is thromboses of the basilar artery involving the posterior portions that are apt to produce 6th nerve paralyses.[597]

Paralysis of the lateral rectus occurs also with lesions that do not affect the other ocular motor nerves. It is occasionally hereditary.[619] A not uncommon congenital defect occurs wherein the lateral rectus is replaced by an inelastic fibrous band; this is characterized clinically by the fact that the eye retracts into the orbit several millimeters on turning medially. Hence, it is called the *retraction syndrome* (Duane's syndrome).

Sixth nerve paralysis occurs occasionally after lumbar anesthesia[988, 173, 864, 1032, 403] or after pantopaque injection for myelography[1138] and may even follow a simple *lumbar puncture*.[311, 180, 403] The paralysis usually comes on a week or more following the spinal puncture and is frequently associated with other signs of meningeal irritation.[311, 238, 149]

Sixth nerve paralyses may occur simply with increased intracranial pressure, presumably through mechanical stretching of the nerves over the crest of the temporal bone. Thus 6th nerve paralysis in the presence of papilledema or of other evidence of increased intracranial pressure has little or no topical significance; failure to recognize this is a frequent source of confusion clinically.

An entity known as *Gradenigo's syndrome* occurs at times following middle-ear infection (Fig. 43). It is characterized by diplopia (6th nerve palsy) with pain on one side of the face (5th nerve involvement) and deafness; it is due to osteitis of the petrous tip of the pyramid.[1056, 714] It usually follows a mastoid or middle-ear infection on the homolateral side, but occasionally the 6th nerve paralysis is on the side opposite the middle-ear disease.[819] The combination of pain in the face and 6th nerve paralysis, but without deafness, occurs with various other lesions in the petrous pyramid; most frequent, perhaps, is metastatic carcinoma.

Wernicke's encephalopathy is usually accompanied by 6th nerve paralysis on one or both sides.[224] This is a disease due specifically to thiamine deficiency and occurs most frequently in alcoholics on a deficient diet. It results in destruction both of nerve cells and nerve fibers with a predilection for the paraventricular regions of

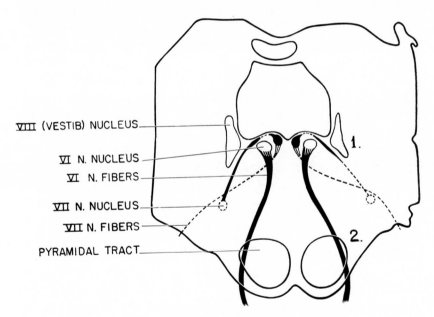

Fig. 44. *Diagram of brain stem through sixth nerve nuclei indicating structures involved by lesions at different levels*

Lesions at level 1 result in homolateral sixth and seventh nerve paralyses with varying degrees of nystagmus and weakness of conjugate gaze to the homolateral side. Lesions at level 2 result in homolateral sixth nerve paralysis and crossed hemiplegia (Millard-Gubler syndrome).

the brain stem. Aside from the 6th nerve palsies, pareses of horizontal conjugate gaze, nystagmus, ataxia, and Korsakoff's psychosis are frequently present and equally characteristic. Diagnosis is made by the history and by the prompt reversal of the ocular signs and symptoms following thiamine administration.[830]

Finally, 6th nerve paralysis occurs along with involvement of the 5th, 7th, and 8th cranial nerves, with lesions of the cerebellopontine angle, and with intramedullary lesions of the brain stem (Fig. 44). Most frequent are the acoustic neuromas producing the characteristic symptomatology of unilateral deafness, facial paralysis, diplopia, and papilledema. Lesions within the pons, of whatever type, may produce 6th nerve paralysis on the homolateral side of the body and pyramidal tract signs on the contralateral side of the body (Millard-Gubler syndrome), for the pyramidal tracts have not decussated at the points where they are in contact with the 6th nerves. For the same reason, there may be 6th nerve paralysis and contralateral hemianesthesia from lesions within the brain stem. These are often associated, as might be expected, with palsies of conjugate gaze to the same side and homolateral 7th nerve paralysis.

SUMMARY

The motor nerves to the extraocular muscles are: the 3rd nerve, running to the levator palpebrae, superior rectus, medial rectus, inferior oblique, and inferior rectus; the 4th neve, running to the superior oblique; and the 6th nerve, running to the lateral rectus. These three motor nerves together with the three sensory branches of the trigeminal nerve are believed to be developed from the three first metameres in the embryo.

The 3rd nerve arises from a paired group of cells in the anterior end of the midbrain. Most of these cells are typical motor cells and presumably connect with the extraocular muscles in an unalterable pattern. In addition, there are smaller cells, not characteristically motor in type, scattered throughout the nuclei and arranged in paired groups between the anterior horns of the 3rd nerve nuclei (Edinger-Westphal nuclei); they are thought to innervate the iris muscles (pupil) and possibly the ciliary muscles (accommodation).

Complete paralysis of the 3rd nerve produces ptosis, inability to turn the eye upward, inward, or downward, and a dilated fixed pupil. If the 6th nerve is intact, the eye is divergent. Lesions of the nerve fibers in the brain stem are usually accompanied by other neurologic signs; for example, anesthesia of the homolateral cornea, tremor of the contralateral limbs, and contralateral hemiplegia.

Third nerve paralysis occurs characteristically with aneurisms of the internal carotid artery, diabetes, herniation of the temporal lobe through the tentorial foramen, and with various focal inflammatory and neoplastic diseases in the region of the interpeduncular fossa and apex of the orbit. Regeneration of the 3rd nerve may result in misdirection of fibers and permanently anomalous eye and lid movements.

The 4th nerves arise from a paired group of motor cells at the posterior end of the 3rd nerve nucleus. The 4th nerve fibers are unique among motor fibers in that they course dorsally to emerge in the central nervous system and decussate completely. Paralysis of the superior oblique produces an extorsion when the eye is directed straight ahead or turned outward, and an inability to look downward when the eye is turned inward. Head tilting is especially characteristic of superior oblique paralysis.

The 6th nerves arise from a paired motor nucleus in the floor of the 4th ventricle adjacent to the vestibular nuclei and in the vicinity of the subcortical centers for conjugate lateral gaze. Paralysis of the 6th nerve results in convergent strabismus, with inability to move the eye laterally. Besides being affected by the inflammatory and degenerative diseases that produce paralysis of the 3rd and 4th nerves, the 6th nerves are especially prone to involvement with increased intracranial pressure, skull fracture, basilar artery thrombosis, suppuration of the sphenoid bone, also following lumbar puncture, and with diseases of the medulla and cerebellopontine angle.

Chapter V

SUPRANUCLEAR CONNECTIONS OF THE OCULAR MOTOR SYSTEM

A N UNDERSTANDING of the higher ocular motor control would be considerably enhanced by a more thorough knowledge than now exists of the development of eye movements in the normal infant. Movements of regard apparently develop before pursuit movements. At two to three weeks the infant turns its eyes to fix an object that attracts its attention[771] but it makes no smooth following movements until three to five months of age.[555] It is therefore assumed that the tracts responsible for the pursuit movements are not myelinated until relatively late. The eye movements made in following an object are at first cogwheel (saccadic) in type; only after several months do they become smooth.

A. MEDIAL LONGITUDINAL FASCICULUS

This tract coordinates the nuclei for the extraocular muscles with each other and with other nuclei in the brain stem; it is therefore appropriately considered with the central connections of the ocular motor nuclei. Phylogenetically, it is one of the oldest tracts in the central nervous system, and embryologically, it is one of the first to be myelinated. Extending on either side of the midline from the optic thalamus anteriorly to the anterior horn cells of the spinal cord posteriorly, it is especially well developed in the region between the nuclei of the oculomotor and the vestibular nerves and is made up in considerable measure by fibers from the vestibular nuclei[1141, 391, 753] (Fig. 45). The medial longitudinal fasciculus serves not only to coordinate motor nerves of the eye with each other and with the vestibular apparatus but also to relay the impulses for conjugate lateral gaze from the pontine centers to the ocular motor nuclei. The important tracts relaying impulses from the pontine center on one side to the medial rectus on the other side are situated on the inner portions of the medial longitudinal fasciculi.[116] Thus, stimulation of the medial fibers results in adduction[105] of the eye, and circumscribed lesions of the medial longitudinal fasciculus on one side produce a selective paralysis of the homolateral medial rectus on attempted conjugate lateral gaze.[573, 105] The lateral rectus, which is innervated by fibers coming directly from the pontine centers without traversing the medial longitudinal fasciculus, is not affected by lesions in this region.

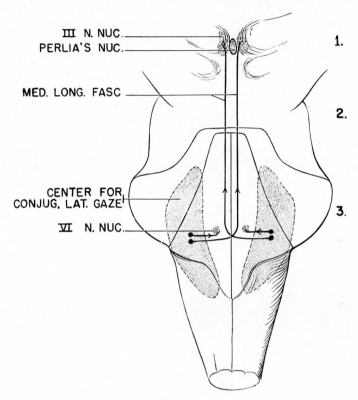

Fig. 45. *Diagrammatic representation of dorsal surface of the brain stem showing the connection of the pointine centers for conjugate lateral gaze with the abducens nuclei and with the oculomotor nuclei by way of the medial longitudinal fasciculus*

Internuclear ophthalmoplegia, characterized by paralysis of the medial recti on attempted conjugate lateral gaze, is due to lesions of the medial longitudinal fasciculus. The internuclear ophthalmoplegia is accompanied by paresis of convergence with anterior lesions (1) and by weakness of conjugate gaze and nystagmus with posterior lesions (3), while there may be normal convergence and normal excursions of the abducting eye with midzone lesions (2).

Since each pontine center represents conjugate lateral gaze to the homolateral side, its innervation must be distributed to the corresponding lateral rectus nucleus and to the contralateral medial rectus nucleus. This latter decussation is thought to occur posteriorly by some [222] and anteriorly by others. [984, 428, 252, 249]

Lesions of the medial longitudinal fasciculi produce a characteristic clinical picture, known as *internuclear ophthalmoplegia,*[645] consisting of paresis of the medial rectus on attempted conjugate lateral gaze (Fig. 46). One medial rectus only may be involved but usually it is bilateral. To the paresis of the medial rectus on attempted conjugate lateral gaze are added other signs which vary

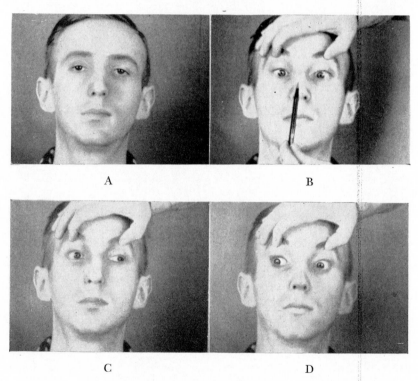

FIG. 46. *Internuclear ophthalmoplegia due to multiple sclerosis*
The patient was a twenty-year-old man who had had diplopia of one week's duration. In the primary position (A) the eyes are directed straight ahead and (B) convergence is good. On gazing to either side (C and D), there is a relative lag of the adducting eye and a predominately monocular nystagmus of the abducting eye.

according to what portions of the tract are involved. With lesions in the posterior part of the tract (medullary portion), the ability to converge the eyes is retained, but there is nystagmus and occasionally paresis of the lateral rectus as well as of the medial rectus on attempted conjugate lateral gaze. With lesions in the anterior part of the tract (midbrain portion), the ability to converge the eyes is decreased or abolished, but there is no limitation of the lateral rectus on lateral gaze. Nystagmus is also present with lesions in the anterior portion of the tract but it is less conspicuous than with lesions in the posterior portion.

Despite the paralysis of the medial recti on attempted conjugate gaze the eyes are usually orthotropic in the primary position. If, however, the nuclei or nerves of the lateral recti are also involved, there will be a superimposed esotropia; conversely, if the nuclei of the medial recti are involved, there will be a superimposed exotropia.

The nystagmus found with internuclear ophthalmoplegia may be vertical, horizontal, or rotary but owing to the weakness of the medial rectus, the horizontal nystagmus is characteristically more marked in the abducted eye than in the adducted eye on gaze to either side. This asymmetric nystagmus is highly characteristic of internuclear ophthalmoplegia.

Accompanying lesions of the posterior portion of the medial longitudinal fasciculus, there may be a limitation of the lateral rectus owing to involvement of the pontine centers for lateral gaze or owing to involvement of the 6th nerves. The latter is inferred to be the case only when there is a convergent strabismus on attempted gaze straight ahead. With lesions of the lateral gaze centers, the eyes are approximately straight in the primary position of gaze.

Bilateral internuclear ophthalmoplegia, wherein both eyes are involved is most frequently seen, by far, with multiple sclerosis[746, 445] but some cases have been reported following epidemics of encephalitis lethargica[645, 520] and it is not uncommon as a complication, of diverse lesions of the brain stem (tumors, Wernicke's encephalopathy, syringobulbia, etc.). Nevertheless, when bilateral internuclear ophthalmoplegia is present alone, or when it is the most conspicuous abnormality, the underlying condition is almost invariably multiple sclerosis. Conversely, the most common ocular motor manifestation of multiple sclerosis is internuclear ophthalmoplegia. Only rarely is it combined with the ocular sensory manifestation (retrobulbar neuritis) of multiple sclerosis. Few cases of internuclear ophthalmoplegia have been examined histologically wherein the lesions were sufficiently discrete to be informative.[991, 902, 909]

Internuclear ophthalmoplegia was originally subdivided into anterior and posterior types according to whether the medial rectus or lateral rectus failed on attempted conjugate lateral gaze.[670] This subdivision is based on the assumption that the brain stem center for conjugate lateral gaze is situated *between* the 3rd and 6th nerve nuclei and that the anterior part of the medial longitudinal fasciculus conveys the fibers to the medial rectus and the posterior part conveys the fibers to the lateral rectus. This assumption is not, however, borne out by any firm anatomic evidence and seems unlikely in view of what pathologic evidence is available.[222, 194] Nor have any cases of the so-called posterior variety been reported. It has therefore seemed more correct, to the present author at least, to consider *anterior internuclear ophthalmoplegia* as that condition in which there is associated involvement of convergence, along with the paralysis of the medial recti on attempted lateral gaze, and *posterior internuclear ophthalmoplegia* as that condition in which convergence is normal but in which there is also some limitation of conjugate lateral gaze or involvement of other functions represented in the medulla. In both cases, there is of course, the essential paralysis of the medial rectus on attempted horizontal gaze and a predominately monocular nystagmus of the abducting eye. Aspects of both the anterior and posterior variety may be present, and usually are, in the same patient. In the anterior type, however, the evidence indicates principal involvement of the midbrain whereas in the posterior type the evidence indicts chiefly the region of the medulla.

Unilateral internuclear ophthalmoplegia wherein only one eye is affected may represent a mild form of the bilateral variety, but when the medial rectus of one eye is completely paralyzed while that of the other eye is normal, the condition has a different etiology and clinical significance.[222] This true unilateral variety is practically always due to an infarct of a small branch of the basilar artery (Figs. 47, 48, and 49). It occurs precipitously with vertigo

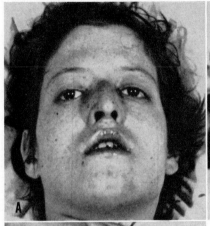

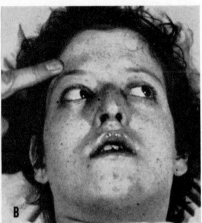

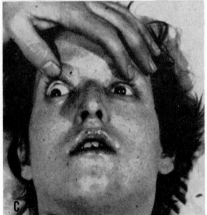

FIG. 47. *Photographs of patient with unilateral internuclear ophthalmoplegia showing:*
(A) eyes in primary position with gaze directed straight ahead; (B) normal conjugate movements on levoversion; but (C) lag of the adducting eye on dextroversion. The patient, who had lupus erythematosus, had developed diplopia suddenly two days prior to the time when the present photographs, reprinted from movie film, were taken. She died ten days later with ascites and pulmonary edema. (Cogan, Kubik & Smith.[222])

and, often, with other brain stem signs. Like the bilateral variety it is associated with predominately asymmetric nystagmus of the abducting eye on horizontal gaze but unlike the bilateral variety it resolves more slowly and is often accompanied by a vertical separation of the images (see Skew Deviation. p. 134). Pathologic

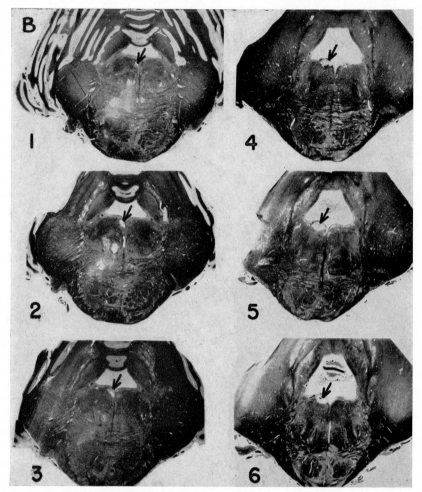

Fig. 48. *Serial sections through the brain stem of the foregoing case showing the small infarct (indicated by arrows) in the region of the left medial longitudinal fasciculus.* (Cogan, Kubik, and Smith.[222])

examination of these cases has shown discrete areas of softening in the medial longitudinal fasciculus on the side corresponding to the paralyzed medial rectus muscle.[222, 194]

The syndrome of internuclear ophthalmoplegia has been produced experimentally in cats by making discrete lesions on either side of the midline between the 3rd and 6th nerve nuclei.[573] The eye on the side of the lesion showed paresis of the medial rectus on conjugate gaze, even with lesions situated as far back as the 6th nerve nuclei. The nystagmus produced by the rotation was, as in patients with internuclear ophthalmoplegia, weaker in the eye on the side of the lesion and could be abolished altogether in this eye by removal of the lateral rectus and retractor bulbi muscles. It appears from this that the pathways from one vestibular nucleus

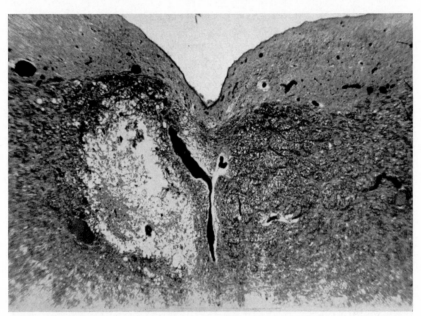

FIG. 49. *Higher magnification of the infarct showing practically complete necrosis of the left medial longitudinal fasciculus with a normal or near-normal fasciculus on the right side.* (Cogan, Kubik, and Smith.[222])

to the opposite medial rectus nucleus cross far back in the medial longitudinal fasciculus. The nystagmus present is due to the intermittent lateral rectus relaxation. Owing to the paralysis of the medial rectus it is weaker on the side of the lesion. Recently the clinical syndrome has been reproduced in the monkey by destruction of the medial fibers of the medial longitudinal fasciculus.[105]

B. LATERAL CONJUGATE MOVEMENTS

According to a principle first clearly enunciated by Hughlings Jackson,[512] the supranuclear centers and pathways for all types of motor activity represent functions rather than individual muscles. Applied to the eyes, this means that the supranuclear mechanisms are concerned with the function of elevation of the eyes or that of horizontal movements or that of torsion, and not with the individual muscles that are used to effect these movements. From the practical point of view this means that stimulation or extirpation of these centers will involve the movements of the two eyes equally; diplopia will not occur. This is important since without diplopia the patient may not be aware of any ocular difficulty; thus in spite of gross disturbance of eye movements supranuclear lesions are often overlooked.

The present knowledge of conjugate centers and pathways in the central nervous system is far from complete. The present concepts are based on information from the following sources: from the eye movements produced by stimulation and ablation of various portions of the brain; from the histologic characteristics of the cortex and pathways before and after experimentally induced lesions; and from the disturbances of eye movements produced by clinical lesions in various portions of the brain. The following areas have been sufficiently well shown to be associated with conjugate lateral movements to be called supranuclear ocular motor centers.

1. Cerebral Centers

(a) *Frontal.* That the frontal lobe, or some portion of it, exerts a tonic innervation tending to turn the eyes to the opposite side has been know since the early experimental work in which conjugate deviation of the eyes to one side occurred following stimulation of the opposite frontal lobe or extirpation of portions of the homolateral frontal lobe. These original observations have been abundantly corroborated in a variety of animals and in man,[82, 346, 858] and the responsible area for deviation of the eyes has been precisely localized in area 8, according to Brodmann's classification. This is at the posterior end of the second frontal convolution,[346, 550, 202, 255, 253] but separated from the motor cortex by a strip of unexcitable cortex[85, 644] (Fig. 50).

Since the current necessary to produce deviation of the eyes is considerably greater than that necessary to excite other motor areas in the cortex,[644] the criticism has been raised that the eye movements are due to spread of stimulus to the basal ganglia rather than due to stimulation of an ocular motor center.[752] This interpretation is, however, vitiated by the observation that section of the corticofugal tract abolishes the reaction of the eyes on stimulation.[980]

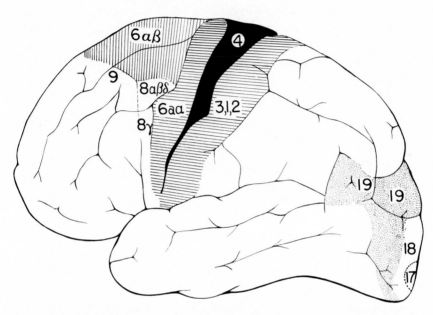

Fig. 50. *Divisions of the human cerebral cortex indicating especially those areas concerned with ocular motor function (Foerster)*

Area 4 represents motor function; its cells give rise to the pyramidal tract. Excitation of any point in area 4 results in isolated movements of a part of the body.

Area 6aα also represents motor function, and excitation of any point results in isolated movements; but the stimulus threshold is high and the effects are mediated through area 4.

Area 6aβ represents mass movements. Excitation results in a turning of the head, eyes, and trunk and the contraction of the arm and leg on the opposite side of the body. The threshold is relatively high.

Area 8aβδ represents conjugate movement of the eyes to the opposite side and, occasionally, dilatation of the pupil. Excitation of this area (and of 8γ and 9) also causes opening of the eyelids.

Areas 3, 1, and 2 represent sensation.

Areas 17, 18, and 19 represent primarily visual sensation; excitation causes not only visual hallucinations but also conjugate deviation of the eyes to the opposite side.

From the cytologic point of view, area 8, which is presumably the cortical region for eye movements in the frontal lobe, is a transitional zone between the purely *motor* cortex posteriorly (area 6), containing large Betz cells, and the *associational* cortex anteriorly (area 9), containing a predominance of granular cells. It is one of the few regions in the prefrontal lobe where there is a correlation between morphologic differentiation and function.[30]

The frontal area is thought to mediate impulses for the *voluntary* movements of the eyes that do not depend on visual stimuli. These are commonly referred to as movements on *command,* since they can be elicited by instructing the subject to look to the right or left.[169] They are often associated with head and sometimes with body movements.[253] This area is also thought to mediate impulses coming from the sensory cortex, especially from that portion representing facial sensation in the postrolandic cortex,[670, 86] and also impulses arising in the neck muscles.[202] The movements on command are to be differentiated from movements elicited by having the subject *follow* a moving object. Because they are characteristically rapid or jerky they are called *saccadic* movements[273, 1101] and are to be differentiated from the slower *pursuit* movements that characterize following a moving stimulus. However, the command movements may be slowed down under sedation and thereby simulate pursuit movements.

Acute loss of the frontal center or of its efferent pathways on one side is said to result in a transient inability to look voluntarily toward the contralateral side although the following movement is retained.[670, 482]

The frontal center for conjugate gaze is situated close to the cortical area (Area 6) which on stimulation produces turning of the head.[346, 168, 550, 202] Both the ocular motor and head-turning centers are presumably acted on by impulses coming from the whole frontal area anteriorly and from some of the somesthetic cortex posteriorly. There appears to be no direct connection between the two frontal centers, but each of them is connected with the homolateral occipital lobe by superficial association fibers.[202] The occipital lobe exerts a tonic depressant effect on the frontal eye centers, for cocainization of the occipital lobe increases the excitability of the frontal lobe, and conversely, electrical stimulation of the occipital lobe decreases the excitability of the frontal eye centers.[202] Despite the connection between the front and hind portions of the brain, the suggestion that all optomotor impulses arising in the occipital cortex are mediated through the frontal center[358] is incorrect, since both frontal lobes, and indeed the whole cerebrum with the exception of the occipital lobes and occipito-pontine pathways, may be separated from the rest of the brain without abolishing the conjugate eye movements on occipital stimulation.[912, 883, 748, 781, 634, 639, 44] The inferior longitudinal fasciculus of Burdach, which was at one time thought to connect the occipital and frontal lobes, is now known to be part of the visual radiation and not an association pathway within the cerebrum.[848]

Whereas the foregoing description represents the frontal eye fields as inferred from the consensus of experimental and clinical observations, significant variations from this basic pattern have been described. Although stimulation of one frontal area in man usually causes a conjugate deviation of the eyes to the opposite side, there is occasionally a deviation of the eyes to the same side.[858]

In addition to the ocular movements that have occurred repeatedly from stimulation of the prefrontal area (Area 8), similar deviations have been reported to occur in man[823] and in the monkey[255] from stimulation of adjacent portions of the central area (Area 4). These are thought to represent automatic associated movements of the eyes such as accompany face and limb movements[644] rather than true voluntary movements of the eyes.

Finally, each frontal area in the monkey appears to have two foci, one above and one below the horizontal sulcus, stimulation either one of which induces deviation of the eyes to the opposite side.[253]

The *fibers* running from the frontal area to the subcortical nuclei are less accessible to experimental demarcation than are the cortical centers because they lose their identity in the undifferentiated maze of fibers coming from all portions of the precentral cortex. However, an extensive extrapyramidal projection has been traced from the eye area in the frontal cortex to the striatum,[470] to the thalamus,[900] to the midbrain[255] and to the pons,[470, 401, 1006, 255] so that there is no dearth of possible connections. The efferent ocular motor fibers probably pass through the anterior arm of the internal capsule occupying the medial segment not far from the elbow of the internal capsule, in apposition to the supranuclear fibers for the facial muscles. Thence they course through the basal ganglia, with or without synapsing, and terminate in the rostral part of the pons, chiefly about the dorsal and medial portions of the pontine nucleus. The decussation of the fibers for conjugate lateral gaze takes place before the decussation of the face fibers. This is of some diagnostic importance in the exact localization of lesions involving these pathways. Lesions between the capsule and the point of decussation in the pons may be expected to involve the face and conjugate eye movements concomitantly, whereas lesions below this involve the face without affecting the conjugate eye movements.

(b) **Occipital.** As was the case with the frontal lobe, an occipital center for conjugate deviation of the eyes was first suspected from the fact that stimulation of one occipital lobe produced conjugate eye movements to the opposite side. This original observation has been repeatedly confirmed and corroborated by the observation that acute paralytic lesions of the occipital lobe may produce transient deviation of the eyes to the homolateral side.

Unlike Area 8 in the frontal lobe, no one area in the occipital lobe has been found that is exclusively productive of conjugate movements. Conjugate gaze to the opposite side has been produced by stimulation over a wide occipital area (Fig. 50). In monkeys the lowest threshold is to be found about the calcarine fissure (Area 17),[644, 168] where voltages as low as 1.0 volt are just sufficient to cause conjugate deviation.[1064] The parastriate region (Area 18) and peristriate region (Area 19) require respectively larger potentials, despite the fact that these portion of the cortex contain more motorlike cells (optomotor field)[304] than is the case with the striate region. The conjugate eye movements with occipital stimulation do not depend on secondary stimulation of the underlying fibers from other areas, as has been suggested,[662, 593a] since eye movements are still produced by stimulation of this region even after the underlying fibers have degenerated.[1064]

Stimulation of the angular gyrus was at one time thought to produce eye movements,[748] but it is now believed that turning of the eyes from stimulation of this region is due to secondary transmission of the impulses to the underlying fibers. If the stimulation is confined to the cortex of the angular gyrus, no eye movements occur; nor are any abnormalities of the eye movements produced by isolated removal of the cortex of the angular gyrus.[811]

The opportunities for stimulation of the occipital cortex in man have not been so great as those for stimulation in the frontal lobe.[344] While phosphene is usually the only response elicited in man on stimulating the occipital cortex,[662, 593a] all other evidence indicates that the ocular motor activity of the occipital lobe in man is not basically different from that in monkeys, in which conjugate ocular movements may be produced with adequate stimuli.

Recently a most significant series of cases has been reported in which ocular deviations were induced by stimulation of the paracalcarine area;[823] although predominately contralateral, the direction of deviation was occasionally ipsilateral. This bilaterality in representation in the occipital lobe may, as in the case of the frontal area, have considerable significance in compensating for unilateral loss of one of the cerebral ocular motor centers (see p. 103).

Various portions of the occipital cortex are intimately connected with each other in an orderly way. Stimulation of Area 17 by strychnine results in electrical disturbances that are propagated only as far as Area 18; stimulation of Area 18 produces disturbances that extend to Areas 17 and 19.[294] Stimulation of Area 19, on the other hand, does not extend to Areas 17 or 18 but does induce a suppression of the electrical activity of the entire cortex. This suggests that Area 19 determines associational activities of the occipital cortex with the rest of the cerebrum.[715]

There can be little doubt that the occipital centers for conjugate lateral movements of the eyes are closely associated with the sensory functions of this portion of the brain and mediate the visual reflexes. Just as the frontal centers are thought to serve the nonoptic, voluntary movements of the eyes elicited by the stimuli of command, the occipital centers may be assumed to serve movements of the eyes induced by the visual stimuli in following a moving object[242, 985, 86] and other reflex visual movements.[118] These pursuit movements are largely involuntary; they do not develop in the infant until some time after the voluntary movements, and cannot be produced by stimulation of the occiput until some time after birth.[109]

In lower animals the superior colliculi serve much of the function that in the higher animals is served by the occipital lobes, not only for the visual but also for the optomotor activities. Removal of the superior colliculi in cats and guinea pigs has much the same effect as removal of the occipital lobes in man. Unilateral lesions of the superior colliculi in lower animals impair the following movement toward the operated side, whereas ablation of both superior colliculi abolishes it toward both sides.[962]

The connection between the ocular motor centers in the occipital area and those in the frontal area has already been discussed (p. 94). A connection is evident encephalographically also, for lesions of the occipital lobe produce confusing disturbances in the electrical activity of the frontal area. The frontal centers appear to *dominate* the occipital centers to the extent that simultaneous excitation with equipotential stimuli of one frontal and the opposite occipital center results in a deviation of the eyes in the direction determined by the frontal area.[742, 109] This observation is occasionally advanced to account for the known functional dominance of the voluntary movements over the following movements. Unlike the frontal centers, which have no apparent effect on one another, the occipital lobes are connected with each other through the corpus callosum[847, 242, 723] and appear to inhibit one another. Cocainization of one occipital lobe increases the optomotor excitability of the other, and stimulation of one occipital lobe inhibits the motor activity of the other.[202]

The threshold for excitation of the occipital lobe is higher than that for excitation of the frontal lobe,[634, 168] and the latent period before a reaction is elicited is longer.[914] Moreover, the eye movements are less quick and regular than is the case with frontal lobe stimulation.[44, 242] This is consistent with the familiar observation that voluntary movements on command are more rapidly executed than are those in response to visual stimuli such as occur in the pursuit reaction.

Efferent fibers connecting the occipital cortex with the lower centers arise as axones of the large ganglion cells of the 4th lamina and of large solitary cells in the 6th lamina.[207] These cells undergo a partial degeneration when the subcortical connections of the area striata are sectioned, whereas other cellular elements in the cortex show little change. The efferent fibers from the occipital cortex form a well defined fasciculus and course parallel with and medial to the visual radiation. Passing through the posterior end of the internal capsule, these fibers have been traced to the thalamus,[723, 752] pons,[833, 55, 1006] superior colliculi,[847, 84, 130, 206, 834, 52, 254, 827, 628] and other portions of the mesencephalon.[723] They occupy a position in the lateral segment of the cerebral peduncle and are thought to terminate chiefly about the ventral and lateral aspects of the rostral three fifths of the pontine nucleus.[1006] While these efferent fibers may be differentiated from the afferent visual fibers by their smaller size, by differential staining,[767] and by the fact that they are myelinated later in the embryo,[340] there is no way of determining precisely which ones are concerned with lateral conjugate movements of the eyes. For what it is worth, however, it does appear that fibers projecting from the occipital lobe to the pontine nucleus come from that portion of the cortex representing peripheral rather than macular function.[723]

It would be of considerable clinical interest to know the precise anatomic relation between the efferent pathways for ocular motor function from the frontal and occipital centers. The two tracts are presumably separate, since the ocular movements on command may be dissociated from those in the pursuit reaction (pseudo-ophthalmoplegia), but the exact course of each is unknown. The fact, however, that section of the medulla abolishes the conjugate lateral movements of the eyes from frontal stimulation but not from occipital stimulation[202] and, conversely, that elimination of the superior colliculi abolishes conjugate lateral movements from occipital stimulation but not from frontal stimulation[80, 981] suggest that the efferent fibers from the occipital lobe are mediated through higher levels in the brain stem (perhaps by way of the superior colliculi) than are the efferent fibers from the frontal lobe. Further, the common absence of ocular movements on command with the retention of the following movements, due to bilateral lesions of the basal ganglia suggests that the efferent fibers from the frontal lobe are mediated through the basal ganglia (see discussion of opticokinetic response, p. 196). In summary, one may tentatively infer from the scant evidence now available that the occipital ocular motor fibers are relayed through the superior colliculi, whereas the frontal ocular motor fibers are relayed through the basal ganglia.

(c) ***Other cortical centers.*** Conjugate deviation of the eyes has followed stimulation of other portions of the cortex, especially those concerned with hearing,[331, 344, 879, 398] and epileptiform attacks from lesions of hearing centers result in a turning of the eyes toward the imagined sound.[822] Since these movements in animals are accompanied by retraction of the ear on the side opposite the stimulus, this portion of the cortex has naturally been assumed to serve the acoustic eye reflexes.[1029] But whether the eye movements result from stimulation of the cortex itself or of the underlying fibers, and whether in the former case the impulses are transmitted directly to the lower centers or through some other cortical center, has not been demonstrated. It is known, however, that cocainization of the auditory cortex decreases the reactivity of the ocular motor center in the frontal lobe.[202] In all probability the disturbances in the ocular following movements reported in human beings with parietal lesions[1093, 16] are attributable to involvement of the underlying optomotor fibers.

2. Subcortical Centers for Conjugate Lateral Gaze

The present knowledge of subcortical centers for conjugate lateral gaze is still fragmentary, and much of it is contradictory. The previous discussion of corticofugal fibers might lead one to assume the existence of subcortical centers in the basal ganglia, in the superior colliculi, and in the brain stem.

The evidence for subcortical centers of conjugate lateral gaze is least substantial for the *basal ganglia*. What evidence there is rests partly on *anatomic findings,* fibers having been traced on the one hand to the ganglia from the occipital lobe[848, 833] and on the other hand from the ganglia to the general region of the ocular motor nuclei,[751, 738] and partly on *clinical findings,* various oculo-gyral crises being attributed to the basal ganglia. Neither form of evidence is conclusive. Perhaps the strongest evidence for a center in the basal ganglia is the old observation that *stimulation* of the ganglia results in a deviation of head and eyes to the opposite side[5] even after the fibers from the cortex have been abolished.[879]

The superior colliculi are intimately associated with vertical conjugate movements of the eyes, but they appear to play a subordinate role in the mediation of horizontal movements in man. Stimulation of the colliculi has not given rise to horizontal movements and ablation of the colliculi has, with one exception,[80] not resulted in gross disturbance of horizontal movements in animals. Nevertheless, there is in the lower animals reliable evidence that the retina projects to the superior colliculi[234] and reveals a correlation of ocular motor activity with retinal representation.[17, 18] It would be surprising, therefore, if some of the visuomotor reflexes were not mediated through this region but the only evidence that *horizontal* movements in man are normally mediated through the superior colliculi is the impairment of the opticokinetic response in some patients with lesions in this region.[212] It may be noted, however, that infants with hydranencephaly may have surprisingly normal ocular movements including intact gaze reflexes despite the absence of effectively functioning cerebral cortex. This does not necessarily imply that comparable reflex areas are present in the normal adult.

The evidence for a *pontine center* for conjugate lateral gaze is abundantly proved by physiologic and clinical evidence, but its actual anatomic position is subject to controversy. It is probably in the vicinity of the abducens nuclei whence it is sometimes called the paraabducens center.[253]

> Although the reticular substance of the pons receives fibers directly from the frontal lobes,[401] it probably does not contain the centers for lateral eye movements, as has been supposed,[661] since lesions of the reticular substance do not result in degeneration of fibers running to the ocular motor nuclei.[815]

The portion of the *vestibular* nucleus that is concerned with eye movements may be the center for conjugate gaze.[751, 70, 795] There is considerable evidence that this is so. Experimental destruction of the vestibular nucleus abolishes all lateral (not vertical) conjugate movements from stimulation of the frontal[986] and occipital cortex.[974] The centers are presumably near the midline, since complete paralysis of conjugate gaze to both sides has been reported with midline lesions.[1096, 116]

It is sometimes held that the pontine center for lateral gaze is identical with the 6th nerve nucleus.[355, 1092, 295, 418, 383] But the cellular components of this nucleus are not extensive enough to account for the conjugate function,[695] and the nucleus may degenerate without impairment of medial rotation in the contralateral eye[955] or without degeneration in the 3rd nerve nuclei.[502, 387]

Each pontine center receives impulses from the contralateral cerebral hemisphere and transmits impulses to the lateral rectus nucleus on the same side and by way of the medial longitudinal fasciculus to the medial rectus on the opposite side (Fig. 57). Stimulation of these subcortical centers results, therefore, in a turning of the eyes to the side of the stimulus, in contrast to stimulation of the cortical centers, which results in a turning of the eyes to the opposite side.

3. Lesions Involving Conjugate Lateral Movements

As already pointed out, supranuclear lesions do not produce diplopia, for movements of both eyes are affected equally. This is of the utmost clinical importance since, in the absence of diplopia, the patient usually volunteers no complaint in reference to his eyes and gross palsies of conjugate gaze may in consequence be overlooked.

It is also important to remember that the difference between the so-called nystagmoid movements, most types of jerk nystagmus, and gross palsies of conjugate gaze is only quantitative.[906] Slight palsies of excentric gaze to one side result in a slow drifting of the eye away from the excentric position. This is frequently corrected by a quick jerklike movement in the direction of the gaze; the combination of movements makes up the cycle of nystagmus or nystagmoid movements. Thus, it is not uncommon to see during successive stages of recovery a complete paralysis of conjugate lateral gaze become merely a nystagmus on excentric fixation, a nystagmus that finally can be scarcely differentiated from the normal movements on extreme conjugate gaze (see p. 223). Conversely, during the stages of a progressive lesion nystagmoid jerks at the outset become a true nystagmus and finally a gross palsy to one side.

(a) **Cerebral.** With *unilateral* lesions of the cortical centers and cerebral pathways, the eyes tend to deviate conjugately toward the homolateral side. But this deviation is ordinarily apparent only during stupor and, unlike other motor phenomena, it disappears within a few hours after the patient regains consciousness; it is then manifest only by a nystagmus on conjugate gaze to the opposite side. But even when not grossly evident a latent deviation persists, for if the patient again loses consciousness or is deeply narcotized, the deviation reappears. This compensation is probably effected through corresponding centers in the opposite hemisphere.

More subtle manifestations of unilateral cerebral lesions are: jerky pursuit movements toward the side of the lesion; reduction in, or abolition of, the opticokinetic response on rotation of the field toward the side of the lesion; and a conjugate deviation of the eyes, on attempted closure of the lids, to the side opposite the lesion. Nevertheless, the chief basis for localization of lesions within the cerebrum causing ocular motor disturbances is the associated signs and symptoms outside the ocular system.

In most respects palsies of conjugate lateral gaze of cerebral origin are analogous to hemiplegia of cerebral origin. They are predominately contralateral so far as can be determined by ordinary testing. The asymmetric tonus which produces spasticity of the limbs is manifest in the ocular motor system by deviation of the eyes to the side opposite the lesion with forced closure of the lids; thus it is opposite to the paralytic deviation.[845, 35, 216] Ordinarily this latent deviation is obscured by the fixational reflexes and can be evoked only when these reflexes are abolished by attempted closure of the lids. This "spacticity of conjugate gaze," as it may be called, probably accounts also for the saccadic following movements toward the side of the lesion and possibly for the deficiency in the opticokinetic response.

Frontal area. Lesions involving the eye field in the frontal area may be irritative or paralytic.

Irritative lesions are characterized by a clonic turning of the eyes and head toward the side opposite the lesion, usually followed by a generalized convulsion (Jacksonian epilepsy) (Fig. 51). With lesions in Area 8, the turning of the eyes precedes that of the head, whereas with lesions in Areas 6 and 9, the turning of the head precedes that of the eyes.[345]

Acute paralytic lesions in the region of the frontal eye field show a transient deviation of the eyes (with or without turning of the head) to the side of the lesion. This is seen with vascular accidents,

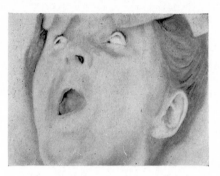

injuries, and subdural empyema[596] of the frontal region and is accompanied by stupor and coma. With *chronic* lesions such as tumors and abscesses,[725] spontaneous deviation of the eyes is seen not at all or to only a slight extent unless accompanied by coma (Fig. 52). The deviation disappears shortly after the patient regains consciousness and shows either no residuum or only nystagmus on conjugate gaze to the contralateral side. The nystagmus is of the neuromuscular-insufficiency type and is scarcely distinguishable from that seen normally, although it is said to be characteristically intermittent.[117]

Fig. 51. *Conjugate deviation of the eyes to the right with an irritative lesion in the left frontal area*
At the time the picture was taken the patient was having a convulsive seizure characterized by clonic turning of the head and eyes to the right, blinking of both lids (but more marked on the right), a pulling of the mouth to the right and a clonic jerking of the right arm (but not of the leg). In the interim between the convulsive episodes the ocular motility was normal except for slight horizontal nystagmus on extreme conjugate gaze to the right and to a less extent to the left.

With lesions of the frontal eye field, there is usually some hemiplegia affecting chiefly the head and upper extremity on the side opposite the lesion.

With acute cerebral lesions the defect of conjugate gaze is on the *same* side of the body as the hemiplegia, whereas with pontine lesions the defect of conjugate gaze is to the side opposite that of the hemiplegia. This differentiation may be of crucial significance in localizing the lesion of unconscious patients.

The curious *pseudohemianopsia* observed in monkeys[120, 471, 730, 121, 550, 548, 205] with lesions of the frontal eye field has also been observed

in human beings with acute frontal lesions.[45, 956] The patients show
no blink reflex as objects are thrust at them from the affected side,
grope for objects on the affected side, and show unilateral disturbance of counting and reversal of spelling. While not blind in any
part of the field, it is as though the patients (and monkeys) had

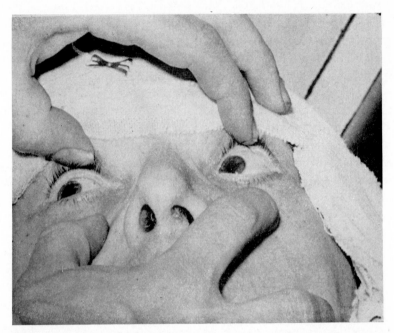

FIG. 52. *Spontaneous conjugate deviation of the eyes to the right in an unconscious patient with a right frontal lobe lesion*
  This patient had a glioblastoma multiforme of the right frontal lobe. The
picture was taken two days following exploratory craniotomy. While conscious the patient showed full excursion of his eyes and the eyes were held
in the primary position, but on losing consciousness the eyes deviated to the
extreme right.

lost the motor responses and some of the other higher functions
which are usually associated with visual perception. There results
an immobility of the eyes and loss of blinking which strongly suggests the clinical picture of parkinsonism.
  An especially interesting and informative syndrome occurs with
bilateral lesions in the frontal eye fields or with a lesion in one eye
field and its connection with the opposite hemisphere. In contrast to the unilateral lesions, compensation does not readily occur

and such patients have a persistent palsy of voluntary gaze to one or both sides. Yet random movements of the eyes may be retained whence one variant of the condition has been called *ocular motor apraxia*[219] (also Balint's Syndrome[32, 450, 451]). There is usually an associated apraxia of the head and sometimes of the limbs. The paradoxic preservation of random movements with loss of purposive movements often gives rise to the erroneous impression of hysteria or blindness in such patients.

The significance of persistent palsies after bilateral lesions is, aside from the diagnostic importance, its physiologic implication as to the mechanism of compensation. It suggests that the facile compensation which follows unilateral cerebral lesions and which is characteristic of the ocular motor system depends on participation of the corresponding region in the opposite hemisphere. This is seen strikingly in persons who, having had a lesion on one side with transient ocular motor deviation, develop a corresponding lesion at some later date on the opposite side; these patients then have a persistent palsy for which they have little or no compensation.

Although the center for lateral gaze to one side has an obvious analogy with that for the limbs, the facility with which one ocular motor area can compensate for that of the opposite hemisphere is in contrast with that for the limb area. Thus conjugate palsies resolve in a matter of hours whereas the simultaneous hemiplegia may resolve only in a matter of weeks; indeed, after a hemispherectomy, the hemiplegia will be permanent while the eye movements return essentially to normal.

The neuroanatomic basis for this compensation may be a *bilateral* representation for ocular movements in the cerebral hemispheres; although stimulation of one motor area induces a predominantly contralateral deviation, a homolateral deviation occasionally occurs. Stimulation of the limb area, on the other hand, always produces a contralateral effect.*

A congenital variety of ocular motor apraxia has been described.[217] Unlike the acquired variety, there is no associated

---

* In this respect cerebral representation of ocular motor innervation is more like that of sensory innervation for, during the first years of life at least, one sensory cortex appears to be able to take over many of the functions of the other.

apraxia of the head. In consequence, the patient develops head thrusts that compensate for the deficiency of eye movements, and comprise the most striking feature of the clinical syndrome (Figs. 53 and 54). Such patients also have an obligate turning of their eyes on rotation of the body (the Roth-Bielschowsky deviation, see

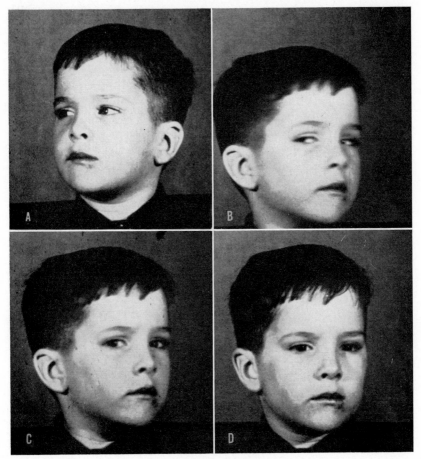

Fig. 53. *Photograph of a patient with congenital ocular motor apraxia*
    The patient was gazing to the right (A) when he was asked to look at the camera. A turn of the head was accompanied by a closure of the lids, as in the normal person, but when the lids opened the eyes were seen to be in the position of extreme dextroversion (B). As a result the patient had to overshoot the mark with his head to attain fixation straight ahead (C). Once the eyes fixated, the head returned to the approximately primary position (D). (Cogan.[217])

p. 221f) as occurs in other forms of pseudo-ophthalmoplegia, but the condition is differentiated from these by the presence of normal random movements.

Occipital area. Irritative lesions of the occipital area produce a turning of the eyes and head toward the opposite side, but the

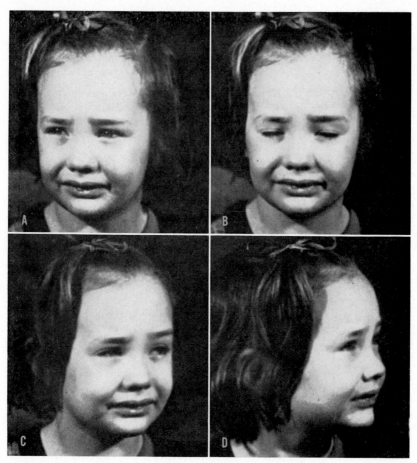

Fig. 54. *Photograph of normal head-eye movements to be compared with the foregoing apractic movements*

The subject who happened to be looking to the right (A) was asked to fixate an object on her left. The lids closed momentarily as the head began to turn to the left (B). When the lids opened, the eyes were seen to be fully turned to the left (C). The turning of the head had lagged behind that of the eyes. Finally, both head and eyes were turned to the left for final fixation (D). (Cogan.[217])

syndrome is unlike that of the frontal area in being usually accompanied by subjective visual phenomena, formed and unformed images, and in being less likely to be accompanied by generalized convulsions.

Acute paralytic lesions of the occipital area may be accompanied by transient conjugate deviation of the eyes[486, 119] to the side of the lesion[119] and, as in the case of frontal lesions, leave as residuum only a nystagmus on directing the gaze toward the side opposite the lesion. These signs are less conspicuous than is the case with frontal lesions.[65, 811] Lesions of the occipital area produce a cogwheel movement of the eyes in following an object toward the side of the lesion[133, 246, 482] and often a defect in the opticokinetic response when the drum is rotated toward the side of the lesion[242, 356] (see p. 200).

Occipital lesions are usually accompanied by defects of the visual field, and with *chronic* lesions these field defects are more conspicuous than are the ocular motor disturbances. Rarely are the motor disturbances present without visual field loss.[242] Lesions of the angular gyrus in the dominant half of the brain are characteristically accompanied by agnosia and alexia.

Noteworthy is a curious syndrome known as pseudo-ophthmoplegia,[1093] in which movements for command and for following a moving object are unequally affected or in which command and following movements are abolished but the vestibular deviation is preserved. The former, also called dissociated paralysis, is characterized by the fact that the patients are unable to move their eyes voluntarily in one or more directions on command and usually are unable to fixate an object in the peripheral field, but the eyes may follow a slowly moved object and may show full ocular excursions with stimulation of the labyrinth (Fig. 60). They always tend to lose fixation, however, and return to the primary position. A particularly vivid description of this syndrome is furnished by a case in which the patient could read an entire line only by letting his eyes wander aimlessly about and in this way eventually perceive all the words.[521] In order to get to the beginning of the next line, he had to follow his finger back across the page.

First predicted on theoretical grounds by Wernicke,[1093] this syndrome has been observed often since that time, producing different clinical pictures in various patients. It usually occurs in association with *pseudo-bulbar palsy,* whence its name, and is then thought to be due to involvement of the corticofugal fibers from the frontal centers to a greater extent than those from the occipital centers.[127] It usually involves both horizontal and vertical movements, but either may be affected alone. It may even be unilateral.

Few pathologic studies have been done on patients with pseudo-ophthalmoplegia,[1019, 1025, 886] and the diffuseness of the process in most of the cases reported makes the significance of these studies questionable. Although the lesion in most of the instances has undoubtedly been primarily cerebral, cases of pseudo-ophthalmoplegia have been reported with lesions in the pons and in the superior colliculi.[127] Thus, while the syndrome is of considerable physiologic and clinical interest, indicating the separate representation of eye movements for command, for following, and for vestibular movements, it has, nevertheless, little localizing significance at the present time.

The opposite condition, in which eye movements are present for command but absent in the following reaction, has been reported only once clinically,[246] but it will be remembered that this is the normal condition for the first few months of life.[555] Here it is presumed that the corticofugal fibers from the occipital centers are not functioning, whereas those from the frontal centers are.

Efferent fibers. As with lesions of the cerebral cortex, acute lesions of the corticofugal pathways produce a transient deviation of the eyes to the same side. But the accompanying hemiplegia and other signs are more profound in the case of lesions of the pathways especially when, as is often the case, the lesion is in the internal capsule.

The spontaneous oscillations of the eyes that have been reported with lesions in the region of the angular gyrus[959] probably reflect the patient's unconscious state rather than the site of the lesion.

With chronic lesions involving the efferent pathways, the only ocular motor residuum may be saccadic following movement and a deficit in the opticokinetic response (see p. 200).

(b) **Subcortical.** *Basal ganglia—reticular substance.* The evidence for correlating certain ophthalmologic and neurologic syndromes with lesions in the basal ganglia and reticular substance is no better than the evidence of ocular motor centers in these regions.

However, there is an irritative syndome and a nonirritative syndrome that, according to the best evidence at the present time is
due to lesions in these regions.

The *irritative syndrome* goes by the name of *oculogyral crises.*
It is characterized by spasmodic and involuntary deviation of the
eyes, usually upward, although deviation in any direction is possible. The spasms may last for a few minutes or a few hours and
usually recur at increasing frequencies. Oculogyral crises occur
most frequently in association with parkinsonism,[481, 397] occurring
as a late manifestation of encephalitis (approximately 20 per cent
of all patients with this disease) but the crises also result from
neurosyphilis[592, 454, 768] and occasionally from trauma.[541]

The *nonirritative syndrome* that is currently attributed to the
basal ganglia or reticular substance is Parkinson's disease. This condition resulting from arteriosclerosis or encephalitis shows a characteristic rigidity of the eye movements; although the patient can
look fully to either side, the eye movements are jerky.[245, 242, 251] Vertical gaze is also characteristically affected showing either a gross
paresis of upward gaze or a vertical nystagmus on looking upward.

> The similarity of eye movements and other signs in monkeys
> that have had bilateral ablation of the frontal eye fields and in
> human beings with postencephalitic Parkinson's disease, together
> with the known anatomic and physiologic connections of this
> portion of the cortex with the striatum, naturally suggests that the
> striatal syndrome is due to an interruption of these corticofugal
> pathways.[550] Restricted lesions in the basal ganglia of monkeys
> do not in themselves produce abnormal eye signs, but they do
> enhance those produced by lesions of the frontal eye field and
> make the disturbances more lasting.[549]

Pons. Palsies of conjugate gaze from lesions in the pons (Foville's
syndrome[355]) are more often seen than are palsies from cerebral
lesions, partly because they last longer but chiefly because they are
usually accompanied by diplopia from associated peripheral nerve
involvement.

Pontine disease is caused by a wide variety of lesions. Most frequent are the vascular accidents (especially thrombosis of the
basilar artery), but tumors, multiple sclerosis, abscess, tuberculomas, and encephalitis contribute a considerable number of cases.

Although occurring sporadically with poliomyelitis[637, 828] some epidemics of encephalitis are said to involve the lateral conjugate mechanisms preferentially.[70] Less common are the palsies of conjugate lateral gaze with platybasia[220] and with Wernicke's disease.[224] Paralysis of lateral conjugate gaze with facial paralysis also occurs

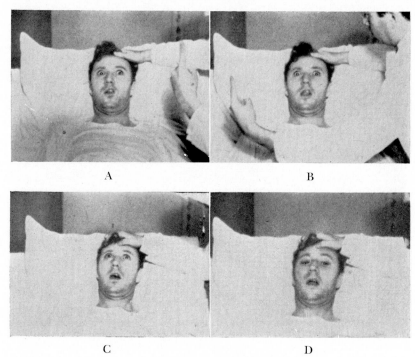

Fig. 55. *Complete paralysis of conjugate lateral gaze to either side (A and B) with normal upward (C) and downward movements (D) due to a lesion of the pons*

This patient had an extensive glioblastoma multiforme of the pons.

as a congenital abnormality.[465, 267a] Of great practical importance is the fact that typical ocular motor signs of pontine disease may result from pressure on the brain stem by expansive lesions of the cerebellum. Such signs do not, therefore, necessarily indicate lesions within the pons.[638, 185]

The symptoms produced by pontine lesions are characterized by a paralysis of conjugate horizontal gaze combined with nystagmus and involvement of the ocular motor and other cranial nerves. The

conjugate paralysis varies all the way from nystagmus on deviation
of the eyes to one side to a total inability to turn the eyes past the
midline. The palsy is greatest on the side of the lesion. Unlike
cerebral lesions, those in the pons usually produce bilateral involvement of conjugate gaze, since the pontine centers are located
near the midline (Fig. 55) but this involvement is not necessarily
symmetric. Also unlike the cerebral palsies of conjugate gaze, the

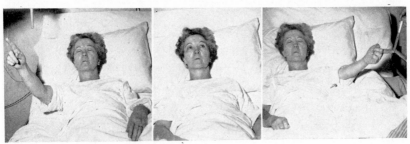

FIG. 56. *Past-pointing to the right with paresis of conjugate gaze to the right*
    The patient was a fifty-four-year-old woman with a history of dizziness and
    numbness of the left side of the body of two weeks' duration, thought to be
    due to a thrombosis in the pons. Examination showed anesthesia of the right
    cornea, hemianesthesia of the left side of the entire body, and a paresis of
    conjugate gaze to the right. The patient lay in bed with eyes deviated ap-
    proximately 15 degrees to the left; any attempt to look to the right resulted
    in a coarse nystagmus to the right. When the patient looked at an object
    placed on either side and then attempted to point at the object with eyes
    closed, she showed correct pointing to the left side but distinct past-point-
    ing to the right.

pontine palsies last as long as the lesion is present and are accompanied by compensatory turning of the head toward the side
of the paralysis and past-pointing on the side of the lesion (Fig. 56).

    Caloric irrigation of the ears is especially instructive with
pontine lesions.[40, 125] The fast phase of the nystagmus is commonly
abolished, so that one or both eyes show a maintained deviation
to one side following the irrigation, frequently toward the side to
which the patient was unable to turn his eyes voluntarily. When
only one eye shows the deviation, there is presumably an internuclear lesion (medial longitudinal fasciculus) as well as pontine
lesion. If, in spite of an intact 8th nerve, no deviation occurs on
irrigation, the conjugate center is presumably entirely out of

function. When conjugate deviation occurs with irrigation but cannot be executed voluntarily, the lesion is presumably higher than the pontine conjugate center.

As already stated the chief distinguishing feature of pontine conjugate palsies is the association with them of cranial nerve involvement. The nerves involved are, like the conjugate palsy, on the same side as the lesion. Most frequently affected are the 6th nerves, but the 5th nerve (paresthesias and numbness of the face and corneal insensitivity), 7th nerve (facial paralysis), and 8th nerve (deafness, usually on the opposite side [363]) are often affected. Even the 3rd nerve is frequently involved owing to the extension of the lesion into the mesencephalon. Convergence is usually preserved.[865, 363] Associated with the conjugate ocular and cranial nerve palsy there is often involvement of the pyramidal tract and vestibular nuclei, producing hemiparesis and various types of nystagmus. Paresthesias are also common, owing to involvement of the lemnisci. Lesions in the lateral portions of the pons are frequently associated with miosis owing to involvement of the sympathetic pathways. In fact, it is the wide diversity of manifestations that characterizes the pontine syndrome. Yet the clinical symptoms develop relatively late, and the histologic changes are considerably more extensive than would be expected from the signs and symptoms.[763, 905]

The nystagmus with lesions of the pons may be horizontal, vertical, or rotary, or any combination of these. The horizontal nystagmus has a characteristic drifting quality and is poorly sustained. But the vertical nystagmus is the most significant for only with brain stem lesions does vertical nystagmus occur (see p. 218).

When pontine lesions are combined with mid-brain lesions there may be practically complete fixation of the eyes and consequent confusion with the myopathic ophthalmoplegias. With the latter, however, the lids are much more commonly affected and the pupils spared; also, the involvement of other pontine centers or tracts is of prime importance in the differentiation.

The type of lesion determines to some extent the clinical manifestations. With *thrombosis of the basilar artery* there is usually a sudden onset, progression for several days followed by remission and then coma, often with a high temperature, and death. In addition to the conjugate palsies, cranial nerve involvement, nystagmus, and pyramidal signs, there is a characteristic *miosis* of the pupils. *Aneurisms* of the vertebral artery or of the basilar artery may produce conjugate gaze palsy, 6th nerve palsy, nystagmus and other pontine signs. Unlike those causing 3rd nerve paralysis, aneurisms in the pontine region may induce ocular motor symptoms without rupturing. In consequence, they may produce brain stem signs intermittently for long periods of time; eventually death may occur from thrombosis of the basilar artery. *Tumors* of the pons show varying combinations of weakness of conjugate gaze and peripheral nerve palsies, frequently with cerebellar signs.[184, 13] Curiously, increased intracranial pressure is not a characteristic feature of intramedullary pontine tumors. Pontine tumors are most often confused with *cerebellar tumors* and *acoustic neuromas,* either of which may produce weakness of conjugate gaze. Pontine tumors can usually be differentiated from pure cerebellar tumors by the relatively extensive involvement of the cranial nerves in the former, and from acoustic neuromas by the characteristic chronology of the latter, which invariably begin with marked 8th nerve involvement.[494] Of the three types of tumors (pontine, cerebellar, and acoustic) pontine tumors are usually the ones that produce diplopia at the onset.

SUMMARY

Connecting the ocular motor nuclei with each other and with other brain stem nuclei is the *medial longitudinal fasciculus.* This tract relays the impulses for conjugate lateral gaze from the subcortical centers on one side of the medulla to the medial rectus nucleus on the opposite side. Lesions of the medial longitudinal fasciculus produce an entity known as *internuclear ophthalmoplegia* characterized by selective paralysis of the medial rectus on horizontal gaze and by predominantly monocular nystagmus of the abducting eye. When the lesion is situated anteriorly so as to involve the convergence mechanism it is arbitrarily called *anterior* internuclear ophthalmoplegia; when situated posteriorly so as to involve the pontine centers for conjugate gaze it is arbitrarily called

posterior internuclear ophthalmoplegia. *Bilateral* internuclear
ophthalmoplegia is most frequently caused by multiple sclerosis
and conversely it is the most frequent ocular motor manifestation
of multiple sclerosis. *Unilateral* internuclear ophthalmoplegia, on
the other hand, is almost always due to a vascular accident arising
in a small branch of the basilar artery.

In the cerebrum *lateral* gaze is represented in both the frontal
and occipital lobes. The *frontal* ocular motor zone corresponds to
Brodmann's Area 8. Excitation of this region produces deviation
of the eyes to the opposite side, whereas ablation results in deviation to the same side. The *occipital* ocular motor zone, which on
excitation similarly produces a deviation of the eyes, is scattered
over Areas 17, 18, and 19 without any sharp localization. The
frontal center is believed to mediate impulses in response to
ideational and somesthetic stimuli, whereas the occipital center is
thought to mediate impulses in response to visual stimuli. Efferent fibers connect these cerebral areas with the subcortical centers
in the basal ganglia, superior colliculi, and pons, but their exact
course is not known.

In the brain stem of man the most important subcortical
centers for conjugate lateral gaze are in the pons adjacent to, or
possibly identical with, the vestibular nuclei. Each center receives
impulses from the opposite cerebral hemisphere and relays them to
the homolateral lateral rectus nucleus and to the contralateral
medial rectus nucleus.

Lesions of the supranuclear centers and pathways in the cerebrum produce irritative and paralytic manifestations. *Irritative*
lesions of the frontal eye center produce a clonic turning of the
eyes to the opposite side, with convulsive phenomena in other
parts of the body, whereas *paralytic* lesions produce slight weakness of conjugate gaze, sometimes manifest as a nystagmus, with
variable degrees of hemiplegia. Attempted closure of the lids frequently results in a deviation of the eyes to the side opposite the
lesion. Unlike the phenomena of hemiplegia, the ocular motor
signs of unilateral frontal lesions are rapidly corrected in the conscious patient. This facile compensation is believed to occur
through the mediation of corresponding eye centers in the opposite hemisphere, for it does not occur with bilateral frontal lobe

lesions. *Irritative* lesions of the *occipital* motor center produce some deviation of the eyes accompanied by visual hallucinations; *paralytic* lesions produce some weakness of gaze, with a defect in the opticokinetic response and varying degrees of hemianopsia. Dissociation of the effects of the frontal from those of the occipital centers is thought to produce the syndrome of pseudo-ophthal-moplegia. Paralytic lesions in either the frontal or occipital area produce jerky following movements toward the side of the lesion. This, together with the conjugate deviation of the eyes on closure of the lids, and possibly the defective opticokinetic response, are interpreted as manifestations of "spasm of conjugate gaze" analogous to spastic hemiplegia.

Lesions of the supranuclear centers in the brain stem differ from those in the cerebrum in producing more marked and more enduring signs and symptoms. Lesions of the basal ganglia are usually irritative, producing various oculogyral crises, but as with lesions of the superior colliculi, the disturbance is primarily one of vertical eye movements. Lesions of the pontine center are usually paralytic, producing weakness of gaze to the homolateral side and being accompanied by other characteristic signs of brain stem involvement.

Chapter VI

SUPRANUCLEAR CONNECTIONS OF THE OCULAR MOTOR SYSTEM (Continued)

A. VERTICAL CONJUGATE MOVEMENTS

1. Cerebral Centers

VERTICAL conjugate movements are represented in the cerebrum as integral parts of the centers for lateral gaze. The upper portions of these centers represent downward gaze, along with the representation for the lateral movements, while the lower portions represent upward gaze. Thus, with rare exceptions,[1064] stimulation of the upper or lower portions of the frontal and occipital centers results in a movement of the eyes not only to the contralateral side but downward or upward as well.[742, 748, 730, 1064] *Purely* upward or downward movements can be produced with cerebral stimulation only by: (1) section of the lateral rotating muscles;[894] (2) destruction of the centers for lateral gaze;[986, 974] (3) total transverse section of the brain stem behind the midbrain,[987] or (4) equipotential stimulation of corresponding points in both cerebral hemispheres at the same time.[742, 894, 255]

The descending pathways carrying impulses for vertical movements of the eyes from the cortex to the lower centers have not been identified histologically, but their intracerebral course is probably the same as that inferred for the fibers representing lateral movements.

It has been suggested that the corticofugal fibers for lateral and vertical gaze are distinct within the cerebrum because lesions of the internal capsule produce paralysis of lateral gaze only,[86, 485] but a lesion involving all of one center or all its efferent pathways would produce purely horizontal effects, inasmuch as both upward and downward impulses are equally abolished; the evidence cited does not necessarily indicate a separate representation.

Having passed through the internal capsule, the corticofugal fibers for vertical gaze divide from those for horizontal gaze (Fig.

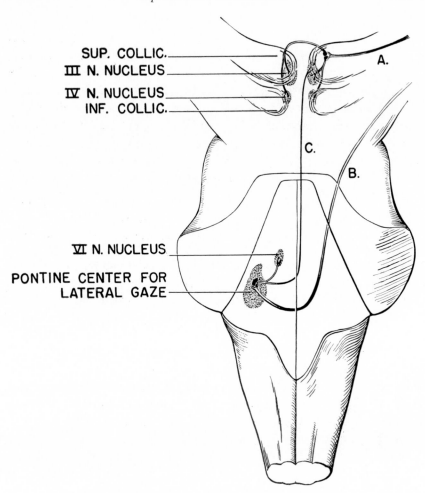

SUP. COLLIC.

III N. NUCLEUS

IV N. NUCLEUS

INF. COLLIC.

A.

C.

B.

VI N. NUCLEUS

PONTINE CENTER FOR
LATERAL GAZE

FIG. 57. *Diagrammatic representation of the dorsal surface of the brain stem showing the chief ocular motor centers and their supranuclear connections*

The main pathway from the cerebrum for conjugate lateral gaze (B) is by way of the cerebral peduncle to the opposite pontine center for lateral gaze and thence to the homolateral sixth nerve and opposite third nerve nuclei. The main pathway for conjugate vertical gaze (A) and for convergence is by way of the brachium to the superior colliculi and thence to the third and fourth nerve nuclei of both sides. Thus lesions in the anterior portion of the midbrain will affect primarily conjugate vertical movements and convergence, while lesions in the posterior portion will affect primarily conjugate lateral movements. Lesions in between will produce internuclear ophthalmoplegia from involvement of the medial longitudinal fasciculus (C).

57). While most of the fibers for *horizontal* movements course caudally to the pons, most of the fibers for *vertical* movements are believed to travel along the brachium toward the superior colliculi. This course is inferred from the fact that lesions of the pons produce disturbances predominantly of the lateral movements, whereas lesions of the superior colliculi produce disturbances predominantly of the vertical movements. In the higher animals and especially in man, in whom mobility of the eyes assumes increasing importance, the brachia contain an increasingly large proportion of corticofugal fibers.

> This dichotomy of efferent fibers in the brain stem of man applies to voluntary gaze and probably to most pursuit movements. It does not necessarily apply to some of the more subtle movements in man nor to some of the reflex movements in animals. Thus there is some clinical evidence that *all* opticokinetic responses (including those for horizontal gaze) are mediated through the anterior midbrain rather than simply through the pontine centers.

2. Subcortical Centers

There may be representation of vertical movements in the basal ganglia and reticular substance, for palsies of vertical gaze are frequent in Parkinson's disease and Huntington's chorea. Moreover vertical oculogyral crises are frequent following encephalitis, but no further evidence for the assumption of centers for vertical gaze in the basal ganglia is available at the present time.

Especial interest attaches to the *superior colliculi* as subcortical centers for vertical movements of the eyes. Fibers have been traced not only from the occipital lobe to the superior colliculi[847, 110, 635, 52] but, in turn, from the latter to the ocular motor nuclei.[196] Moreover stimulation of the superior colliculi or of the regional gray substance about the aqueduct has been shown to result in vertical eye movements.[5]

It has been observed that destruction of the superior colliculi does not appreciably affect vertical movements from frontal stimulation but does abolish or markedly diminish the vertical component from occipital stimulation.[80, 981] This observation has an obvious bearing on the clinical dissociation of vertical movements with different stimuli (pseudo-ophthalmoplegia).

Although the suggestion has been made that the effects reported from stimulation and destruction of the superior colliculi are actually due to involvement of the underlying 3rd nerve nuclei,[838] the weight of evidence is overwhelmingly in favor of supranuclear involvement. Not only is the paralysis usually symmetrical in the two eyes, which would be difficult to explain on the basis of nuclear lesions, but with supranuclear lesions the upward movements of the globe may be normal with some stimuli (for example, on closure of the lids) while completely paralyzed with other stimuli, indicating that the nucleus must be intact.

In the tectum, representation for upward gaze is probably distinct from that for downward gaze, since either may be affected clinically without the other, but there is scant and contradictory knowledge of the relative anatomic positions of the two. By electrical stimulation, it has been found possible to produce upward movements in cats with the electrode in the roof of the superior colliculi, whereas downward movements occur when the electrode is placed ventrally in the central gray substance beneath or behind the posterior commissure.[981] By strychninization of various points in the superior colliculi of cats it has been shown that impulses for upward movements of the eyes in response to a photic stimulus are mediated through the medial portions of the colliculi while the impulses for downward movements are mediated through the lateral portions.[18] It has also been suggested on clinical grounds that upward gaze is represented in the superior colliculi and downward gaze anteriorly in the posterior colliculi, since tumors in the tectal region produce first a paralysis of upward gaze and then a paralysis of downward gaze.[694, 485] Needless to say, further studies on the localization of vertical ocular movements in the superior colliculi of primates are needed.

Although there is strong evidence for the belief that vertical conjugate movements are mediated through the *superior colliculi,* there is also reason to believe that some regulation of vertical movement occurs in the *medulla* and possibly in the vestibular nuclei. Not only is vertical nystagmus frequent with lesions in this region, but vertical movements of the eyes may be induced by labyrinthine stimulation in patients who, on account of lesions of the tectum, cannot otherwise move their eyes vertically. The medullary center for *vertical* movements is thus purely a vestibular reflex center.

3. Lesions Involving Conjugate Vertical Movements

Cerebral lesions, especially if irritative, may show a vertical component with the disturbance of conjugate lateral gaze, but the vertical phase is relatively insignificant.

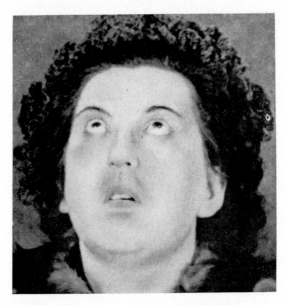

Fig. 58. *Oculogyral crisis in a patient with parkinsonism*
The patient is presumed to have had encephalitis in the past, but no definite history of this could be obtained. Oculogyral crises have occurred intermittently during the previous year, usually at noon, and were characterized by involuntary upward deviation of the eyes. The attacks lasted several hours and were preceded by faintness.

Lesions of the subcortical regions producing disturbances of conjugate vertical gaze are relatively common and are clinically important from the point of view of localization, since the vertical and horizontal functions are separately represented in the brain stem. The lesions are both irritative and paralytic.

Irritative lesions manifested by vertical oculogyral crises (Fig. 58) occur almost exclusively following encephalitis and, curiously, after some particular epidemics.[56] The deviation of the eyes is generally upward (see p. 111). The curious occurrence of these crises at specific times or with specific activities suggests a strong functional overlay.

Paralytic lesions resulting in vertical palsies occur with involvement of the subcortical centers and pathways. Especially noteworthy is the paralysis of upward gaze (Parinaud's syndrome) and to a lesser extent that of downward gaze, which is found with lesions in the vicinity of the superior colliculi (Fig. 59). This occurs most frequently with tumors of the pineal gland, but it is also seen with lesions within the superior colliculi[1120, 12] and in the thalamus,[930] with neurosyphilis,[694] encephalitis,[610] multiple sclerosis, gliomas, trauma,[25] vascular lesions,[15, 903] and as a congenital defect.[288] Along with the paralysis of vertical gaze, there are practically always pupillary disturbances and frequently absence of convergence. The pupils characteristically do not react to light but do react to near focusing and differ from the Argyll-Robertson pupil only in so far as they are not miotic. The absence of convergence is a common finding when downward gaze is affected, but convergence is often retained when only upward gaze is involved.[86, 486] Diplopia is present when the oculomotor nuclei are also involved.

The paralysis of vertical gaze with pinealomas does not necessarily indicate infiltration of the superior colliculi. It may merely be a pressure effect; full gaze movements may be restored simply by relief of the hydrocephalus through a shunt operation.

> Weakness of upward gaze should be evaluated cautiously in stuporous or uncooperative patients. Being the least comfortable of the conjugate movements, it is the first to show a deficit in generalized depression of function. Failure to recognize this has often led to an erroneous diagnosis of paresis of upward gaze.

Paralysis of vertical gaze shows curious variations when different stimuli are used. These are given the comprehensive name of *pseudo-ophthalmoplegia* because of their obvious analogy to, and frequent association with, pseudobulbar palsy.[810, 1095] Vertical movements on *command* are most profoundly affected, but a

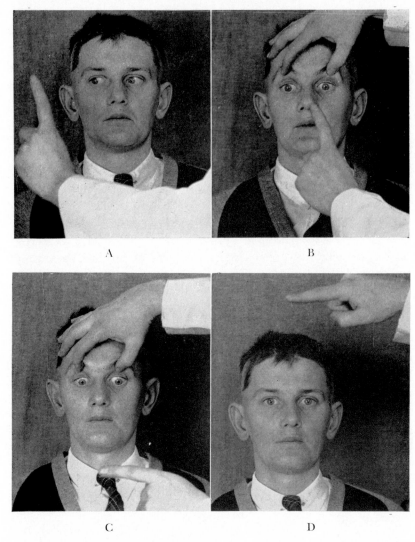

FIG. 59. *Paralysis of upward gaze and areflexic pupils (Parinaud's syndrome) in a patient with a pinealoma*

The patient was a twenty-six-year-old man whose presenting complaints were intermittent headaches and nausea of one year's duration. Examination showed normal lateral excursions of eyes (A) in both directions but an absence of convergence (B), a slightly diminished downward gaze (C), and an absence of upward gaze (D). The pupils were 5 mm. in size and did not react to light but did react fairly well to near focusing.

patient who cannot volun-
tarily move his eyes up or
down may be able to *follow*
a slowly moved object or may
be able to move the eyes up
or down by looking at separate objects placed close together in a vertical line[127] (one
form of pseudo-ophthalmoplegia). Again a patient with complete paralysis of vertical gaze
for both voluntary and following movements may show full
vertical rotation of the eyes
on closure of the lids and on
passive bending of the head
or other forms of labyrinthine
stimulation[994] (another form
of pseudo-ophthalmople-
gia, Fig. 60). Indeed, in such
cases the vertical movements
of the eyes with passive movements of the head are often
uncontrollable, acting in all
respects like those of the eyes
of mechanical dolls, upward
rotation of the head causing

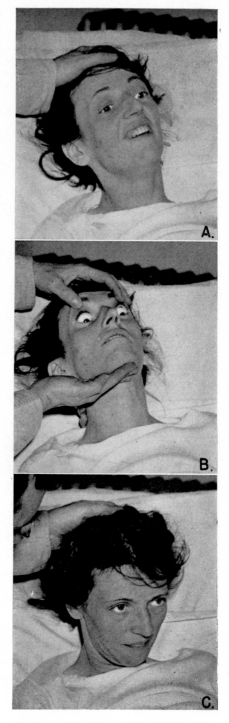

⟫→

FIG. 60. *Pseudo-ophthalmoplegia
("doll's head movements") showing
full ocular excursions with passive
movements of the head despite absence of voluntary control of the eyes*
    The patient was an eighteen-
year-old-girl with Huntington's
chorea. She was able to look conjugately to either side to full extent but could not voluntarily look
upward or downward. On passive
extension (B) or flexion (C) of the
head the eyes turned upward and
downward to full extent involuntarily.

movements of the eyes downward and vice versa.[352] Once the eyes
are rotated upward, they often cannot be brought down by voluntary effort; they remain deviated upward for a matter of seconds (depending on the amount of labyrinthine stimulation), and
in order to keep his gaze fixed on an object in front, the patient
must bend his head forward.

Thus the head movements in patients with pseudo-ophthalmoplegia compensate for the defective eye movements and constitute the only means by which such patients can fixate an object
effectively. But it should be noted that the head movement per
se induces a vestibulogenic deviation of the eyes in the direction
opposite to that of intended gaze. Thus it is necessary for the patient to "overshoot" with the head, producing the characteristic
thrust. This same thrust of the head, occurring in the vertical
direction for patients with pseudo-ophthalmoplegia, has been
noted in the horizontal direction for patients with congenital
apraxia (see p. 107). The basis for both is a paralysis of voluntary
gaze with preservation of vestibulogenic movements. It is not seen
in patients who also have involvement of their vestibular mechanism (brain stem lesions) or of the peripheral neuromuscular
system (cranial nerve palsies and myopathic ophthalmoplegia).

While palsies of vertical gaze result most frequently from lesions of the superior colliculi or its immediate environs they
may also arise from lesions elsewhere. Selective paralysis of conjugate vertical eye movements has been reported in cases wherein
the superior colliculi were found to be histologically normal.[989, 646]
Parkinson's disease, Huntington's chorea, and congenital cerebro-
spastic palsy, which are not ordinarily thought to be associated
with tectal lesions, affect upward movements of the eyes to a much
greater extent than horizontal movements (Fig. 60). These diseases
are frequently associated with the neurologic entity of pseudobulbar palsy involving the basal ganglia and other regions higher
than the brain stem. Multiple cerebro-vascular accidents may also
result in pseudo-ophthalmoplegia, and other signs of pseudobulbar
palsy, with preferential involvement of vertical gaze.

Paralysis of upward gaze has been reported with tumors of the
thalamus, and this cannot always be accounted for by extension
of the tumor toward the colliculus;[964] it may have some bearing

on the reported representation of vertical movements (in animals) in the thalamic nuclei.[901] Vertical palsies, vertical nystagmus, and spasms of vertical gaze also occur with lesions of the 4th ventricle and cerebellum, especially with lesions of the flocculus.[698] The signs produced by these lesions differ from those occurring with lesions of the colliculi in the retention of normal pupillary reactions and, usually, in the presence of nystagmus. Paralysis of upward gaze has also been attributed, rightly or wrongly, to lesions in the nucleus of Darkschewitsch[1121, 390, 392] and in the posterior commissure.[809]

B. TORSIONAL CONJUGATE MOVEMENTS

Of all the conjugate ocular movements in man, those involved in torsion, i.e., clockwise and counterclockwise rotations, are unique in not being under voluntary control and, so far as is known, having no representation in the frontal lobe. It is to be presumed that there is some torsional representation in the occipital lobe, since torsional following movements can be induced by a rotation of the field of vision, but there is no anatomic or physiologic evidence of the site of this representation at the present time. Judging from the meager clinical evidence available no disturbance of torsion occurs with lesions of the superior colliculi.[590]

On the other hand, conjugate torsional movements *are* regularly produced by appropriate vestibular and postural stimuli. Among the first to observe the effect of head posture on the rotation of the eyes was Javal (1866),[522] who discovered that when his head was tilted to one side, the cylindrical lenses he was wearing no longer corrected his astigmatism. When the head is tilted to one side, the eyes undergo a conjugate rolling in the opposite direction. This torsion tends to maintain the original orientation of the eyes in relation to the environment. The compensation is, however, far from complete.[587, 4]

The stimulus for this postural torsion comes in part from the neck muscles but chiefly from the labyrinth.[1029] The maintained torsion is maximal with head tilting of approximately 60 degrees, at which angle the otoliths are thought to be in a position to produce maximal gravitational pull;[1029] a transient torsion occurs with sudden rotation of the head and the amount of torsion varies with the speed of the head tilting. Removal of one labyrinth diminishes primarily the torsion induced by tilting the head to the opposite side,[414] whereas removal of both labyrinths abolishes torsion of the eyes almost completely.[587, 4]

Aside from rotary nystagmus, disturbances of the conjugate torsional mechanism have not been reported clinically. In the presence of a superior oblique paralysis of one eye, however, advantage is taken of the normal conjugate movements on head tilting to produce a torsion of the other eye and thereby avoid diplopia (see p. 75).

> Because of the almost exclusive control of torsional movements by the labyrinths, rotary nystagmus is prima-facie evidence for involvement of the vestibular mechanism. Rotary nystagmus is especially frequent with lesions of the vestibular nuclei in the floor of the 4th ventricle and is oftenest seen with multiple sclerosis (see p. 220).

C. DISJUNCTIVE MOVEMENTS

1. Convergence

Convergence is the act wherein the optic axes of the two eyes are aligned on some relatively near point. It is effected through the predominant action of the medial recti. These muscles are presumed to be equally innervated in the act of convergence just as are conjugate pairs of muscles on lateral gaze (Hering's Law).[703] But there are reasons to believe that the adduction is effected by different muscle groups for convergence as compared with conjugate gaze. Not only is the adductive amplitude less for convergent than for conjugate movements, but convergence induces an associated intorsion whereas conjugate movements induce an extorsion of the adducted eye.[1052] Further studies on these differences should yield interesting and important information.

(a) *Cerebral centers.* Although convergence has on occasion been noted to occur with stimulation of one cerebral hemisphere,[634, 644, 858] it is bilateral stimulation that is characteristically associated with convergence. Convergence has been produced by bilateral stimulation of the frontal[742, 894] and occipital lobes,[913, 742, 781, 109, 634] but the observations have been too few and too inexact to permit localization other than in the general eye fields of both the frontal and occipital ocular motor centers. Weakness of convergence has followed bilateral occipital lobe injuries.[826, 449, 118, 1042, 562, 325] Ablation of the cortex in the region of the angular gyri has been reported to result in a paralysis of convergence with a disturbance of depth perception.[747, 872, 484]

Since no laboratory animal has an amplitude of convergence comparable to that in man, the experimental approach is necessarily handicapped. But it is clear that convergence is, like pure vertical movements, represented in the cerebrum as a bilateral function, and the higher centers for convergence are intimately associated with those for conjugate lateral gaze.

Convergence is both a voluntary and an involuntary function. One can voluntarily converge the eyes, but unless there is some object on which to fix one's gaze, the amount of voluntary convergence can be varied only roughly. While it is possible to converge one's eyes at random, it is practically impossible without practice to converge on an imaginary point in space if an object is placed in the line of vision near, but not at, the point of intended convergence. In other words, the visual (presumably the occipital) impulses dominate the purely voluntary (presumably frontal) impulses for convergence.

Under normal conditions the act of convergence is inseparably associated with miosis and accommodation. This triad is the *near reflex,* but where in the brain the three components become associated is not known. The totally involuntary nature of the pupillary reaction suggests that the association occurs in the midbrain. In any case, the components are mutually independent to the extent that if, for any reason, one component is prevented from acting normally, the others act independently. It is variously reported that the pupillary and accommodative functions are more intimately associated with each other than either is with the function of convergence[621] but also, by other criteria, that the pupillary functions are more closely associated with convergence than with accommodation.[869]

The pathways for convergence by which impulses pass from the cortex to the ocular motor nuclei are as ill understood as are the cortical centers themselves. But it can be shown experimentally that convergence is retained after transection of the brain stem at the posterior end of the midbrain,[981] and it has been abundantly shown on clinical grounds that convergence may be retained with extensive lesions of the pons and of the medial longitudinal fasciculus. Hence, it is reasonable to infer that the corticofugal paths for convergence reach the ocular motor nuclei along the anterior brachia and superior colliculi rather than by way of the pons (Fig. 57). This accounts for the frequent dissociation of convergence and conjugate lateral movements with lesions in various parts of the brain stem [865] and the paradoxic preservation of medial rectus function on convergence despite its loss on conjugate gaze (or vice versa).

(b) **Subcortical centers.** The frequency with which lesions in the vicinity of the superior colliculi are accompanied by paralysis of convergence (along with fixed pupils and palsies of conjugate vertical gaze) leads one to suspect a subcortical center for convergence or a conjugation of convergence fibers in the superior colliculi. It does not seem likely that these lesions produce a convergence paralysis through pressure transmitted to the underlying 3rd nerve nucleus, since the convergence paralysis is often unaccompanied by other evidence of 3rd nerve involvement.

Perlia's nucleus, the unpaired group of motor cells lying between the 3rd nerve nuclei, is generally supposed to be a center for convergence, since it develops phylogenetically along with the function of convergence (p. 57). There is, however, no direct evidence that it serves convergence exclusively.

(c) **Lesions of the convergence mechanism.** Paralysis of convergence is an inability to converge (with consequent diplopia) on an object ordinarily within the distance of a meter or so. But this diagnosis should be made only with a great deal of caution, since the amplitude of convergence normally depends on numerous factors, including the effort that the patient makes, the presence of binocular vision, the visual acuity in each eye, the sense of nearness,[1052, 23] the adaptive[831] and refractive status of the eyes and the attention value of the object used to elicit convergence.* An

---

* In testing the convergence function, it is important to use an object which adequately holds the patient's attention. A finger or a light is often insufficient. A convenient object is a watch, the patient's attention being held on the object by instructing him to state where the little hand is as the watch is moved closer toward him.

abnormality in any of these may produce an apparent decrease or absence of convergence on functional grounds and should not be confused with a true paralysis of convergence caused by organic disease. Suggestive of a *true* paralysis are the history of sudden onset of diplopia, the presence of a known intracranial lesion, and the constancy of the findings on successive trials.[127] With simple paralysis of convergence either eye may be rotated inward to the full extent on conjugate lateral movements, showing that there is no true paralysis of the medial recti.

While disturbances of convergence occur with occipital lesions,[826, 449, 1042, 325] it is with lesions in the region of the superior colliculi that paralysis of convergence occurs characteristically. Aside from discrete lesions in this region (tumors or aneurisms) diffuse lesions such as occur with encephalitis, multiple sclerosis, Parkinson's disease (post-encephalitic variety), and vascular lesions also cause a paralysis or weakness of convergence. Usually, but not invariably, there is also a concomitant absence of accommodation and of miosis on looking at a near object.

> The diplopia associated with alcoholic intoxication,[227, 842] or altitude hypoxia[1043, 8, 289] is due to an increased esophoria (for distance). The reason for this is not apparent, but the net result is that those persons who are esophoric to begin with develop diplopia with slight intoxication or slight hypoxia whereas those who are exophoric may approach orthophoria (euphoria?) and never develop diplopia. Despite the increase in esophoria for distance, the near point of convergence may actually be diminished.[131]

Spasm of convergence occurs along with spasm of accommodation and miosis, and is therefore more comprehensively designated *spasm of the near reflex*. The spasm is usually intermittent and occurs when attention is directed to the eyes, as by asking the patient to look at an object, by shining a light in the eye, or by holding open the lids. It has been reported following *encephalitis*,[700, 143, 593] (when it is usually accompanied by nystagmus), with *tabes dorsalis*,[260] with *labyrinthine fistulas*,[147] and with *trauma*.[740] But spasm of the near reflex is especially common with *hysteria*[1111, 971, 490, 1074, 221] (Fig. 61). It is most often confused with lateral rectus paralysis, since the patient complains of the diplopia

and is found to have a convergent strabismus. It may be differentiated from this condition, however, by the accompanying pupillary
and accommodative spasm and by the preservation of normal

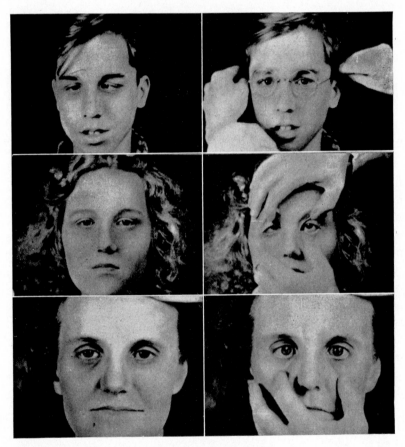

FIG. 61. *Spasm of the near reflex of functional origin*
    The convergence in all patients was intermittent and accompanied by
marked miosis and spasm of accommodation (5-7 diopters). The first patient
shows an apparent cure by minus (!) lenses. The second and third patients
show elicitation of the syndrome by manipulation of the lids.

lateral excursions of the eyes. Aside from the usual therapy directed
toward the psychiatric background, minus lenses that compensate
for the accommodative spasm may also be effective in correcting
the convergence. Atropinization has at times the same effect.
    A compensatory spasm of the near reflex occurs occasionally in

patients with paralysis of horizontal gaze and may lead to a per-
plexing clinical picture. This is a purposive movement by which
patients can fixate an excentric object through the adduction of
convergence when the adduction of conjugate horizontal gaze is
lacking. It is not common, however, as most such patients prefer to
fixate through head turning and thereby avoid the blurring of the
associated accommodation and the diplopia of the associated convergence. But if the patient's head is held still, or immobilized for
any other reason, the spasm of the near reflex may be invoked as
the only means for excentric fixation.

2. Divergence

Divergence functions comprise a controversial subject. Centers
for divergence in the cerebrum and in the brain stem are commonly postulated[171] and some pathologic evidence suggests localization in the medulla and in the tectum.[104] Stimulation of the
ocular motor area in the frontal lobe has also been reported to produce divergence in monkeys.[253] But the total evidence is meager and
one cannot deny that divergence may be brought about simply by
relaxation of the medial recti through inhibition of the convergence center.[115, 933, 1052] The matter must await further observation
from clinicians; animal experimentation is limited by the fact that
divergence of significant magnitude is present only in man and in
the higher primates.

Whether or not divergence centers exist, there is a clinical syndrome, properly called *divergence paralysis,* in which convergent
strabismus suddenly develops with diplopia and with full function
of the lateral recti on conjugate gaze. Homonymous diplopia is
then present for all objects that are farther than one-quarter or one-
third meter away; and for any one distance the diplopia is essentially the same for all directions of gaze.[127] As an object is brought
nearer, the patient is able to unify the images over a certain range,
but frequently there is also an associated convergence insufficiency
so that crossed diplopia is present for near objects.

Divergence paralysis is caused by many of the same pathologic
processes that have been noted to cause convergence paralysis;[171]
for example, encephalitis (including poliomyelitis), tabes dorsalis,
multiple sclerosis, and head trauma.[907, 642] It has also been reported

with tumors and cysts of the cerebellum[881, 652, 908] and with acoustic neuromas,[908] (all of which may conceivably have exerted their effect through pressure on the 4th ventricle). It also may occur with simple increase in intracranial pressure.[198] Difficult to explain is the occasional occurrence of divergence paralysis with generalized polyneuritis. Interesting from the point of view of localization is the occasional occurrence of alternating divergence and convergence with migraine[1051] and alternating palsies of these two functions with Wernicke's disease,[224] suggesting that the convergence and divergence centers or tracts are closely associated in at least some portion of the central nervous system. On the other hand, divergence paralysis may appear during the resolving stages of a Foville syndrome suggesting that the divergence center of tracts are close by the centers for conjugate lateral gaze. It is of course entirely possible that divergence centers are present both anteriorly in the tectum *and* posteriorly in the medulla.

Divergence paralysis may be differentiated from bilateral 6th nerve paralysis by the normal excursions of the eyes on lateral gaze, and from spasm of convergence by its constancy, by the absence of other spastic phenomena of the near reflex, and by the normal or diminished amplitude of the convergence. In any case this is a diagnosis to be made only with considerable caution, since a latent esotropia (divergence insufficiency) may produce the same syndrome without evident neurologic disease.[1040]

3. Skew Deviation

By skew deviation is meant a hypertropia that is referable to neither a peripheral neuromuscular lesion nor to a local mechanical factor in the orbit. It is the human counterpart of the Magendie-Hertwig syndrome* in animals and is often so-called in man. Abundant evidence indicates that lesions within the central nervous system will cause skew deviation but evidence is scanty for localization, other than in the general region of the posterior fossa.

Skew deviation is characterized by a maintained deviation of one eye above the other, frequently fixed for all directions of gaze but

---

* Ohm (*Arch. f. Ophth.*, *149*:364, 1949) calls attention to the common, and erroneous, inversion of these names. Magendie described the deviation in 1825 and Hertwig described it in 1826.

equally often variable for different directions of gaze. Thus it may be a right hypertropia on looking to one side and a left hypertropia on looking to the other side. It may simulate palsies of individual vertically-acting muscles and be differentiated from these only through the associated signs of brain stem disease and the absence of mid-brain or peripheral nerve disease.

Skew deviation may occur with any lesion of the brain stem or cerebellum. It is more common with unilateral than with bilateral lesions; thus it is characteristically present with unilateral internuclear ophthalmoplegia and absent with bilateral internuclear ophthalmoplegia.[222] The eye on the side of the lesion is usually hypotropic. The fact that a vertical divergence occurs on stimulating the labyrinth or with unilateral labyrinthine disease[55, 342, 1024] suggests that the pathogenesis of skew deviation is linked up with the vestibulo-ocular pathways and most of the clinical cases are compatible with such an assumption.[801] It is found with cerebellar tumors, acoustic neuromas, compressive lesions (platybasia) and vascular accidents of the pons and cerebellum (especially thrombosis of the cerebellar and pontine arteries). It is, nevertheless, surprisingly infrequent with demyelinative lesions.

> Skew deviation has been produced experimentally in animals with lesions of the middle cerebellar peduncle,[607, 676, 919, 1061] of the cerebellum itself,[489, 460] of the restiform body,[77] and of the inferior olive,[77] and especially with lesions of the vestibular nuclei and of their connections with the ocular motor nuclei.[808] Since, however, vertical divergence is a normal conjugate act for animals with laterally placed eyes and has no counterpart in man, the above experimental results cannot be directly applied to human beings.

The clinical importance of skew deviation resides chiefly in its recognition as a cognate sign of lesions in the brain stem and cerebellum; it does not necessarily indicate involvement of the ocular motor nerves.

4. Fusional Movements (Unification)

While the two eyes receive equal innervation for all the foregoing conjugate and disjunctive movements (Hering's Law), there is still another movement serving the function commonly known as fusion or unification.[1049] which may or may not result from symmetrical innervation of the two eyes. The *sensory* component or stimulus for this reflex is disparateness of the retinal images and the *motor* component is called duction. The duction power is usually measured by prisms or by moving the field of vision separately before the two eyes. The ability to diverge the eyes horizontally is called abduction; ability to converge them, adduction; ability to diverge them vertically, sursumduction; and ability to rotate them clockwise or counterclockwise in opposite directions, cycloduction. Duction movements differ from other eye movements in being executed more slowly and in a persistence of the induced position of the eyes for some time after the stimulus has been removed.

The question of what neurologic centers and pathways are used for duction is subject to dispute. The fact that stimulation of the rolandic area just posterior to the frontal eye field of the dog's brain has resulted in unilateral, vertical, and horizontal movements of the opposite eye[472, 287, 880] has led to the assumption of a cortical center for monocular movements such as are seen in duction.[126] Although in the anthropoid species these movements have not been observed to result from electrical stimulation, a center similar to that in the dog is thought to be present because of the similarity of the rolandic representation in other respects.[927] Moreover, this supposedly unilateral center is held to account for the ocular motor disturbances limited to one eye seen occasionally in man; for example, unilateral nystagmus after local skull injuries, unilateral vertical and torsional movements in sleep and in narcosis, and unilateral movements with one-sided amblyopia.[1029]

Contrary to the foregoing concept of a *cerebral* center for duction, it has been maintained that since duction is involuntary, the impulses for it are relayed directly from the retina to the superior colliculi and ocular motor nuclei without traversing the cerebrum.[1108, 1110] In apparent support of this it has been reported that patients with hemianopsia from an intracerebral lesion show normal duction, whereas those with tract hemianopsia do not have duction.[90] This has, however, not been confirmed,[585, 595, 129, 526, 1063] and patients who have been blinded by a bilateral cortical lesion have been shown to have no duction power, indicating that the impulse for duction must be mediated through the occipital lobes.[127]

It seems reasonably certain that the neural connections for duction in the horizontal plane are allied to the convergence-divergence mechanism and not to the conjugate mechanism. Conjugate palsies may show complete paralysis of the medial recti for associated lateral movements but so long as the convergence-divergence mechanism is intact there is no abnormal phoria and the duction power is normal. The duction power may also be normal in patients with internuclear ophthalmoplegia so long as convergence is normal, despite the fact that both medial recti are paralyzed for conjugate movements.

SUMMARY

In the cerebral hemispheres vertical conjugate movements of the eyes are represented as integral parts of the centers for conjugate lateral movements. Downward gaze is represented in the upper portions of the centers, while upward gaze is represented in the lower portions, but in both cases the vertical movements are indissociable from the lateral movement. In the brain stem of man, however, the vertical and lateral movements are represented separately. Vertical movements are mediated almost exclusively through the superior colliculi, whereas lateral movements are mediated for the most part through the pons. From the clinical standpoint this means that cerebral lesions result in a defect that has both a lateral and a vertical component, whereas brain stem lesions may result in a dissociation of lateral and vertical movements. Lesions in the region of the superior colliculi produce a disturbance of upward or rarely downward gaze, while lesions of the pons produce disturbances of lateral gaze.

Conjugate torsional movements of the eyes are produced exclusively by vestibular or fixational reflexes. The common clinical disturbance of the conjugate torsional mechanism is rotary nystagmus, and this is prima facie evidence of a lesion of the vestibular mechanism.

Disjunctive movements of the eyes are convergence, divergence skew deviation, and various duction movements. Convergence is presumably represented bilaterally in the cerebrum and is mediated through the 3rd nerve complex (possibly Perlia's nucleus). Together with miosis and accommodation, convergence forms the triad known as the near reflex. Spasm of the near reflex occurs most frequently as a manifestation of hysteria. Paralysis of convergence, with or without paralysis of the other components of the near reflex, occurs with various lesions in the anterior portions of the midbrain.

Divergence may or may not be represented in the central nervous system as is convergence; no one group of cells has been identified as the significant group. Paralysis of divergence occurs with the same type of lesions as produces paralysis of convergence but also with lesions more posteriorly situated in the brain stem and cerebellum.

Skew deviation is a static or variable hypertropia resulting from lesions in the posterior fossa and presumably due to involvement of the vestibulo-ocular pathways.

Chapter VII

SUPRANUCLEAR CONNECTIONS OF THE OCULAR MOTOR SYSTEM (Continued)

LID MOVEMENTS

THE MUSCLES controlling the eyelids are the levator palpebrae including Müller's muscle) which opens the palpebral fissure, and the orbicularis oculi, which closes it. The levator is innervated jointly by the 3rd nerve and the sympathetic; the orbicularis is innervated by the 7th nerve, and possibly by the parasympathetic as well.[97, 641] Despite earlier statements to the contrary,[942, 947] the levator and orbicularis oculi show the same type of reciprocal contraction and relaxation (in the blink reflex at least) as shown by the extraocular muscles.[945, 411, 136]

Actually, the reciprocal relationships between the levator and orbicularis oculi have never been subjected to the study which their importance merits and for which methods of investigation are available. It does appear, however, that voluntary closure of the lids, as in the act of winking, is executed through the chief, and possibly exclusive, means of orbicularis contraction whereas the closure of the lids in sleep or in the act of downward gaze is executed through the chief, and possibly exclusive, relaxation of the levator. The blink reflex, on the other hand, invokes both the contraction of the orbicularis and relaxation of the levator. This conjecture is, however, subject to subsequent evaluation by electrophysiologic means and is also subject to variation among individuals. It is a recognized fact that some persons have voluntary control of levator relaxation and can, for instance, wink without causing any of the lid wrinkling that is characteristic of orbicularis contraction.

The lid-closing and lid-opening mechanisms are served by different neural arcs, some of which are mediated through the cerebrum and some of which are purely subcortical.

1. Cerebral Centers

Opening of the lids has been produced experimentally by stimulating zones in the frontal[331, 83, 496, 429, 634, 644] and occipital[1064] lobes in close proximity to the centers previously described for conjugate lateral movements of the eyes (Fig. 50).

While the opening of the lids from *frontal* lobe stimulation usually occurs *with* conjugate turning of the eyes and head to the opposite side and with simultaneous dilatation of the pupils, the lid reaction may be the *primary* effect with stimulation of an area in the first frontal convolution just above the frontal eye field.[169] Both lids are raised, but the lid on the side opposite the stimulus is raised more than that on the same side. Conversely, *lesions* in the frontal areas have been reported to produce ptosis of the lids. This cortical ptosis is usually bilateral and symmetrical.[117]

Raising of the lids from stimulation of the *occipital* lobe has been less regularly produced than that from stimulation of the *frontal* lobe. Elevation of the lids has been reported, however, to occur with stimulation of the inferolateral surface of the occipital lobe.[1064]

Although *stimulation* of areas other than those just noted has not been reported to produce opening of the eyelids, *lesions* of the *angular gyrus*[747, 733] and of the *temporal lobe*[404] have been reported to produce ptosis.

Closing of the eyelids has also been reported with stimulation of the frontal and occipital lobes in proximity to the centers for conjugate lateral gaze.

In regard to the frontal lobe, *stimulation of the rolandic area* and of the precentral gyrus[823] have produced lid closure,[83, 748, 471, 1058, 634] especially stimulation of the region adjacent to centers for the thumb and in the vicinity of centers for movement of the ear, nostril, neck, and lip[317, 429] and just below that representing the thumb.[823] The lids of both eyes close, but those of the contralateral eye close more vigorously.[85, 345, 858] *Lesions* of the frontal area, specifically Area 8, have been reported to produce a deficiency of the lid closing mechanism.[548]

Closing of the lids has also been produced by a stimulus applied to the *occipito-parietal* region.[333] This closure occurs with stimulation of the anterolateral occipital surface in a region not far from the lid-opening centers and is accompanied by movements of the eyes to the opposite side and by narrowing of the pupil.[1064]

By analogy with ocular motor representation in the cerebrum, it may be assumed that the frontal centers for lid movements respond to *voluntary* impulses, and it is noteworthy that, in contrast to the *following* movements of the eyes, movements induced by volition are usually accompanied by a blink of the lids. It also occasionally happens, especially in blind patients, that the *fast* phase of a jerk nystagmus, that is the phase which is related to voluntary movements (p. 213), is regularly accompanied by a blink of the lids. The frontal area also mediates, in all probability, lid closure in response to painful stimuli in and about the eye since stimulation of this frontal area, and of the corresponding post-rolandic region, results in pain referred to the eyes.[823]

While there are no experimental data on lid closure from stimulation of other portions of the cerebrum, it is possible that reflex closure in response to loud noises or to painful stimuli is mediated through other cerebral centers.[81, 93, 321, 384]

One may also expect a close association of the centers for lid movements with those for vertical movements of the eyes since these functions are intimately correlated but there is scant experimental evidence to indicate where this association takes place.

Clinical disturbances of the lid musculature are manifest by either a ptosis and insufficient raising of the lids (with lesions involving the *opening* mechanism) or an abnormal widening of the palpebral fissure and inadequate closing reflexes (with lesions involving the *closing* mechanism). It is to be expected with cerebral lesions that the lids on the side *opposite* the lesions will be the more profoundly affected (Fig. 62). Abnormalities of lid movements from cerebral lesions are not conspicuous and are usually masked by other disturbances of the eye movements. However, a ptosis that is more marked in the contralateral eye has been reported clinically with lesions in the parieto-temporal lobes and about the angular gyrus.[1109] Lesions of the frontal lobe are less productive of ptosis. Disturbances of the closing mechanism, manifested by abnormal widening of the palpebral fissure, infrequency of blinking, and a persistent closure of the lids on tapping or other stimuli applied to the forehead[756] are seen with Parkinson's disease and may be interpreted as bearing on the supranuclear representation of lid function, but in the present state of knowledge it has little localizing significance.

That the failure of the blink reflex in Parkinson's disease, attributed to the striatal lesion, may in fact be due to a bilateral frontal lesion or interruption of the corticofugal pathways is suggested by the analogous lid condition in monkeys following bilateral ablation of Area 8.[548]

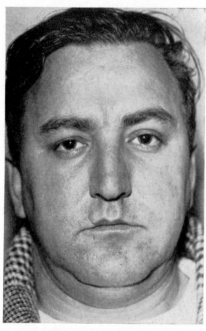

Fig. 62. *Slight ptosis on left associated with a right sided temporo-occipital lesion*

The patient had seizures consisting of formed visual hallucinations and left homonymous hemianopsia.

The *pathways* from the cortex to the nuclei mediating the impulses for lid movements are not known, but they are apparently separate from the pathways for conjugate lateral and vertical movements, since either of these may be separately abolished by pontine or tectal lesions without affecting the lid movements.

The pathway for relaying impulses from the cerebrum to the *facial* nuclei, and thence to the orbicularis, apparently undergoes complete decussation in the medulla, for midline incision of the brain stem abolishes the lid closure on cerebral stimulation. That the corticofugal fibers to the facial nuclei do not pass through the tectum is evident from the facts that removal of the superior colliculi and section of the posterior commissure are without effect on the lid closing function.[317]

2. Subcortical Centers

Subcortical centers for opening and for closing of the lids exist in animals, and possibly in man, since decerebrate animals show a narrowing of the palpebral fissure in reponse to light and other stimuli. Even a reflex closing that is conditioned in the normal animal in response to visual stimuli may be elicited when, following the conditioning, the occipital lobes are removed.[707]

There are at least two afferent arcs relaying the impulses to the lower motor centers for lid movement which in animals are *independent of the cerebrum*. One is the *trigeminal* route, by which impulses are relayed in response to irritative stimuli applied locally to the eye or adnexa and transversing that portion of the trigeminal nucleus that lies in the floor of the 4th ventricle.[317, 765] The other afferent arc is by way of the *optic nerve,* and this, of course, relays the impulses in response to light. In animals, most or all of this latter afferent pathway is subcortical, the impulses passing by way of the superior colliculi[302, 303] to the facial nuclei, but the absence of the blink reflex in patients with complete occipital softening is presumptive evidence that in man the impulses are mediated through the occipital lobes. Yet even in man, preservation of the blink reflex has been reported on occasion with complete cortical blindness[633, 636] and in anencephaly.[307, 890]

It would appear that impulses for the blink reflex are relayed in part through the mid-brain for even when there is an effective transection of the brain stem that involves the supranuclear pathways to the orbicularis the blink reflex may be retained.[212] This retention of the blink reflex despite involvement of the facial fibers may, of course, be effected through inhibition of the levator rather than through contraction of the orbicularis.

An abnormal *widening* of the palpebral fissure, known as "tucked lids," is said to be characteristic of lesions in the region of the superior colliculi[225] but this widening is probably secondary to the weakness of upward gaze.

Other subcortical reflexes such as the auropalpebral reflex for lid closing are thought to be mediated through the brain stem, and because of their independence of the cerebrum they have been said to have some clinical value in coma.[322] A particularly interesting reflex opening of the lids may sometimes be demonstrated in comatose patients by raising of the head or turning of the head from side to side. This phenomenon, which does not appear to have been previously described, is obviously analogous to the doll's head movements of the eyes in pseudo-ophthalmoplegia (see p. 223). Whether it is attributable to afferent impulses arising in the neck muscles or in the vestibular end organs has yet to be determined.

Clinical disturbances of lid movements from subcortical lesions occur frequently. Ptosis is a conspicuous feature of several of the myopathies (myasthenia gravis and abiotrophic ophthalmoplegia). It is also a cognate part of 3rd nerve palsies and may, on occasion, be the sole manifestation of a 3rd nerve paresis. Similarly weakness of the orbicularis oculi occurs commonly with 7th nerve palsies but may be the only demonstrable weakness of facial function with the ocular myopathies (myasthenia gravis and abiotrophic ophthalmoplegia). In these conditions the orbicularis oculi may be weak despite the presence of ptosis!

A curious and not uncommon disturbance is the Marcus Gunn[432] or jaw-winking phenomenon, in which the upper lid of one eye retracts when the jaws are opened or when the lower jaw is moved to the opposite side (Fig. 63).

The Marcus Gunn phenomenon is a congenital and sometimes hereditary[320] anomaly. One eye only is affected. The typical jaw-winker has at rest what appears to be a paresis of the levator muscle, with consequent ptosis, and frequently a paralysis of the superior rectus muscle. But when the mouth is opened, the lid that was ptotic becomes momentarily retracted. It sometimes retracts merely with the act of swallowing. Contrary to the name jaw-winking, the patient shows the opposite of winking; that is, raising of the lid. The retraction is especially striking when, and may be present only when, the patient is looking down at the time the mouth is opened. The lid then snaps open but remains elevated only momentarily even though the jaws are kept open. A similar elevation of the lid is produced by moving the lower jaw to the opposite side. Since in this movement and also in that of opening the jaws the external pterygoid is contracting, the phenomenon of jaw-winking is usually attributed to an anomalous connection between the nuclei of the external pterygoid muscle (innervated by the mesencephalic root of the 5th nerve) and of the levator muscle (innervated by the 3rd nerve). It is somewhat akin to the anomalous innervation of the extraocular muscles in the phenomenon of aberrant regeneration of the oculomotor nerve (see p. 71). It is unlike this phenomenon, however, in that the lid is not kept open, and for this reason the lid retraction may be thought to be due to spread of stimulus rather than to any anomalous connection between the nuclei. An alternative explanation based on antidromic impulses is suggested by the fact that sec-

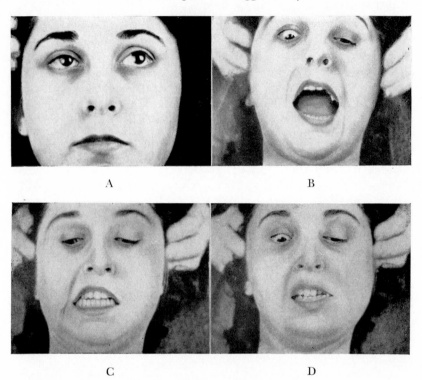

A   B

C   D

FIG. 63. *Marcus Gunn (jaw-winking) phenomenon*
In the primary position (A) there is a slight ptosis of the right eyelid. On opening the jaw (B) the right upper lid retracts markedly; this is especially striking if the patient is looking down at the same time. On moving the jaw (C) to the right, there is little retraction of the lid, but on moving it to the left (D), the lid snaps up.

tion of the motor division of the trigeminal nerve has abolished the reflex;[417] a somewhat similar reaction can be produced by sensitization of the levator muscle through denervation and subsequent stimulation of the first branch of the trigeminal nerve. Jaw-winking has therefore been likened to the Vulpian phenomenon, in which stimulation of the chorda tympani nerve causes contraction of the tongue muscle.[641]   -

The jaw-winking phenomenon has been produced by stimulat-

ing the cortex over a fairly wide area of the parietal lobe in a patient who had had the syndrome since infancy and who was being
operated upon for epilepsy.[504] This does not, however, indicate a
cerebral origin for the anomaly; it merely reiterates that stimulation of these areas associated with jaw movements result in simultaneous lid retraction.

A substantial proportion of patients with ptosis and jaw-
winking have also a congenital paralysis of the homolateral ele-
vating muscles. Nevertheless, opening the jaw has never been
known to result in elevation of the eye in these patients and one
must assume that there is no spread of the stimulus to the nuclei
of the superior rectus or inferior oblique such as there is to the
levator nucleus.

It may be noteworthy that a somewhat similar phenomenon
consisting of widening of the palpebral fissure of *both* eyes and
opening of the mouth occurs normally as a surprise reaction[1053]
and, indeed, ophthalmic surgeons have long employed the trick
of asking a patient to keep the mouth open to prevent any forced
closure of the lids following an intraocular operation.

Aside from the Marcus Gunn syndrome, disturbance of lid movements occurs with *aberrant regeneration* of 3rd nerve fibers into the
levator nerve, producing the syndrome of the pseudo-Graefe phenomenon (see p. 72 and Fig. 35), and anomalous regeneration of
the 7th nerve fibers following Bell's palsy, producing tics of lid
and mouth movements.[653]

With the pseudo-Graefe phenomenon the lid is usually ptotic
when the eyes are in the primary position, but any attempt to
look in the direction of the paralyzed extraocular muscle results
in a retraction of the upper lid. This is especially conspicuous
when the levator comes to be innervated by fibers originally connected with the inferior rectus or medial rectus. Then any attempt
to look down or inward results in impaired downward or inward
movement of the eye but, instead, elevation of the lid. The phenomenon is permanent.

An analogous condition occurs with anomalous regeneration
of the 7th nerve fibers following Bell's palsy. Fibers originally
connected with the orbicularis of the lids become connected with
the orbicularis about the mouth, and closure of the lids, even
momentarily as in the blink reflex, results in a momentary retrac-

tion of the mouth (a tic).[498] Conversely, but less conspicuously, innervation for retraction of the sides of the mouth, as in the act of smiling, may result in partial closure of the homolateral eye. A particularly curious anomaly occurs when the fibers of the 7th nerve originally connected with the facial muscles regenerate along those pathways originally connected with the lacrimal gland. There will then result anomalous tearing ("crocodile tears") with any attempted innervation of the facial muscles, as in the act of eating. A disturbing abnormality also occurs at times when the portions of the 7th nerve, originally innervating the orbicularis oculi, grow into the sheaths connected with the muscles of the inner ear; then any blink of the lids causes a subjectively audible "click" while maintained closure of the eyes results in a disquieting hum.

Maintained retraction of the upper lid and infrequency of blinking occur with several systemic diseases, especially with thyrotoxicosis, paralysis agitans and myotonia. Whatever the cause of these may be, it is apparently not sympathetic stimulation, since there is no associated mydriasis. A retraction of the upper lid occurs frequently in patients with weakness of upward gaze from whatever cause (for example, severe dysthyroid exophthalmos, tectal lesions, etc.). This type of retraction differs from that often seen in patients

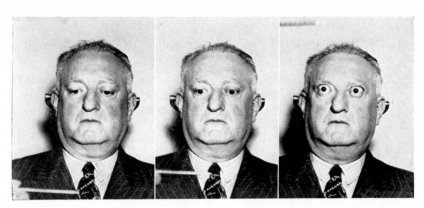

Fig. 64. *Retraction of the upper lids due to weakness of upward gaze*
The patient developed an exophthalmos and associated weakness of ocular movements, especially for upward gaze, following a thyroidectomy. Unlike the usual manifestation with hyperthyroidism, the lid retraction is present here only on attempting to look upward and disappears on downward gaze.

with typical hyperthyroidism in that there is no lid lag in the former on looking down and the retraction disappears on downward gaze (Fig. 64).

Fasciculations of the orbicularis oculi are a common experience related to the vague entity of nervous tension. Ordinarily they have no other neurologic significance, but they occasionally occur with trigeminal neuralgia.[212] Their pathogenesis is obscure but they are believed to be of peripheral origin. They are worsened by neostigmine and relieved by quinine.[400]

Spastic closure of the lids (blepharospasm) occurs frequently with intermittent spasm of the rest of the facial muscles in an entity of obscure but probably functional origin. As with spasm of the near reflex, it is precipitated by attention directed to the eyes; it is usually evoked by shining a light into the eyes or by manipulation of the lids.

SUMMARY

The lids are motivated by the levator muscle, which opens the palpebral fissure, and the orbicularis oculi, which closes it. The levator is innervated by the 3rd nerve and by sympathetic fibers; the orbicularis is innervated by the 7th nerve. The cerebral centers for lid movements are associated with the centers for conjugate movements of the eyes. Subcortical centers for lid movements have not been identified, but there are at least two afferent arcs, the trigeminal nerve and the optic nerve, that relay impulses for lid closing without traversing the cerebrum.

The clinical disturbances of lid movements from *cerebral* lesions are usually masked by the ocular motor disturbances. The disturbances from *subcortical* and *peripheral* lesions result in part from anomalous connections of the nuclei with muscles; for example, raising of the lid with opening of the jaw (Marcus Gunn phenomenon) or raising of the lid on attempting to look down or to the opposite side (aberrant regeneration of the 3rd nerve). Ptosis is an especially conspicuous feature of some of the myopathies (myasthenia gravis and abiotrophic ophthalmoplegia). Anomalous lid movements and lid-induced movements occur also with aberrant regeneration of the 7th nerve. This may result in tics of the mouth, anomalous tearing, and auditory phenomena.

Chapter VIII

SUPRANUCLEAR CONNECTIONS OF THE OCULAR MOTOR SYSTEM

CEREBELLUM

WITH THE FIRST edition of this text it was necessary to say that the paucity of information on functional localization in the cerebellum precluded adequate correlation of clinical findings with anatomic structures. It was further stated that the evidence did not reveal whether the cerebellum acted in unison as an entire organ, as assumed by Luciani[666] and Sherrington,[943] or showed discrete representation of function as assumed by others on the basis of comparative anatomy,[144] isolated lesions,[876] and stimulation experiments.[754] Experimental approach to the cerebellum has always been difficult in comparison with that to the cerebrum insofar as physiologic control of circulation could not be as readily maintained, anesthetic agents had less consistent effects,[966] and less of the cerebellar cortex was accessible for study than in the case of the cerebrum.[438]

Significant advances have recently been made, however, by the use of modern neurophysiologic means so that it is now possible to state categorically that the cerebellum has a somatotopic organization quite as orderly as that for other portions of the nervous system.[438] Action currents have been tapped off the cerebellum during stimulation of peripheral end organs[967] and during minimal stimulation of various sensory areas in the cerebrum.[10, 438] The resultant map represents sensory localization within the cerebellum. Similarly a plot of action currents resulting from stimulation of the motor areas of the cerebrum or of combined focal ablations in the cerebrum and cerebellum[285, 969] represents the motor map of cerebellar localization. Since, however, the motor activity of the cerebellum is largely inhibitory, an equally profitable approach has been the focal inhibition of spasticity (either acutely induced by cerebral stimulation[775] or chronically induced by decerebra-

149

tion[436, 437]) through stimulation of specific areas in the cerebellum. There is now general agreement on the localization of function within the cerebellum and much of the conclusions in the subsequent sections are based on these studies.

A. ANATOMY

The cerebellum is customarily divided for discussion into the median and paramedian lobes, collectively called the *vermis,* and the paired *lateral lobes.*[379] The vermis, comprising for the most part the older portion of the cerebellum, contains most of the paleocerebellum, while the lateral lobes are composed chiefly of neocerebellum. Since the cerebellum arose as an outpouching of the vestibular nuclei[614, 253] and since the two are connected by an abundance of fibers,[857] it is not surprising that the vermis or the portion of it that is the paleocerebellum has functions primarily associated with *equilibration and posture,* whereas the lateral lobes serve *motor coordination.* Accordingly, lesions of the vermis, especially of the posterior central lobules (the nodulus and the associated flocculus), produce profound disequilibrium and ataxia, while lesions of the lateral hemisphere produce hypotonia and asynergia.

The anatomic and physiologic data pertaining to the cerebellar representation of *ocular* function may be similarly divided into a consideration of the midline structures and of the lateral lobe structures. The clinical aspects do not lend themselves readily to such a separation, since clinical lesions of the cerebellum do not ordinarily limit themselves to one anatomic division.

> The cerebellum is connected with the brain stem through three major peduncles called by names that have more historical than anatomic significance. The anterior peduncle, called the brachium conjunctivum, is largely an efferent tract extending from each lateral lobe to the opposite red nucleus in the midbrain (and to the opposite thalamus); the middle peduncle, called the brachium pontis, transmits fibers from the gray matter of the mid-pons to all parts of the cerebellar cortex (with the possible exception of the flocculo-nodular lobes); the posterior peduncle, called the restiform body, transmits fibers from the spinal cord and more especially from the vestibular nuclei to the vermis.

1. Midline Structures

These include the wormlike central lobe called the vermis and a number of medially placed intracerebellar and roof nuclei called the globosus, emboliform, and fastigial nuclei. The vermis is subdivided into a number of lobules that on sagittal section are seen to form an arbor vitae resting on the roof of the 4th ventricle (Fig. 65). In the anteroposterior direction these radiating lobules are

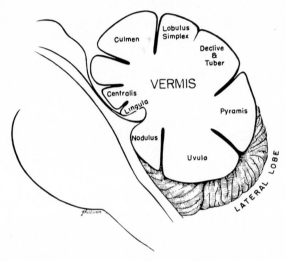

FIG. 65. *Diagram of midline cerebellar structures*

called the lingula, central lobule, culmen, declive, folium, tuber, pyramis, uvula, and nodule. Associated with the vermis but not in the midline are the paired flocculus and paraflocculus. Removal of the antero-dorsal portions of the cerebellum results in a predominately truncal ataxia (inability to sit up or to walk) whereas removal of the postero-ventral portions results in disturbances of equilibrium.[193]

It is noteworthy that the most anterior and posterior lobules are not far from the centers in the floor of the 4th ventricle that are known to be associated with eye movements.

These lobules have been shown to have a dual or mirror-like representation. The greater development of the dorsal lobules (lobulus simplex, declive and tuber) in the human species parallels the increased importance of cephalic and ocular functions in man. The cortex of these lobules projects to the fastigial nuclei which in turn project to the vestibular and ocular motor nuclei in the pons.[993, 754, 379, 381, 853] Excitation of the nucleus fastigius results in deviation of the eyes to the homolateral side and lesions of it result in weakness of gaze to that side with consequent nystagmus.[253] If there is a change from a suppressive to an irritative lesion, the nystagmus is said to show a corresponding reversal in its direction.[923]

Further, there is evidence that a change in frequency of the stimulus, or of intensity, will change the effect from one of inhibition to one of facilitation;[775] and that facilitation and inhibition are represented separately in the cerebellum.[380]

Lateral movements of the eyes have resulted from stimulation of points scattered widely over the vermial cortex[754] but especially from stimulation of the lobulus simplex, declive and tuber.[436] These movements are then associated with movements of the head.

Vertical movements of the eyes have been reported on occasion with stimulation of, or lesions of, the anterior portions of the vermis,[982] middle portion of the vermis,[330, 982] and roof nuclei,[439, 982] and with stimulation of the pyramis,[284] but the results are to be interpreted cautiously, since it is not always apparent that adequate precautions have been taken against spread of the stimulus to the underlying ocular motor centers in the floor of the 4th ventricle.[495, 209, 483, 284] Experimental lesions of the roof nuclei have resulted in conjugate deviations of the eyes upward and falling of the body backward.[751] Torsion of the eyes has been reported with stimulation of the flocculus,[41] but this was not confirmed.[754, 284]

> The most exhaustive study of representation of eye movements in and about the vermis is that of Hoshino,[497] who, by means of stimulation and ablation experiments in the rabbit, found a reactive zone located in the lobus simplex and adjacent cortex of the vermis up to the medial border of the paramedial lobe. Destruction of this region produced several jerks toward the homolateral side, just as did mechanical or electrical stimulation. Reducing the activity of this zone by the local application of cold resulted in a deviation of the eyes to the opposite side. If the lesion was carried forward to the roof of the 4th ventricle, a temporary skew deviation developed. Removal of the vermis

altered the vestibular nystagmus (decreasing the amplitude and increasing the frequency), whence the author concluded that the vermis was essential for the normal mediation of vestibular nystagmus. Previous experiments had shown, however, that although removal of the vermis temporarily lowered the threshold for vestibular nystagmus,[74] the nystagmus could, nevertheless, be elicited after removal of the entire cerebellum.[567] Removal of the vermis and roof nuclei lowered the threshold for the development of nystagmus on rotation of the head.[875]

2. Lateral Lobe Structures

These include the large lateral hemispheres and the intracerebellar dentate nuclei, to which the cortex of the lateral lobe projects and which in turn are connected with the brain stem via the brachium pontis and brachium conjunctivum.

Although the threshold for eliciting an ocular reaction is lower toward the midline, it is nevertheless high relative to motor thresholds elsewhere in the central nervous system. This, together with the fact that direct stimulation of the dentate nucleus causes deviation of the eyes to the homolateral side, has naturally led to the general belief that the eye movements from cerebellar stimulation are actually due to spread of the stimulus to the intracerebellar nuclei.[332, 495, 209, 483] That there is such a spread seems all the more likely since the ocular reaction occurs with stimulation through the dura mater as well as after removal of it.[284] The spread of the stimulus may account for the discrepancy in the results from experimental stimulation. Similarly, the occasional occurrence of nystagmus after experimental lesions of the cerebellum is accounted for by damage to the intracerebellar nuclei and their paths, rather than to damage of the cerebellar cortex itself.[55]

Removal of large portions of the lateral hemispheres produces homolateral hypotonia, weakness, and dysmetria of the skeletal muscles, but in most animals nystagmus is not elicited.[74, 891, 679, 567, 293] Even in monkeys and chimpanzees nystagmus does not occur if the lesions are limited to the cortex of the lateral lobes.[381] Yet in man nystagmus is often found with lesions of the lateral hemispheres.

The impression one obtains from clinical studies is that the lateral lobes of the cerebellum are essential in man for maintenance of excentric conjugate gaze toward the homolateral side and for precise fixation whereas the vermis is essential for the maintenance of vertical gaze. In the presence of unilateral cerebellar lesions, there is an inability to maintain conjugate gaze to the side of the lesion, and the eyes drift back toward the midline. This is corrected by quick, quasi-voluntary movements of the eyes back to the point of fixation. The slow drifting away from the side of the lesion and the quick corrective movement back make up the cycle of jerk nystagmus (see p. 184). Nevertheless it must be conceded that topical representation in the lateral lobes has not been as precisely demonstrated as in the mid-line structures.

B. CLINICAL CONSIDERATIONS

The major ocular motor signs of cerebellar disease in man are nystagmus, skew deviation, dysmetria, and flutter-like oscillations of the eyes. Because of the usual diffuseness of the lesions by the time they are seen pathologically and because of the difficulties in obtaining substantial series of cases for post-mortem examination, there has been little or no attempt to correlate these signs and symptoms with topical localization. Yet this is of the utmost importance and depends entirely on clinicians since the foregoing observations on somatotopic representation was necessarily determined in animals and can only be inferred for human beings.

Nystagmus is a frequent finding with cerebellar disease of man (see p. 214) although infrequent with experimental lesions of animals. It is seen especially often in acute cerebellar disease, but it is common in chronic cerebellar disease as well. It is usually horizontal, although vertical and rarely rotary nystagmus do occur. The horizontal nystagmus has a fast component toward the side of the lesion, and the oscillations are always greatest when the eyes are deviated toward the side of the lesion.[995] The oscillations are said to be enhanced by attempted fixation of the eyes on an object[1117, 489] and have been likened to ataxia of other muscles.[812, 511] The vertical nystagmus is usually greatest when the gaze is directed upward. Associated with the nystagmus there is frequently a jerky rhythm of the eye movements[246] and a gross paresis of conjugate gaze to the side of the lesion,[489, 995.185] so that the head may be habitually turned, as in pontine lesions, to permit the eyes to be deviated in a position of rest 10 to 20 degrees to the side opposite the lesion[489] (Fig. 66). It is reasonable to assume that the nystagmus is a manifestation of a weakness of conjugate gaze, or more strictly, an inability to maintain conjugate gaze to the side of the lesion. The underlying disturbance in conjugate gaze is evident in narcosis or unconsciousness; then the nystagmus is absent and the eyes are deviated continuously to one side. Occasionally there is complete paralysis of conjugate lateral movements of the eyes with cerebellar disease.[185] The rare condition of paralysis of downward gaze[212] and spasms of upward gaze (oculogyral crises)[698] may also occur with cerebellar disease. Perhaps related to the foregoing paresis of conjugate gaze is the fact that some patients with cerebellar disease are unable to hold fixation of the eyes during active and passive turning of the head.[408] So-called divergence paralysis has

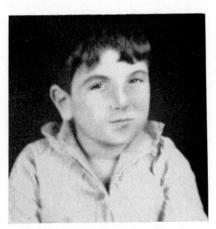

Fig. 66. *Head turning with left cerebellar tumor*

The patient had a weakness of conjugate gaze to the left with consequent coarse nystagmus to the left and compensatory turning of the head to the left. An astrocytoma was found in the left cerebellar hemisphere.

also been occasionally reported with cerebellar disease.[881, 652]

Nystagmus is especially evident in neocerebellar disease and is then associated with homolateral weakness and hypotonia of the rest of the body musculature. The severity of the nystagmus depends on the amount of involvement of the cerebellar nuclei. Nystagmus is less conspicuous with lesions of the vermis. When present the nystagmus is usually vertical and, vice versa, vertical nystagmus from cerebellar disease is usually due to lesions of the vermis.

The nystagmus of cerebellar disease (and vestibular disease) is said to vary characteristically with posture.[811, 777, 937, 714, 898, 368, 649] The nystagmus is reported to be greatest when the patient is lying on his side with the lesion in a dependent position. Standing up may abolish the nystagmus entirely, or conversely the nystagmus may be greatest while the patient is erect. The variation in nystagmus with posture is generally attributed to variation in vestibular tone with different positions of the head[780] or to a varying pressure exerted on the vestibular nuclei. But postural nystagmus has been reported after clearcut removal of the cerebellar hemispheres[957] and also in cases in which the lesion was entirely limited to the vermis with allegedly no pressure on the vestibular nuclei.[982] In the latter case, however, the nystagmus is transient and presumably due to an increased excitability of the vestibular reaction. The positional nystagmus produced experimentally in animals by alcohol poisoning[889] can be shown to depend on the labyrinthine end organ and not on the vestibular nuclei.[569]

A type of nystagmus called *periodic alternating nystagmus* has been described with cerebellar disease[556, 189, 412] but it must be rare. It is described as having cycles of a jerk type of nystagmus for several minutes in one direction and then of a jerk type in the other direction. On the other hand intermittent nystagmus is not uncommon with expansive lesions in the posterior fossa; its intermittent occurrence is presumably attributable to variable compression of the brain stem.

Skew deviation (see p. 134) occasionally occurs as a transient manifestation of acute cerebellar lesions in man. It was present in 5 of a series of 40 cases of gunshot wounds of the cerebellum.[489] It is especially frequent after operations on the cerebellum.[33] Persistent skew deviation has also been reported clinically with lesions of the vestibular nuclei,[643, 841] of the vestibular end organ (labyrinthitis),[69] of the vestibular nerve,[244, 69] and of the medial longitudinal fasciculi and, superior colliculi,[841, 808] (any of which may be secondarily affected with cerebellar disease). Rarely skew deviation with cerebellar disease may take the interesting form of an alternating hypertropia with a right hypertropia on gaze to one side and a left hypertropia on gaze to the opposite side.

Dysmetria of the eye movements[812, 218] and flutter-like oscillations[218] appear to be characteristic of lesions of the cerebellum or cerebellar pathways. Although ocular motor dysmetria may be detected by having the patient look alternately at eccentric points on either side, it is most easily demonstrated by having the subject look from an eccentric point back to the midline. This movement is normally executed with remarkable precision but in the presence of cerebellar disease there is a characteristic overshoot (occasionally an undershoot) with several pendular excursions of the eyes before final fixation is attained. It is obviously analogous to dys-metria of the limbs and, with the possible exception of laby-rinthine deficit, it does not oc-cur with neurologic disease other than that of the cerebel-lum. It may, however, be simu-lated in persons with central visual defects who may show several searching movements when asked to fix an object that is in a blind part of their field. Although the dysmetria may be, and often is, asymmetric on change of fixation from the two sides, this asymmetry has not, as yet, been shown to have lateralizing significance.

Flutter-like oscillations of the eyes is an entity related to dysmetria and equally charac-teristic of cerebellar disease. Instead of occurring only with changes of fixation, however, the flutter-like oscillations in-terrupt maintained fixation. They are characterized by 3-4 rapid pendular cycles with mo-mentary blurring of vision. Like dysmetria, with which it is often associated, it may occur with disease anywhere in the cerebel-lum or cerebellar peduncles but

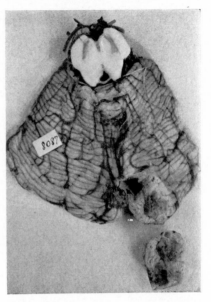

FIG. 67. *Angiomatous cyst (Lindau's disease) of the posteromedial tip of the right cerebellar hemisphere.*

The patient was forty-eight-year-old man, blind from bilateral angi-omatosis retinae. The outstanding ocular motor symptom was coarse nystagmus on looking to the right, that is to the side of the cerebellar lesion, and some vertical nystagmus on looking up. He also had right-sided ataxia, falling to the right, headache, nausea, and vomiting. The patient died postoperatively. Aside from the angiomatous cysts in the retina and cerebellum, there were multiple cysts in the pancreas and kidney.

has not, as yet, been shown to have any further topical significance. It is not to be confused with the continual oscillations of the eyes, called opsoclonus[812] occurring in patients with encephalitic coma.

The commonest lesions of the cerebellum are tumors and abscesses, although vascular lesions (thrombosis, Lindau's disease, etc.), primary degeneration and tuberculomas are not rare (Figs. 67 & 68). The cerebellum or cerebellar pathways are also involved with herniation of the intracranial contents through the foramen magnum in platybasia and the Arnold-Chiari malformation[220] (Figs. 69 & 70).

Two types of *tumors* are especially frequent.[261] They are the astrocytomas and the medulloblastomas. The astrocytomas are relatively slow growing, predisposed to cyst formation, and relatively favorable for surgical eradication. They occur oftenest in children. They produce nystagmus and pareses of conjugate gaze, along with adiadokocinesis and hypotonia of the skeletal muscles. The medulloblastomas are rapidly growing, usually arising in the posterior portions of vermis, and are unfavorable for complete surgical removal. They occur more frequently in males than in females and may be found in twins. They produce primarily disturbances of equilibrium but little if any nystagmus (flocculonodular syndrome).[381] The removal of a midline cerebellar tumor that requires manipulation of the floor of the 4th ventricle may lead to a catastrophic and permanent paralysis of conjugate lateral gaze and skew deviation. This is a prime neuro-ophthalmic complication of neurosurgery in this region.

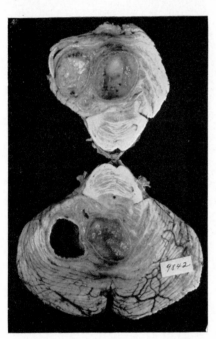

FIG. 68. *Multiple abscesses of the cerebellum*

Three cerebellar abscesses (one in the midline overlying the floor of the fourth ventricle and two in the left hemisphere) in a patient who had had a left mastoidectomy seven weeks previously. Examination shortly before death showed a paralysis of downward gaze, a vertical nystagmus on looking straight ahead or upward, and a horizontal nystagmus on looking to either side.

Cerebellar *abscesses* produce much the same symptoms as do tumors. They are, however, complicated by the fact that there may be a coincident labyrinthitis when, as is usually the case, the abscess comes from middle-ear disease. With labyrinthitis, however, the nystagmus is on the side opposite the lesion (in reference to

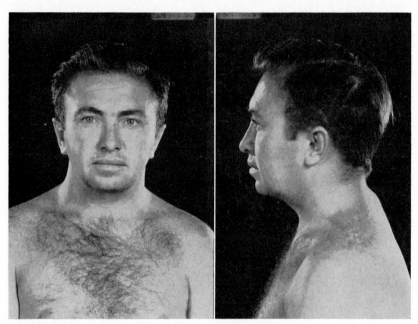

FIG. 69. *Front and side views of patient with platybasia showing the character-istic "bull neck"*
Noteworthy is the abnormally short distance between the occiput and the vertebra prominens (seventh cervical vertebra). The patient had developed, over several years, progressive incoordination, left sided weakness, horizontal nystagmus, ocular motor dysmetria, and illusory movement of the environ-ment. At one time he had been diagnosed as having multiple sclerosis. (Cogan and Barrows.[220])

the fast component) and is exaggerated when the eyes are turned conjugately to the opposite side. It is therefore important to note during the course of a middle-ear disease any *change of nystagmus* from the side opposite the lesion to the side of the lesion. Such a change is presumptive evidence of a cerebellar abscess.[764]

Along with the disturbance of eye movements, cerebellar disease usually produces other signs evident in the eyes. *Papilledema* is especially characteristic, and because the cerebellar lesion may be asymptomatic, it may go for a long time unnoticed. Thus, secondary optic atrophy from papilledema is relatively frequent with tumors of the cerebellum. The elevated intracranial pressure occa-

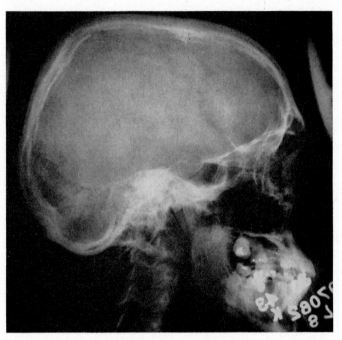

Fig. 70. *Lateral view of the skull of the foregoing patient, showing severe platybasia with invagination of the occipital bone into the posterior fossa*
     The first and practically the entire second cervical vertebra lay above a plane connecting the posterior edge of the foramen magnum with the hard palate. (Cogan and Barrows.[220])

sionally gives rise to *palsies of the 6th nerves. Absence of the corneal reflex* is frequently a feature, and this characteristically varies, as does the nystagmus, with posture.[811] But despite the proximity of the cerebellum to the occipital lobes, hemianopsia from the pressure on the occipital lobes never occurs with cerebellar lesions.

SUMMARY

Recent studies have indicated a well developed somatotopic localization within the cerebellum. The head region (including the eyes) is represented particularly in the dorsal portions of the midline structures (lobulus simplex, declive and tuber). The prime functions of these regions appears to be inhibitory although there is also substantial evidence for facilitatory activity as well. The midline structures (vermis) are concerned primarily with equilibration whereas the lateral structures (lateral lobes) are concerned with motor coordination.

Experimentally, lesions of the cerebellum produce remarkably little ocular motor disturbance. Clinically the signs are variable but often marked. They consist chiefly of nystagmus, palsies of conjugate gaze, skew deviation, dysmetria and flutter. The nystagmus is of the jerk type with fast component in the direction of gaze; vertical nystagmus is especially significant. Variations of the nystagmus with posture is said to be frequent. The palsies of horizontal conjugate gaze (and compensatory head turning) are probably due to secondary pressure effects on the brain stem. The skew deviation may be constant or variable for all directions of gaze. Ocular dysmetria is an overshoot (occasionally an undershoot) of the eyes on changes of fixation, and flutter movements are brief pendular oscillations of the eyes occurring during maintained fixation. Both are highly characteristic of lesions of the cerebellum or cerebellar pathways.

Chapter IX

PUPIL

THE PUPIL is the diaphragm of the eye through which all image forming rays of light gain entrance and out of which relatively little light is re-emitted (whence its apparent blackness). Adapted to serve a variety of purposes, it is especially controlled by the level of illumination, by the sense of nearness, and by the dual influence of the autonomic nervous system. While most will not agree with the determination of personality types on the basis of pupillary size and reactions, as proposed once upon a time, and certainly not with the pseudo-science of iridopathy, nevertheless the pupil may be used as a reliable indicator of retinal photoreceptive processes and of sympathetic-parasympathetic interplay when extraneous factors are sufficiently controlled and the methods of testing are sufficiently quantitative.

For measuring the size of the pupil, pupillometers have been constructed of varied, and often ingenious, design. The simplest and perhaps most useful for the clinician are the diagrams having a series of solid circles of graded sizes which can be compared with the pupils of the patient.[48] For precise studies, especially in research, more quantitative methods are necessary. Simple flash photographs have been widely used but this method is time-consuming, expensive, and gives static pictures only. Cinematography which gives a more dynamic picture has been widely used in the laboratory and in certain clinics.[663, 150, 1089, 1034] The subsequent plot of the pupillary size, recorded as a function of time, is called the pupillograph. To eliminate the effect of light it is necessary to use infra-red illumination and infra-red sensitive film. Other methods employed for specific purposes include the registration of visible or infra-red radiation reflected from the iris surface (an inverse function of pupillary size [709, 1031, 258, 259]), the projection of an infra-red image of the pupil on a fluorescent screen,[589] the doubling of the pupil image by birefringent crystals[1090] or by a split ocular,[230] the measurement of light emitted through the pupil from a source of illumination placed behind or within the eye[689, 200] and, finally, various means dependent on the entoptic visualization of the pupil.[161, 215, 282]

The pupil is operated by the reciprocal action of the sphincter muscle which tends to make the pupil smaller (*miosis*) and the dilator which tends to make it larger (*mydriasis*). The sphincter is a substantial bundle of smooth muscle fibers situated within the iris stroma near, but not at, the pupillary margin. The dilator is made up of unique muscle cells coexistent with, and just anterior to, the pigment epithelium. The sphincter muscle is innervated by the parasympathetic nerves and the dilator by the sympathetic. Those drugs which excite the parasympathetic end-organs (acetylcholine, pilocarpine, mecholyl) or facilitate their spontaneous activity (physostigmine, neostigmine, diisopropyl fluorophosphate, or tetra-ethylfluorophosphate) will constrict the pupil and are, therefore, called miotics while those drugs which excite the sympathetic end organs (epinephrine, benzidrine, ephedrine) or facilitate their spontaneous activity (cocaine) will dilate the pupil and are therefore called mydiatrics. Further, those drugs which paralyze the parasympathetic end organs (atropine, scopolamine, tetra-ethyl ammonium chloride[29, 492]) will be mydriatics while those which paralyze the sympathetic end organs will be miotics (but none of the latter are in common usage).

Nowhere in the body is the mutual antagonism within the autonomic system more perfectly exemplified than in the pupil, and the same basic architecture which governs the autonomic innervation elsewhere applies to the pupil.

The *sympathetic* nervous system is composed of fibers emanating from the central nervous system with the spinal nerves of the thoraco-lumbar region. They then pass to the paravertebral chain of sympathetic ganglia where the fibers undergo synapsis (one synapsis per nerve fiber) before being distributed to the organs of sympathetic innervation. The *parasympathetic* system takes root from the central nervous system in the craniocaudal region but has ganglia nearer to the organ of supply than is the case with the sympathetic system. In both, the sympathetic and parasympathetic systems, the preganglionic fibers are myelinated and the post ganglionic fibers are usually non-myelinated. In both cases there is also a transformer-like step-up in which several post ganglionic fibers are present for each preganglionic fiber.

From a functional point of view the sympathetic system fortifies those activities which are aggressive or alarm reactions (excitement,

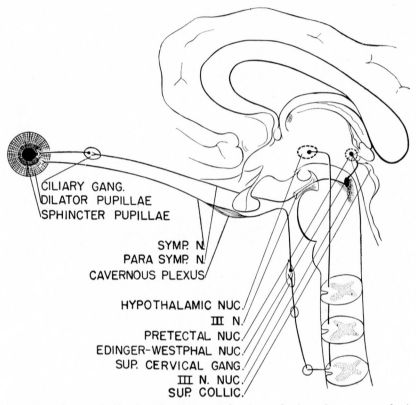

CILIARY GANG.
DILATOR PUPILLAE
SPHINCTER PUPILLAE

SYMP. N.
PARA SYMP. N.
CAVERNOUS PLEXUS

HYPOTHALAMIC NUC.
III N.
PRETECTAL NUC.
EDINGER-WESTPHAL NUC.
SUP. CERVICAL GANG.
III N. NUC.
SUP. COLLIC.

FIG. 71. *Diagram indicating the course of the sympathetic and parasympathetic nerves from the brain stem to the eye*

fear, rage) whereas the parasympathetic system is concerned with re-actions of conservation (homeostasis) designed to maintain the body's economy (nutrition, sleep).

Both systems have centers within and without the central nervous system (Fig. 71). In addition, there are supranuclear pupillary centers concerned with light, near focussing, etc. which are not strictly part of the autonomic system but which utilize the same final common pathway.

A. CENTERS AND TRACTS OUTSIDE THE CENTRAL NERVOUS SYSTEM

1. Miosis

The ciliary ganglion is the *parasympathetic* relay outside the central nervous system for impulses to the sphincter muscle in response to light and parasympathetic tone. The impulses to the sphincter in response to *near focusing* may be relayed partially *outside* the ciliary ganglion, since miosis occurs with accommodation even after removal of the ciliary ganglion.[349] The ciliary ganglion is situated just lateral to the optic nerve in the midorbit. It receives pre-ganglionic parasympathetic nerves via the 3rd nerve, specifically by way of the branch of it that goes to the inferior oblique muscle. Aside from the parasympathetic nerve cells, the ciliary ganglion contains sensory cells and sympathetic fibers but no sympathetic cells. The post-ganglionic parasympathetic fibers leave the ciliary ganglion by some twenty roots, which enter the eye cone-fashion about the optic nerve (ciliary nerves) and run forward in the suprachoroidea to the ciliary body and iris. Unlike post-ganglionic fibers elsewhere, those from the ciliary ganglion are for the most part myelinated, like the pre-ganglionic fibers.

While the effect of stimulating the 3rd nerve is predominantly excitatory and causes a contraction of the sphincter iridis, there is also a weaker inhibitory effect from 3rd nerve stimulation tending to relax the sphincter muscle. The inhibitory effect can be observed only after paralyzing, as by atropine, the excitatory component.[604]

2. Mydriasis

The superior cervical ganglion is the *sympathetic* relay outside the central nervous system for impulses to the dilator muscle. It is situated in the neck adjacent to the carotid artery and at the top of the thoracolumbar chain of sympathetic ganglia. It is the synaptic relay for all sympathetic impulses *to the eye* and, moreover, it is made up for the most part of cells that are exclusively concerned with the eye. It receives pre-ganglionic fibers that have emerged from the central nervous system in the lowermost cervical segment and the first two thoracic segments.[813, 862] The fibers that carry ocular impulses traverse the inferior and middle cervical ganglia without undergoing any synapsis until they reach the superior cervical ganglia. Of the pre-ganglionic fibers going to the superior cervical ganglion, those that are destined to innervate the *pupil* are the largest and accordingly have the lowest threshold.[135]

The post-ganglionic fibers of the superior cervical ganglia are, like most post-ganglionic fibers elsewhere, unmyelinated and therefore do not form discrete nerves. Instead, the fibers are affixed to other structures, especially to the carotid artery, extending cranially. On reaching the base of the skull the sympathetic fibers intertwine to form the carotid and cavernous plexuses and thence are distributed along the ocular motor and trigeminal nerves, as well as other structures, to enter the orbit. Some may pass through the middle ear.[939] Perhaps the greatest number enter with the nasociliary branch of the first division of the trigeminal nerve.

Stimulation of the superior cervical ganglion produces homolateral mydriasis, exophthalmos (in animals), relative hypermetropia,[190, 211, 739, 806, 731] retraction of the upper lid, and contraction of the blood vessels. Since the fibers destined for the pupil have the lowest threshold, it is possible with minimal stimulation of the superior cervical ganglion to produce pupillary dilatation only. The sympathetic fibers that cause flattening of the lens and consequent hypermetropia are said to course with those that produce dilatation of the pupil.[731] The exophthalmos on sympathetic stimulation that is a conspicuous feature in animals does not occur in human beings.[1128, 1078, 369]

B. CENTERS AND TRACTS WITHIN THE BRAIN STEM

1. Miosis

There are apparently subcortical centers for miosis in the pretectal region of the hypothalamus and in the nuclear complex of the 3rd nerve (Fig. 72). The center in the pretectal region has been investigated by electric excitation[506, 856, 685, 683, 203, 464, 1010, 106, 922] and by ablation experiment.[1010] The formerly held concept[732, 540] that afferent pupillary pathways traverse the superior colliculi or form a synapse there is apparently erroneous, for no fibers can be traced from the maculas (which are especially rich in pupillary receptors) to the superior colliculi[163]; furthermore, the superior colliculi may be extensively damaged or removed without significantly affecting the pupillomotor response to light,[334, 631, 113, 978, 547, 682] and excitations confined to the superior colliculi do not produce miosis.[203] That a synapse does occur, however, in the *pretectal zone* is shown by successive stimulation along the pathways from the retina when, after section of the optic nerve or tract, sufficient time has been allowed

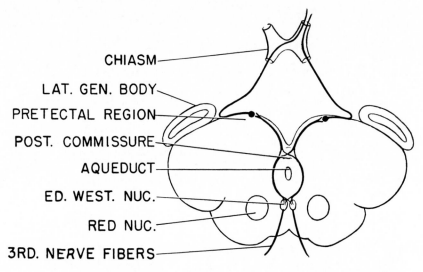

CHIASM

LAT. GEN. BODY

PRETECTAL REGION

POST. COMMISSURE

AQUEDUCT

ED. WEST. NUC.

RED NUC.

3RD. NERVE FIBERS

Fig. 72. *Course of the afferent pupillary fibers from the chiasm to the Edinger-Westphal portion of the third nerve nuclei (modified from Magoun and Ranson)*

for the degeneration of the nerve fibers.[440] It is then found that miosis occurs only when the pretectal zone is reached. Also, after the optic nerve has been cut degenerating fibers can be traced to the pretectum[616, 53] but not to the 3rd nerve complex.[273, 27, 186, 540]

It thus seems likely that that group of small cells situated at the dorsal surface of the tectothalamic junction immediately under cover of the anterior and lateral margin of the superior colliculi, long known to comparative anatomists as the pretectal nuclei, are, in fact, centers for the transmission of afferent pupillary impulses from the retina to the ocular motor nuclei.

The tracts from the pretectal center to the ocular motor centers are presumed to course ventrocaudally about the aqueduct to the

3rd nerve nuclei. Some of the fibers decussate in the posterior commissure, since stimulation of the posterior commissure results in a bilateral miosis, but not all of them decussate here, for section of the posterior commissure results merely in an enfeebling of the light reaction without its abolition.[855, 683, 1010] Nor does cocainization or refrigeration of the posterior commissure abolish the light reaction.[203] Stimulation of the fibers coursing ventrally about the aqueduct results in a miosis that is greatest on the homolateral side.[855, 107]

The portion of the 3rd nerve believed to be concerned with miosis is the *Edinger-Westphal nucleus,* which has been described previously (see p. 167). The pretectal and other centers for miosis are believed to project to this nucleus.

2. Mydriasis

There is evidence of subcortical centers and tracts for mydriasis in the posterior hypothalamus, inferior colliculi, pons, tegmentum, and cervical cord (Fig. 71).

The sympathetic centers and tracts in the *hypothalamus* extend over a considerable area.[537, 950, 505, 948, 856, 464, 473, 922] The hypothalamic centers are made up of neuronal relays and not merely a conjugation of tracts from the cerebrum, since the effects of stimulation in this area may be elicited long after decerebration and consequent degeneration of the centripetal tracts from the cerebrum.[538] Stimulation of one half of the hypothalamus produces predominantly homolateral mydriasis,[950, 76, 464] and its removal produces a homolateral Horner's syndrome.[640, 315] The mydriasis from hypothalamic stimulation is characteristically accompanied by such other sympathomimetic reactions as elevation of the lid, rise of blood pressure, and various manifestations of the fright reaction.[464] From the hypothalamus the fibers run posteriorly in the tegmentum of the midbrain, the reticular substance of the pons and medulla, and probably the medial longitudinal fasciculus,[505] to the cervical cord. In the cervical cord the fibers course in the anterolateral column,[347,348] always on the homolateral side,[500] to the point of emergence in the lower cervical segments. The mydriasis produced by stimulation of the hypothalamus does not occur if the cervical sympathetic is first sectioned,[75] but section of the 3rd nerve has no effect, indicating that the hypothalamic center for mydriasis mediates most of its effect through the sympathetic chain[537, 540] and not by inhibition of the parasympathetic center.

Stimulation of the *superior colliculi* has been reported to produce pupillary dilatation[574, 537, 538, 539, 856] but it does so only when the electrode crosses the tectum and reaches the dorsal limits of the tegmentum or central gray matter. Hence, it is believed that the stimulation is due to spread of the stimulus to tracts in the brain stem rather than to excitation of the superior colliculi.[203] Stimulation of the *inferior colliculi* does cause pupillary dilatation, however, and since these bodies are concerned with acoustic relays, it is assumed that they mediate the impulses for mydriasis in response to sounds.[203] The mydriasis produced by stimulation of the inferior colliculi is bilateral and is probably brought about through inhibition of the sphincter nucleus, since removal of the cervical sympathetic chain does not affect it. It is abolished by cocainization or refrigeration of the inferior colliculi.[203]

Pupillodilator fibers that produce their effect by inhibition of the pupilloconstrictor centers in the midbrain also come from the *spinal cord*.[444] The pathways for these impulses traverse the reticular substance and dorsal tegmentum in the pons and occupy the paramedian position in the midbrain.

C. CENTERS AND TRACTS WITHIN THE CEREBRUM

1. Miosis

Miosis from cerebral stimulation, unlike mydriasis, occurs only when certain localized areas of the cortex in the vicinity of the centers for movements of the eyes are stimulated.[977] Miosis occurs with stimulation of the optomotor field of the frontal lobe[985, 440] and of the occipital lobe.[1081, 53, 440, 52, 1070] The miosis is bilateral although not necessarily symmetrical.[203]

The pathways for pupilloconstriction from the *frontal* ocular motor zone extend directly to the pons or midbrain without undergoing synapses in the basal nuclei.[985] The pathways for pupilloconstriction from the occipital area, at least for the cat in which it has been most thoroughly investigated, form a small fascicle in the lateral wall of the lateral ventricle. The pupillary fibers then course over the geniculate body and are scattered through the stratum zonale of the thalamus; thence they course to the pretectal area, chiefly of the opposite side, where they undergo synapsis.[53, 52] Removal of the pupilloconstrictor zone in one occiput of the cat results in anisocoria, with the larger pupil on the opposite side.[169, 1070]

2. Mydriasis

Bilateral mydriasis occurs with stimulation over a wide area of the cerebral cortex,[539, 540] but it has been especially noted with stimulation of the prefrontal area,[332, 83, 496, 85, 816, 644, 203, 473, 1082] the somesthetic area,[950] and the auditory cortex.[1012] Stimulation of the occipital cortex has given rise to contradictory results,[1081] but stimulation of the intraparietal sulcus causes a dilatation of the pupil.[1064] It is not known whether the cells concerned with pupillodilatation are represented diffusely over the entire cortex or are separated in discrete layers of the cortex.

The pathways by which pupillodilator impulses reach the midbrain from the cortex are not known. They presumably pass through the inferomedial part of the internal capsule, since stimulation in this region (in the cat) results in a bilateral mydriasis.[203] The corticofugal impulses resulting from stimulation of the frontal eye centers apparently excite the sympathetic centers in the brain stem since the resultant mydriasis is abolished by prior sympathectomy.[1087, 1082] The mydriasis from loud noises[516] and emotional stimuli[665] is also largely abolished by prior sympathectomy. Somewhat confusing, therefore, is the fact that the psychosensory mydriasis (resulting from pain) which had been thought to be mediated through the frontal area acts by inhibition of the parasympathetic centers in the brain stem; it is unaffected by prior sympathectomy but prevented by prior section of the 3rd nerve.[1041, 1087, 604] This apparent contradiction may, of course, be due to a species variation. The few experiments on man suggest the psychosensory mydriasis is effected through direct sympathetic stimulation.

Removal of the cerebrum results in a miosis,[545] and removal of one hemisphere is reported to result in a temporary anisocoria, with the pupil on the same side smaller than that on the opposite side.[613] This miosis with decerebration has been compared with the miosis in sleep,[156] and conversely, the mydriasis with stimulation of the frontal area has been compared with that occurring in the normal response of awaking.[963]

As in the case of cerebellar inhibition of extraocular motor activity, there is some evidence for cerebellar inhibition of psychosensory mydriasis. Thus stimulation of one cerebellar hemisphere or of the lateral arm of the lobulus simplex will inhibit mydriasis that is mediated through the contralateral cerebral cortex.[438]

D. CLINICAL SIGNIFICANCE OF PUPILLARY REACTIONS

1. Normal Pupil

The diameter of the normal pupil varies from 2.5 to 7.0 mm., depending on a variety of factors, chief of which are age, refractive status, race, state of light adaptation, and intensity of light reaching the retina. Even the time of day is reported to affect significantly the size of the pupil.[282]

In the newborn the pupils are conspicuously miotic, but at three weeks of age or thereabouts the pupils begin to enlarge and attain a size of approximately one-half that of the cornea. This size is maintained during childhood and most of adulthood. In early senescence the pupils again become miotic.[611]

The pupils of the myopic eye are somewhat larger than those of the hypermetropic eye; those of the blonde eye are larger than those of the brunet eye.

Depending on the state of adaptation and amount of illumination, the pupils show at any one time expected changes in size. In the dark the pupils are dilated and the dark-adapted pupillomotor function shows the same increased sensitivity to light stimuli as does the visual function. In the light the situation is reversed. Furthermore, the pupillomotor sensitivity shows the same Purkinje shift (maximal sensitivity shift from 540 to 500 mu) as does the visual sensitivity in changing from the photopic to scotopic adaptation.[463, 662]

The two pupils are usually equal in size when the eyes are in the primary position, although variations of approximately 1 mm. may occur without pathologic significance. On conjugate deviation of the eyes to either extreme side, the pupil of the abducting eye is usually larger than that of the adducting eye (*Tournay's reaction*).

The pupillary reactions most commonly tested clinically are the direct light reaction, the consensual light reaction, the near reaction, and, less frequently, the reaction on forced closure of the lids. All normally elicit a miosis.

The *direct* light reaction consists of a miosis elicited in one eye by shining a light in that eye, whereas the *consensual* light reaction consists of a miosis resulting from a light shone in the opposite eye. Usually direct and consensual reactions are nearly equal, although the former may be more marked than the latter. The *near reaction* consists of a miosis accompanying a change in focus from a far to a relatively near object and is usually accompanied by convergence and accommodation. The *miosis on forced closure of the lids* (Westphal-Piltz phenomenon) is slight and not easily tested for, except in the presence of a 7th nerve palsy where the lids cannot be closed. This is a low-order reflex mediated through the tegmental fasciculus.[96] When it is present despite loss of other pupillary reactions, one may assume that the lesion is supranuclear and not peripheral.

2. Pupillary Disturbances Occurring with Correlative Visual Disturbances

The *amaurotic pupil* is a syndrome occurring in blind eyes and is characterized by absence of the direct light reaction with preservation of the consensual reaction (provided the other eye is not blind) and preservation of the near reaction. The consensual response in the other eye is, of course, also absent. The amaurotic pupil occurs in all cases where the blindness is due to lesions in the retina or optic nerve, but the pupillary reactions are frequently not affected as soon, or to as great a degree, in the early stages of the disease as are the visual functions.[708] On the other hand lesions within the optic foramen may affect the pupillary fibers more than the visual fibers; this may be due to the predominately nasal position of the pupillary fibers in the optic nerve.

When present to a partial degree only, the amaurotic reaction varies with the amount of blindness. Since the sensitivity for pupillomotor response is greatest in the central portions of the retina and drops precipitously in the extrafoveal region, the amaurotic reaction from local lesions in the retina or optic nerve corresponds roughly to the visual acuity.

The *hemianopic (Wernicke)*[1094] *pupillary reaction** is the abnormality found with lesions of the optic tract and is dependent on the fact that the optic fibers from homonymous halves of the two retinas are conjoined behind the chiasm (Figure 73). The hemianopic reaction is characterized by an absent or diminished pupillary reaction when the light stimulates the retina on one side of the globe, and a normal response on illumination of the opposite side. Various types of apparatus called hemikinesimeters, designed to illuminate only one half of the retina, have been employed for testing the reaction.[463, 91, 1063, 525, 152, 921, 153]

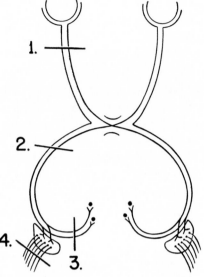

FIG. 73. *Lesions of the afferent pupillary pathway*

Lesions of one optic nerve (1) result in an absence of direct light reaction in that eye and of consensual response in the other eye along with blindness (amaurotic pupil). Lesions of one optic tract (2) result in a hemianopic pupillary response (Wernicke pupil) in both eyes with hemianopic visual field defects. Lesions of one of the brachia of the superior colliculi (3) result in hemianopic pupillary response without visual field defects. Conversely lesions of the visual radiations (4) result in hemianopic visual field defects without hemianopic pupillary disturbances.

In lieu of a hemikinesimeter, a difference in pupillary size may be noticed in patients with tract hemianopsia when the light source (for example, from a window) is alternately on the right and left side.[338, 257]

When the Wernicke reaction is present, the side of the eye that

---

*Actually Heddäeus[452] reported the hemianopic reaction three years prior to Wernicke's description.

on stimulation shows the less excitability corresponds to the side of the tract lesion. There is also usually present a *hemianopsia* of the same side. Indeed, the chief usefulness of the Wernicke reaction has been in the differentiation of tract hemianopsia, in which the reaction is positive, from cerebral hemianopsia in which the pupillary reactions have always been thought to be normal.[807] Recent, and still unconfirmed, evidence, however, has suggested that even in cerebral hemianopsia the pupillary reactions may be defective on stimulating the blind halves.[441, 442] Rarely the Wernicke reaction is present without hemianopsia.[87]

Associated with the Wernicke pupillary reaction and hemianopsia in tract lesions there is usually an *anisocoria,* the pupil on the side opposite the lesion being larger than that on the same side (Behr's sign).[88]

Temporary *anisocoria* and *diminished light reaction* may also be present with *cerebrovascular accidents,* with or without accompanying visual field defects. The anisocoria is more frequent with apoplexy than with cerebral softening. The pupil may be large either on the side opposite the lesion[20] or on the side of the lesion.[837] Anisocoria with these cerebrovascular accidents is said to have ominous portents.[837] Extradural and subdural hemorrhages also cause a homolateral dilatation of the pupil (vide infra).

3. Pupillary Disturbances Occurring Without Correlative Visual Disturbances

Variations in pupillary size and abnormalities in pupillary reactivity may occur from local changes in the iris and are without neurologic significance. Falling into this category is the miosis of old age, the distortion of the pupil with iris atrophy, and probably the relative areflexia of diabetes. This latter may produce a pupil that is indistinguishable from the Argyll-Robertson type.

Paralysis of the parasympathetic nerve supply results in a widely dilated pupil that is nonreactive to the stimuli of light or near focusing, although reactive to most miotic drugs. This paralytic mydriasis, as it may be called, occurs most frequently with 3rd nerve palsies, as the parasympathetic nerve supply accompanies the 3rd nerve fibers (Fig. 74). It may occur, however, *without involvement of the other 3rd nerve functions,* with lesions of the ciliary nerves, or rarely, with selective affections of the nuclei (as is presumed to be the case with diphtheria) or with an entity that is thought to be a ciliary ganglionitis.[272, 873] In this latter case the dilated pupil may be associated with a central scotoma due to a simultaneous retrobulbar neuritis.[873, 690] (For lesions giving rise to 3rd nerve palsies, see p. 63).

Selective dilatation of the pupil, presumably resulting from

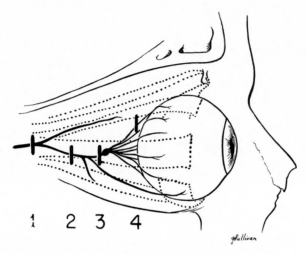

FIG. 74. *Course of the parasympathetic nerves from the apex of the orbit to the eye*

Entering with the third nerve a lesion at (1) would result in a complete third nerve paralysis; a lesion at (2) would result in paralysis of the sphincter iridis and of the inferior oblique and inferior rectus muscles; a lesion at (3) or of the ciliary ganglion would result in paralysis of the sphincter iridis but not of the extraocular muscles; and a lesion at (4), limited to a few of the ciliary nerves, would result in a segmental paralysis of the sphincter iridis and consequent pear-shaped pupil.

partial 3rd nerve involvement, occurs with subdural hematomas, with temporal lobe tumors, and with herniation of brain contents through the tentorium. In their course between the exit from the brain stem and entrance into the cavernous sinus the pupillary fibers are believed to be concentrated in the 3rd nerve close by the temporal lobe and the posterior cerebral and posterior communicating arteries.[1009, 1007, 1008] These fibers are especially vulnerable, therefore, with herniations of the brain stem through the tentorium or with pressure and traction on the 3rd nerve in this region. The same pathogenesis probably underlies the fixed dilated pupil which occurs at times with cerebral concussion.[867a] Mydriasis may be, and frequently is, the only sign with such lesions. Since the mydriasis is almost always on the side of a subdural hematoma, it may constitute a valuable sign to the neurosurgeon in an unconscious patient who otherwise has little neurologic deficit.[402, 749]

The surprising lack of mydriasis despite total paralysis of other functions of the 3rd nerve in lesions about the superior orbital

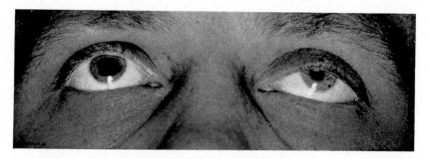

Fig. 75. *Congenital Horner's syndrome of the left eye*
Noteworthy are the ptosis, miosis, and lighter color of the iris on the affected side; actually the right eye is brown and the left eye blue (heterochromia iridis).

fissure and cavernous sinus has already been commented upon (p. 61). It is not always explicable on the basis of coexistent involvement of the sympathetic fibers since the pupillary size and reactions are often normal. It is perhaps attributable to some undetected anatomic feature of the pupillary fibers in the portion of the 3rd nerve within and anterior to the cavernous sinus. Occasionally the pupillary functions are relatively spared only during the early stages of a progressive lesion suggesting merely a delay in response rather than a quantitative difference. Whatever the true explanation, it is as though the pupillary fibers in the cavernous sinus, or in front of it, were less vulnerable while behind the cavernous sinus they were more vulnerable than the rest of the 3rd nerve functions.

Lesions of a *limited* number of the ciliary nerves result in ellipsoid or pear-shaped pupils with asymmetrical pupillary contraction. This is often seen after operative diathermy of the sclera

for separated retina and occasionally following trauma. It is sometimes interpreted as due to sympathetic stimulation.[31]

Paralysis of the sympathetic nerve supply results in a relatively
constricted pupil (paralytic miosis) and is accompanied by a
ptosis of the lid, an apparent enophthalmos, and frequently a dilatation of the vessels, with absence of sweating on the homolateral
side. The entity is known as *Horner's syndrome* (Fig. 75). Al-

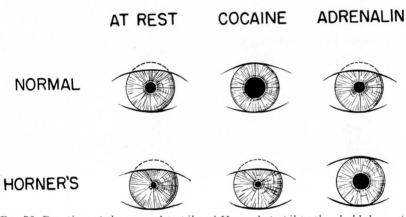

Fig. 76. *Reaction of the normal pupil and Horner's pupil to threshold doses of
cocaine and adrenalin*
    The normal pupil reacts more readily to cocaine but less readily to
adrenalin than does Horner's pupil.

though miotic, the pupil shows normal reactivity to light and near
fixation. While characterized by a *decreased* sensitivity to such
mydriatic drugs as atropine and cocaine, the Horner's pupil shows
hypersensitivity to adrenalin*[836] (Fig. 76).

    This altered reaction to adrenalin (or to its analogues[491]) is the
more marked the farther peripheral is the lesion causing the
sympathetic paralysis.[435, 343, 515, 1135, 517] Thus adrenalin (1 drop of
1:1000 solution instilled three times over several minutes) causes
a mydriasis and lid retraction on the affected side but not on the

---

    * This hypersensitivity of the pupil to adrenalin following sympathectomy is
an example of a general change in sensitivity following denervation[191] and is
called the paradoxical pupillary reaction; it is not to be confused with the inverse
pupillary reaction, referred to in some texts as paradoxical reaction, which consists of a slight dilatation of the pupil, instead of a constriction, on exposure to
light (see Argyll-Robertson pupil, p. 180).

normal side; but when the lesion causing the Horner's syndrome is within the central nervous system, the pupil shows little sensitization to adrenalin. Cocaine (1 drop of 4% solution instilled into the conjunctival sac three times over a period of several minutes) shows a reduced effect on the side of the Horner's syndrome whether the responsible lesion is peripheral or within the central nervous system.

> Since the relative size of the pupil is the most sensitive index of the sympathetic ocular effects, it is possible to have miosis as the *only* sign of a sympathetic lesion, but by the same token it is impossible to have other such signs as ptosis and enophthalmos on a sympathetic basis without involvement of the pupil as well.

Horner's syndrome may result from lesions of the sympathetic pathways *within* the central nervous system or of the pathways, especially in the neck, *outside* it. In either case, the syndrome is on the same side as the lesion. It is especially evident after section of the lower cervical and upper thoracic nerve roots[210] or removal of the superior cervical ganglion.[630] The commonest lesions *within* the central nervous system that produce Horner's syndrome are occlusion of the posterior cerebellar arteries[228, 829, 871, 721, 364, 2] (or of the lateral medullary branch), occlusion of the basilar artery,[597] multiple sclerosis,[363] syringomyelia involving the reticular substance of the pons, and tumor of the cervical cord. The many lesions *outside* the central nervous system that cause this syndrome include apical pulmonary disease, mediastinal tumor, aortic aneurisms, goiter, trauma (occasionally associated with lesions of the cervical plexus in Klumpke's paralysis), and cervical lymphadenopathy.[270]

There is some evidence, both experimental[1070] and clinical,[990, 992, 127] that Horner's syndrome may also occur with cerebral lesions. In this case the signs are on the side opposite the lesion. There is also some experimental evidence that a homolateral Horner's syndrome may be produced by thalamic lesions.[386]

With *congenital* Horner's syndrome there is frequently an accompanying heterochromia of the iris, presumably owing to failure of the pigment to develop in the absence of the sympathetic innervation (Fig. 75). Thus in a brunet the eye on the side of the lesion is blue whereas that on the normal side is brown. Congenital Horner's syndrome may be associated with other congenitally determined abnormalities, particularly facial hemiatrophy.

With *combined paralysis* of the sympathetic and parasympathetic nerve supply as occurs with lesions in the cavernous sinus or retro-orbital region, the pupil is fixed and semidilated.

Miosis with lesions of the pons is a constant finding and is characteristic of acute pontine lesions, both clinical and experi-

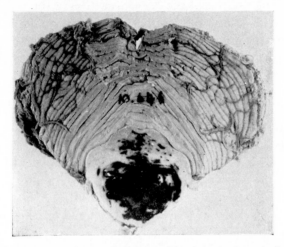

Fig. 77. *Cross section of the cerebellum and brain stem (pons) of a patient in whom the conspicuous eye finding was pinpoint pupils*
The patient was a fifty-three-year-old hypertensive man who suddenly lost consciousness and died within a few hours. The outstanding clinical finding in the eyes was extreme miosis and apparent absence of the light reflex of the pupils, resembling the Argyll-Robertson type. The pathologic examination showed massive hemorrhage in the pons.

mental.[546] The miosis is marked and is usually associated with disturbances of the conjugate ocular mechanism. Occasionally a further miosis can be elicited with the near reflex whence its similarity to the Argyll-Robertson pupil. The pathogenesis of the miosis with acute pontine lesions is presumably involvement of the sympathetic fibers within the brain stem since experimental destruction of this region results in Horner's syndrome.[950] When the lesion is unilateral the miosis is limited to the same side,[989] but the lesion is usually bilateral and so is the miosis. The more frequent lesions causing a pontine miosis are vascular accidents, multiple sclerosis, and tumor (Fig. 77).

Miosis may occur along with pain in the face, epiphora, and paralyses of the pterygoid muscles in an entity called the *para-trigeminal syndrome*[850] due to lesions of the trigeminal ganglion (tumors, trauma). The miosis is presumably due to involvement of the sympathetic fibers which course with, or in close proximity to, the trigeminal nerves.

The *Argyll-Robertson pupil* is a syndrome characterized by an absence or sluggishness of the miotic reaction of the pupil to light, either direct or consensual, with preservation of the miotic reaction to near stimulus. Occasionally there is a slight dilatation of the pupil when a light is shone in the eye, the inverse pupillary reaction. The typical Argyll-Robertson pupil is miotic in both eyes but not necessarily to the same degree in the two eyes and frequently the pupils are irregular. The sensitivity of the pupil to atropine and cocaine is reduced as in Horner's syndrome.

The importance of the Argyll-Robertson pupil lies in the frequency with which it is found in syphilis of the central nervous system. It is the one sign oftenest found in this disease, and syphilis of the central nervous system is the one disease oftenest found with it. The site of the lesion has been variously suggested, but presumably there is involvement of the afferent pupillary pathways, and the lesion is most probably in the vicinity of the tectum.[1118, 507, 722]

The Argyll-Robertson pupil has also been reported with encephalitis,[1118] meningitis, and alcoholism,[934] but the commonest entity other than syphilis in which there is an absence of pupillary reaction to light with preservation of the near reflex is produced by *lesions in the region of the tectum;* for example, encephalitis[1118] and tumors of the pineal gland (Fig. 59), of the mesencephalon,[1120, 1119] and of the thalamus.[964] Here the pupillary disturbance may be differentiated from a true Argyll-Robertson pupil by the absence of miosis and by the associated paresis of upward gaze and frequently by paresis of convergence.

Adie's pupil is a syndrome consisting of absent or retarded constriction of the pupil with light or near stimulus; once constricted, the pupil also dilates more slowly than normal in the dark or on looking into the distance (Fig. 78). Accommodation of the lens may or may not be affected.[487] Since the pupil may attain the full

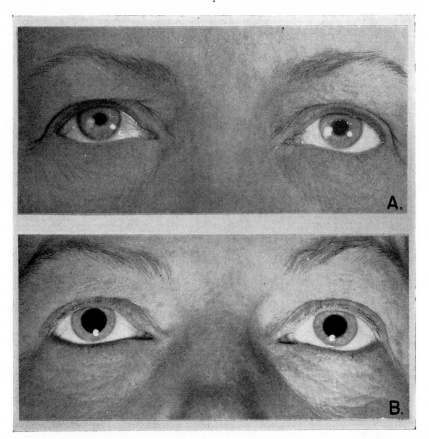

Fig. 78. *Adie's pupil (left)*
The patient was a healthy woman of thirty-five years who noticed that her pupils were of unequal size. Knee jerks were normal. In the light (A) the right pupil constricted promptly and fully, but the left pupil reacted slowly and incompletely. In the dark (B) the right pupil dilated promptly but the left pupil dilated slowly and somewhat less fully than the right pupil.

amount of reaction but at a much slower rate, it has been called in this syndrome the *myotonic pupil*. However, the syndrome is not sharply defined, and in many of the cases that are properly included under this heading there is no reaction to light and little if any reaction to near stimulus. Adie's pupil is subject to spontaneous variations in size, but at no time does it react promptly to light. It is usually (but not always) unilateral, generally occurs in young women, frequently with absent knee or ankle reflexes, and is present for life without being accompanied by other neurologic disease. It does not occur with generalized myotonia but like generalized myotonia it is said to respond to quinine therapy.[359] Its importance lies chiefly in the confusion that in the past has arisen from failure to differentiate it from the true Argyll-Robertson pupil.[6, 7] Of considerable theoretic and practical importance is the characteristic sensitivity of Adie's pupil to some parasympathomimetic drugs. Thus fresh $2\frac{1}{2}\%$ mecholyl instilled into the conjunctival sac will cause a miosis of Adie's pupil but have no effect on the normal pupil.[916, 606] This has been interpreted as evidence for parasympathetic sensitization[916, 1085, 29, 762] pointing to a lesion in the ciliary ganglion or in the post-ganglionic fibers. Others have postulated lesions in the central sympathetic centers[664] and in the iris itself.[543]

Anomalous pupillary reactions occur with the aberrant regeneration of the 3rd nerve.[377, 127, 100, 353, 972] Frequently, the pupil in this condition is fixed to light and occasionally to near stimulus, but when the patient looks to the opposite side or downwards, the pupil constricts (see p. 71f). Since this occurs after a 3rd nerve palsy, and since the constriction occurs on attempting to look in the direction of a muscle that is paralyzed (usually the medial rectus or inferior rectus), it is presumed that the sphincter of the iris receives the nerve fibers that were originally connected with the paralyzed rectus muscle instead of the original pupillary fibers.

SUMMARY

The muscles and nerve supply controlling the pupil are the sphincter, innervated by parympathetic nerves, and the dilator, innervated by sympathetic nerves. Contraction of the former produces miosis, whereas contraction of the latter produces mydriasis. As with autonomic functions elsewhere in the body, the parasympathetic and sympathetic nerve supply to the eye is relayed through centers both outside and within the central nervous system.

The chief parasympathetic center for the pupil *outside* the central nervous system is the ciliary ganglion; the corresponding sympathetic center is the superior cervical ganglion. The chief subcortical centers *within* the central nervous system for miosis are believed to be the pretectal nuclei of the hypothalamus and the Edinger-Westphal nucleus of the 3rd nerve complex. The chief center for mydriasis is a group of cells in the hypothalamus. The fibers relaying impulses from the Edinger-Westphal nucleus presumably join the 3rd nerve fibers and go directly to the ciliary ganglion; the fibers relaying impulses from the hypothalamic nuclei to the superior cervical ganglion take the circuitous course of descending in the cervical cord, to leave the central nervous system in the upper thoracic segments and ascend in the cervical sympathetic chain. In the cerebrum miosis is represented in the vicinity of the ocular motor centers, while mydriasis is represented diffusely over most of the rest of the cortex. Cerebral centers differ from subcortical centers in that they project to *both* pupils and some cerebral effects occur through *inhibition* rather than through stimulation.

The size of the normal pupil depends on light adaptation, age, refractive status, sense of nearness, and race. The outstanding *normal* reactions are the miosis from light (direct and consensual), the miosis on near gaze, and the miosis with forced closure of the lids. Abnormal pupillary reactions may be divided into those *accompanied* by correlative visual defects where the responsible lesion involves the afferent arc and those occurring *without* correlative visual defects. Noteworthy among the former are the amaurotic reaction, the hemianopic reaction, and anisocoria from various cerebrovascular accidents. Among those occurring without correlative visual defects are paralytic mydriasis (usually 3rd nerve paralysis), paralytic miosis (Horner's syndrome), miosis with acute pontine lesions, the Argyll-Robertson pupil, Adie's pupil, and anomalous pupillary reactions following aberrant regeneration of the 3rd nerve fibers.

Chapter X

NYSTAGMUS

A. DEFINITION

AS APPLIED to the eyes, nystagmus is a disorder of eye movements characterized by involuntary oscillations that are to a certain extent rhythmic. This definition is not very precise but neither is the entity of nystagmus.

B. GENERAL CONSIDERATIONS

1. Relation of Nystagmus to Tonus

The position of the eyes at any one time represents the sum total of innervation from all sources. As long as the tendency to turn the eyes is equal in all directions, they are directed straight ahead, but if there is an increase or decrease of tone to one side greater than to the other side, the eyes show a corresponding deviation.

Increase in the tone of one set of yoke muscles, as from excitation of the cortical centers, results in deviation of the eyes in one direction. Conversely, decrease in tone of one set of muscles results in a drifting of the eyes in the opposite direction; that is, toward the side corresponding to the normal tonic innervation. In this latter case if the patient is unconscious or if for any reason cerebral activity is abolished, the eyes remain deviated to that side and no nystagmus results, but if the patient is conscious, this drifting away from the object of fixation is corrected by a movement in the opposite direction. The continual repetition of these oscillations makes up the cycle of nystagmus.

Nystagmus may thus be considered to result from a disturbance in the symmetry of tonic innervation plus the corrective movements. The origin of the nystagmus may be referred to any of the centers or pathways relaying tonic innervation; for example, the retina, labyrinth, brain stem, and cerebrum. That lesions so differently situated produce nystagmus does not necessarily invalidate the localizing value of nystagmus, since its character, as will be subsequently pointed out, varies with the site of the lesion.

Finally, it is worth noting that, as might be expected from the previous discussion on tone, the actual movement of the eyes in nystagmus results from simultaneous contraction of one set of muscles and relaxation of the antagonists. This has been shown experimentally by connecting the lateral and medial recti muscles with recording levers while the semicircular canals are stimulated.[67, 713, 718, 674]

2. Relation of Nystagmus to Illusory Movement of the Environment

With turning of the eyes and consequent displacement of the image on the retina, the environment may or may not appear to move. Some have assumed that the false appearance of movement of the environment occurs when the eyes move too rapidly;[584, 423] others have assumed that the eyes are blind while in motion. That speed of movement is not the determining factor and that the eye is not blind in motion is shown by the observation that when suitable stimuli are used, objects can be seen while the eyes *are* in motion. Thus, the individual flashes from a light such as the stroboscope flickering above the critical fusion frequency can be seen and counted while the eye is moving.[1053] When the eye is stationary, the flashes occurring at a rate above the critical flicker frequency cannot be recognized as separate.

On the other hand, the presence or absence of illusory movement of the environment does have some relation to the innervational background. *Voluntary* turning of the eyes is not accompanied by any sensation of movement of the environment, whereas *passive* turning of the eyes as from displacement of the eye with one's finger or rotation of the globe with forceps, does produce an illusory movement of the environment. The sweep of the image over the retina may be identical in the two cases but in the one, the environment is interpreted as being stationary whereas in the other it gives the illusion of movement. With nystagmus from artificial stimulation of the labyrinth, an illusory movement of the environment occurs during the slow phase only, giving rise to the sensation that the environment is continually moving in one direction (the so-called oculogyral illusion[424]).

The presence or absence of illusory movement of the environment appears to be determined by the information sent to the higher centers. According to a scheme (Fig. 79), which, however, has no known anatomic basis, one may imagine that any attempt

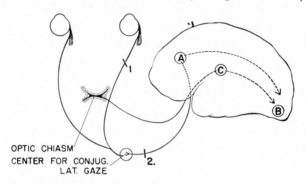

OPTIC CHIASM
CENTER FOR CONJUG.
LAT. GAZE

FIG. 79. *Diagram illustrating possible connections for the interpretation of movement of the environment*

Area A represents the frontal center for lateral conjugate gaze. As efferent impulses are sent down to the subcortical center for movement of the eyes, corresponding impulses are sent to Area B, indicating that a definite amount of image movement on the retina is to be expected. If there is a block at 2 in the efferent pathways (or at 1 in case one eye is used for fixation), the impulses from A will get to B but the eyes (or eye) will not move and the absence of the expected displacement of the image will result in an illusory movement of the environment in the opposite direction. Similarly, when the eyes are moved passively the displacement of the image on the retina will be transmitted to the visual centers by way of C, but since no information has been received from A indicating that the eyes have been moved, the image displacement will be interpreted as movement (illusory) of the environment.

to turn voluntarily the eyes in one direction is accompanied by a corresponding innervation to the coordinating centers indicating that so much displacement of the image on the retina is to be expected and such expected displacement is not to be interpreted as movement of the environment.[413] If, however, the eyes are moved passively (as by one's finger) or by some low-order reflex (such as occurs in the slow phase of labyrinthine nystagmus), no information is sent to the higher centers that a movement of the eyes is to be expected, and the brain interprets the displacement of the image on the retina as movement of the environment. Thus, active movements of the eye mediated through the higher centers, presumably the frontal cerebral centers, are not accompanied by illusory movement of the environment, whereas passive movements, or those mediated through the lower centers only (presumably the brain stem), are accompanied by a false sensation of movement of the environment. This is an old thesis[594, 453] that has recently acquired added support.[510, 668]

An applied corollary of this is to be found with acute lesions of the subcortical pathways to the eye muscles or a block in the eye muscles themselves.[591] Here information is sent to the visual centers indicating that so much displacement of the image on the retina is to be expected, but owing to the block in the subcortical pathways, this displacement does not occur at all or not to the extent that was expected. In consequence, the brain interprets the *absence* of displacement as a movement of the environment in the *opposite* direction, and the subject shows the phenomenon of past pointing (Fig. 56).

In alleged contradiction to this thesis are the observations that fixation of the ocular muscles from curare or from curare-like substances induces illusory movement only during the prodromal stages (or when the head is moved); complete paralysis of the muscles by curare is accompanied by a conscious sensation of limitation in movements of the eyes with no illusory movement of the environment.[951, 952] Similarly, patients with peripheral muscle palsies who have developed a conscious awareness of their limited eye excursions will not have illusory movement of the environment. How this conscious awareness is developed is obscure. That it is a correction imposed by a peripheral muscle sense, as proposed,[952] seems unlikely in view of the persistent past pointing and in view of the fact that it does not apply when both eyes are open. It may well be simply a matter of conditioned learning.

The phenomenon of illusory movement of the environment, but in reverse, can be demonstrated in the dark or with the eyes closed, by means of the afterimage.[274, 584, 476] With passive movements of the eyes, the afterimage appears to remain stationary, since the voluntary centers are not activated, but with voluntary movements or movements in which the coordinating centers are informed of movements of the eyes, the afterimage moves in accord with the innervation. This latter displacement of the afterimage on attempted conjugate gaze occurs even though the eye does not actually move (for example, owing to a recently acquired peripheral paralysis or to a lesion of the subcortical pathways).[413, 476]

Illusory movement of the environment with nystagmus possesses some localizing value. It indicates a lesion of the lower centers (for example, the labyrinth) or of their pathways and is said to be especially frequent with multiple sclerosis.[158] Absence of illusory movement of the environment does not, however, indicate that the causative lesion is in the higher centers, since lesions in various positions of the brain stem and cerebellum may result in nystagmus without the subject being aware of the apparent movement.

C. CLASSIFCATION

Nystagmus has been variously classified. On the basis of *etiology* it is classified as neurologic, otologic or ocular, or merely as labyrinthine or ocular. On the basis of *severity* it is classified as Grades I, II, or III.[11] Nystagmus of Grade I is that in which there is nystagmus on conjugate gaze to one side only; in Grade II, there is nystagmus on conjugate gaze to one side and straight ahead; in Grade III, there is nystagmus on conjugate gaze to both sides and straight ahead. On the basis of the *direction of the fast component,* the disorder is described as nystagmus to the right or left or up or down. Nystagmus is also loosely classified as *physiologic or pathologic,* depending on whether it is the normal result of an extraneous artificial stimulus or is the result of some organic lesion.

In the following simple classification primary emphasis is placed on the *objective* characteristics of eye movements rather than on the conditions that are believed to produce them.

1. Pendular nystagmus
2. Jerk nystagmus
   a. Opticokinetic type
   b. Vestibular type
   c. Nystagmus from neuromuscular insufficiency
   d. Congenital nystagmus*
   e. Latent nystagmus

D. PENDULAR NYSTAGMUS

Pendular nystagmus is characterized by oscillations that, in some position of gaze, are approximately *equal* in rate for the two directions. The oscillations may be fine or coarse, and vary from moment to moment. The direction of the nystagmus is almost always horizontal when both eyes are involved but may be vertical when the nystagmus is limited to one eye. On conjugate gaze to either side the pendular nystagmus becomes converted into a jerk type, with the fast component to the side of the gaze.

A convenient method of recording the eye movements in nystagmus has been employed in which the difference in potential between the front and the back of the eye is utilized.[925, 726, 513, 745, 328, 533, 825] One electrode is placed on each outer canthus and connected to an amplifier-recorder system. As the eyes move conjugately from one side to the other the difference in potential produces a record of the amplitude, frequency, and direction of the eye movements. This not only provides a method for analyzing the movements more accurately than can be done by visual examination but permits study of eye movements under conditions in which the eyes cannot be seen; for instance, in the dark and with the lids closed.

1. Pathogenesis

Absence of central vision is the rule in pendular nystagmus and is generally held to be the *cause* of the nystagmus. The central vision must be lost in early infancy, before the fixation reflexes are developed, or nystagmus will not appear.[58] Some nystagmus practically always develops when central vision is lost in both eyes before the age of two years. Between the ages of two and six, loss of central vision generally results in irregular and unsustained movements of fixation but not a true nystagmus; after six years of age, loss of central vision generally results in no abnormal eye movements.

It is held by some that nystagmus is an attempt to compensate

---

* By congenital nystagmus is meant congenitally predetermined nystagmus and includes those cases caused by lesions sustained in utero or at the time of birth as well as those which have an hereditary basis. Rarely is the nystagmus apparent, however, until several weeks after birth.

for the central scotoma.[271] As evidence of this, it is pointed out that the greater the visual loss, the greater are the excursions of the nystagmus;[68, 609] the excursions are fine and do not differ markedly from the normal fixation tremor when the visual loss is slight, whereas they are coarse (the "searching movements of the blind") when the visual loss is extensive. According to this explanation, it is assumed that in the absence of central vision the sweeping movements of the eye prevent an otherwise blind area in the central visual field. The nystagmus is thought to be analogous to the exaggeration of the fixation tremor that normally occurs in the dark with certain animals,[859, 800, 572, 61, 140] and with human beings when an object having a luminous image less than that necessary to stimulate the macula is viewed.[280] But as will be pointed out, all this is subject to other possible interpretations.

According to the concept that the pendular nystagmus serves a compensatory function, one would expect that any arrest of the eyes or any stabilization of them relative to the object looked at would make the vision worse. This does not appear to be the case. Actually, the oscillations of the eyes are a handicap to visual acuity.

> Thus, the head nodding that usually occurs when patients with pendular nystagmus attempt to fixate an object intently can be shown to compensate for the nystagmus. By means of slow-motion moving-picture photography, the head movements can be seen to be *opposite* those of the eyes and thereby to stabilize the eyes in relation to the object looked at. If the head is held stationary, the nystagmus appears to be worse and so is the vision.

> Some patients with pendular nystagmus find that they can improve their vision by looking toward one side or by converging and are found on examination to show a relative cessation of the nystagmus in these positions of election. Occasionally, patients with pendular nystagmus discover that after rapid pivoting to one or the other side their vision temporarily improves, and their eyes can be seen to be relatively quiet. All these effects are presumably due to superimposing other innervational complexes (voluntary gaze, labyrinthine impulses, etc.) on the eye muscles and thus stabilizing the nystagmus. The important thing is that the vision is *improved* by this stabilization. Similarly, vision is improved in patients with nystagmus when the excursions of the eyes are reduced by barbiturates.[760]

Finally, it is occasionally possible to oscillate a test card from side to side in front of a patient and attain the same frequency as the nystagmus. The acuity is then improved.

This cumulative evidence is taken to indicate that the nystagmus not only does not compensate for the loss of vision but, in most cases, makes the vision worse.

An alternative and more tenable hypothesis is to consider the nystagmus that occurs with absence of central vision to result from the failure of the normal tonic innervation from the macula. It has previously been noted that the extraocular muscles possess no proprioceptive end organs in the usual sense, and the retina, especially the macula, provides the analogous function of a positional sense for the eyes. In the absence of this normal positional information, the eyes do not "learn" adequate fixation, and pendular nystagmus may accordingly be considered true *ataxia* of the eye movements. In the absence of impulses from the macula, there is no dampening effect for the various conjugate impulses that act on the extraocular muscles[68 863] and that are ordinarily held in check by tonic innervation coming from the macula.

2. Conditions in Which Pendular Nystagmus Is Present

Pendular nystagmus is found in a variety of conditions in which central vision is lost early in life. It is typically present in bilateral chorioretinal lesions involving the maculas in early infancy, in albinism where the macula does not develop,[370, 310, 396] and similarly in aniridia,[935] total color blindness (monochromatism),[588, 313] and high myopia of early life. Pendular nystagmus is also present with opacities of the media such as congenital cataracts or corneal scars where the macula may be present but prevented from functioning adequately. There are also several specific types in which the pendular oscillations are a characteristic feature (vide infra).

In all types of pendular nystagmus there is a gross irregularity and inconstancy of the eye movements. On relaxation of attention the ocular excursions become less; they disappear entirely in sleep or when the eyes are closed. In general, the greater the visual defect the coarser and more irregular are the movements.

Pendular nystagmus may be compensated for, to some extent, by synchronous contraversive and rhythmic movements of the head. The excursions may also be lessened occasionally by head tilting whence some patients with pendular nystagmus develop a torticollis.[851]

Spasmus nutans is one type of pendular nystagmus. In its full form it is accompanied by head nodding, chiefly up and down, with occasionally wry positions of the neck. It is a characteristically rapid nystagmus and frequently asymmetric in the two eyes. It often varies with different directions of gaze;[1002, 1003, 774] thus, it may appear in one eye on looking in one direction and in the other eye on looking in the opposite direction. Or it may be entirely monocular;[839, 22] indeed, it is the commonest, if not the only, cause of unilateral horizontal nystagmus in infancy.

Spasmus nutans comes on usually during the first two years of life and lasts a matter of weeks or months. Its etiology is obscure. At one time it was thought to be due to the rearing of infants under inadequate illumination[575, 818, 803] and it was likened to the nystagmus in some young animals which are brought up in the dark[109, 859, 860, 800, 61, 57, 170] but no corroborative history has been obtained in cases that are currently seen in this country. The vestibular nuclei and vestibular nerves play no role in its genesis.[572, 573] The important consideration is that it does not signify organic disease and the prognosis is good.

Miners' nystagmus is also a pendular nystagmus, an exceptionally fine and rapid one,[796] occurring in persons who work in poorly lighted mines for long periods of time. It is much less frequent now that mines are better illuminated. The nystagmus is accompanied by an impairment of vision that varies according to the degree of nystagmus and occasionally by an illusory movement of the environment.[609] As in the case of spasmus nutans, but with possibly more relevance, the condition has been likened to that occurring in animals reared in the dark.[803] The prognosis is favorable when the patient is removed to quarters having adequate illumination.

> The amount of light at the coal face necessary to prevent nystagmus must be of the order of 0.01 candle per square foot or, assuming an 8 per cent reflection from the coal surface, an illumination of 0.4 foot candle.[941] Where power lines are not available this light is adequately supplied by cap lamps, and where these are used, as in the United States, miners' nystagmus is practically nonexistent.

Congenital nystagmus may be of the pendular or jerk type and will be more fully discussed under the latter heading (see p. 225). When of the pendular type, it is frequently accompanied by head nodding and becomes converted into the jerk type on deviation of the gaze to either side. Hereditary nystagmus is usually transmitted either as a dominant or sex-linked recessive trait. In the absence of any histologic observations, it is still unknown whether the primary defect in hereditary nystagmus is absence of macular development or disturbance of motor innervation. In the type of congenital nystagmus to be described subsequently under jerk nystagmus, however, macular function is normal, for in those posisions of gaze where the nystagmus is of lowest degree, the vision is usually normal or near normal.

Voluntary nystagmus is a special case of pendular nystagmus in which the subject can at will cause his eyes to make extremely fine and rapid horizontal oscillations (500-600/min.).[728, 1102] This is likened to tetanic contractions[172, 728] and, unlike other forms of nystagmus, cannot be maintained for more than a few minutes without considerable fatigue. It usually has no clinical importance and is considered more of an acrobatic feat than a diagnostic sign. Rarely a nystagmus, identical with the voluntary variety, may occur as a manifestation of hysteria. It is then likewise transitory and accompanied by tetanic rigidity of the head.

Not to be confused with nystagmus are the chaotic movements called opsoclonus.[812, 218] These are totally irregular, non-rhythmic, oscillations of the eyes in the horizontal and vertical directions occurring almost exclusively in unconscious patients with encephalitis or other brain stem disease.

E. JERK NYSTAGMUS

The oscillations of jerk nystagmus are sufficiently faster in one direction than in the other direction so that the combined cycle has a characteristically jerky rhythm.

The *direction* of the nystagmus (right, left, up, or down) is named according to the direction of the *fast* component, since this component is the more conspicuous one. It would perhaps have been more appropriate to name the nystagmus according to the slow component, since, as we shall see, there is reason to believe that the slow component is the primary one from an etiologic point of view, whereas the fast component is a corrective movement.

Jerk nystagmus is subdivided into five distinct types: opticokinetic nystagmus, vestibular nystagmus, nystagmus from neuromuscular insufficiency, congenital nystagmus, and latent nystagmus.

1. Opticokinetic Nystagmus

(a) *Characteristics.* Opticokinetic nystagmus is a manifestation of the following reaction and may be elicited in all persons possessing a normal visual mechanism although not necessarily a high degree of visual acuity.[146] The usual method of producing it clinically is to have the patient look at the rotating drum on which are a series of figures or alternate black and white lines (Fig. 80). The eyes involuntarily follow one or more of the figures to the edge of the drum or to the limit of comfortable conjugate gaze. They then make a quick corrective movement in the opposite direction and fixate another set of figures. The result is a jerk nystagmus. The slow component corresponds in speed and direction to the rotating drum, while the fast component is independent of the drum.

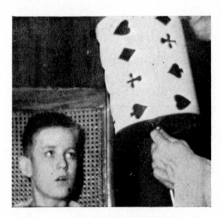

Fig. 80. *Simple device for eliciting opticokinetic nystagmus*

The drum is actually a tin cylinder that rotates on an axial rod held in the hand. The above patient, who had intermittent left-sided convulsions, showed no opticokinetic response with rotation of the drum to his right but normal response on rotation to his left. This is compatible with a right-sided cerebral lesion.

Numerous types of apparatus have been constructed for producing opticokinetic nystagmus;[43, 179, 794, 1097, 533] all are basically similar to the rotating drum, and the nystagmus produced is actually nothing more nor less than that which occurs when one looks out of the window of a moving car, familiarity known as "train nystagmus."

Opticokinetic nystagmus is usually produced in the horizontal plane. It is less well sustained in the vertical plane.[785, 793, 788] Rotary opticokinetic nystagmus, as from the observation of a pinwheel-type test object, is elicited with difficulty or not at all.[794, 770, 155]

The frequency and magnitude of the opticokinetic cycles depend on the speed of rotation of the drum, the size of the field, the distance separating the figures of the test object, attention on the part of the observer,[21] and other factors.[882] If the speed of rotating the drum is too fast or the visual angle subtended by the stripes and the interval between the stripes is too small, nystagmus does not occur.

The fact that opticokinetc nystagmus disappears when the visual angle subtended by the lines becomes less than the visual acuity has permitted its use for the objective determination of the acuity of animals[1127, 461, 134] and of human beings.[617, 26, 789, 405, 766] In the test the distance between the lines is gradually decreased until the subject no longer shows opticokinetic nystagmus. The visual acuity is then a function of the angle subtended by the lines. By varying the intensity of illumination, the opticokinetic response can also be used to measure dark adaptation objectively.[874, 787]

An estimate of acuity can also be obtained by superimposing small test objects[804] or letters[501] in front of the moving screen and determining the size of the object which will be just sufficient to prevent the opticokinetic response.

The opticokinetic response is also conveniently employed for the detection of malingerers who simulate complete blindness in one or both eyes, since the test depends on vision, and the eye movements cannot be voluntarily inhibited.[965, 802, 94] It may also be used for a determination of the approximate visual acuity in hysterical or simulated blindness.

The slow and fast phases of opticokinetic nystagmus are distinct and separable. The slow phase is involuntary in the sense that the eyes cannot voluntarily be kept stationary while the gaze is fixated on the drum. With various lesions of the ocular motor pathways, the slow or fast phase only may be present. When only the slow phase is present, the eyes maintain a conjugate deviation to the side toward which the drum is being rotated, and no nystagmus develops. When the slow phase is absent, no movement occurs.

The opticokinetic response is often said to be subject to voluntary inhibition[557, 1074, 458] but this opinion is based on an artifact of testing. It is true that when a small drum is used, there may be some rivalry between the moving and stationary portions of the field and the observer may feel he can "look through" the drum; or he may be able to immobilize his eyes by fixating a stationary reflex on the surface of the drum. If, however, the whole field is made to rotate and there are no surface reflections, as in the ideal test, the opticokinetic response cannot be voluntarily inhibited.

The normal opticokinetic cycle is a complex process served by a minimum of three neural arcs. There is: (1) the fixation reflex necessitating the integrity of at least some of the visual tracts; (2) the following reflex mediated through the centripetal pathways and resulting in the slow phase; and (3) the corrective reflex, also mediated through centripetal ocular motor pathways but different from those used in the following reflex and resulting in the fast phase.[43] The actual pathways involved in opticokinetic nystagmus have not been identified anatomically. The fact that the slow phase depends on the visual act is evidence that in man, at least, the *area striata* of the occipital cortex is essential.[1044] At the same time, the fact that the movement of the eyes with opticokinetic nystagmus cannot be voluntarily inhibited and that the eyes cannot voluntarily make such smooth slow movements as are made in the slow phase of opticokinetic nystagmus indicates that the slow phase, at least, is an involuntary act. It is reasonable to assume, therefore, that the following reaction (*slow* phase) is mediated through the optomotor field of the occipital lobe; the impulses would then be expected to pass downward medial to the visual radiation and through the posterior portion of the internal capsule to the basal ganglia and lower conjugate centers.[242] As in the case of the visual fibers, the centripetal optomotor pathways would be expected to pass beneath the cortex of the angular gyrus, but there is no good evidence for the assumption that the optomotor impulses are relayed *through* the angular gyrus.

The pathways serving the *fast* phase (corrective movement) in opticokinetic nystagmus are less apparent. Being closely allied to volition and possibly identical with voluntary gaze,[145] the impulse may be mediated through the higher centers, possibly through the optomotor area of the frontal lobe. Since lesions of either the frontal or occipital lobe can cause a defect, of the opticokinetic nystagmus, it has been assumed that the normal opticokinetic arc consists of a centripetal pathway to the occipital lobe and a centrifugal pathway from the frontal lobe with an intercortical connection between the two.[243, 999, 358] There is, however, no direct evidence of this.

The role of the cerebellum in opticokinetic nystagmus is a subject of controversy. Clinically one finds bilateral alteration in the opticokinetic response with cerebellar lesions, but this may be due to pressure effects on the floor of the 4th ventricle rather than to a direct effect of the cerebellum. The labyrinthine end organ plays no role in the opticokinetic response so long as the head remains fixed; removal of the labyrinths or destruction of the 8th nerves has no effect on it.

Opticokinetic nystagmus has been extensively studied in animals, but the results can be applied to human beings only with reservations because of certain inherent differences between animals and human beings. In the first place, an image falling on the macula in man has such a high attention value that it dominates the sum total of images falling on the rest of the retina. Thus, opticokinetic nystagmus is elicited in man when only a small portion of the field is rotated, provided that this small portion corresponds to macular fixation or to whatever portion of the retina has the highest acuity. In animals, however, with more nearly equipotential attention value of all points on the retina, a comparable effect is elicited only when the whole field is rotated;[154] if any considerable portion of the field is stationary, the images from this portion inhibit those from the portion with the moving images, and no opticokinetic nystagmus results.

A second and more serious objection to applying the results of the animal studies of opticokinetic nystagmus to those in human beings is the difference in localization of the visual centers. It is well known that the subprimate animals,[615, 704, 1013, 706] and to a less extent the primates themselves,[707] have considerable visual discrimination in the tectal regions (superior colliculi), which is not

the case in man.[705] It is not surprising, therefore, that opticokinetic nystagmus can be produced in animals after decerebra-
tion,[743, 1014, 910, 911, 961] and conversely that it may be rendered abnormal by lesions of the superior colliculi in animals.[1014, 910, 911]
Man, on the other hand, has no such lower centers for visual
discrimination and, therefore, does not have opticokinetic nystagmus independent of the cerebrum.[122] An attempt to apply the
conclusions based on animal experimentation to human beings
has thus given rise to a conflict between those who, basing their
conclusions on animal experimentation, believe that opticokinetic
nystagmus is a subcortical function[69, 961] and those who, reasoning
from clinical observations, conclude that it is a cortical function.[242, 790, 122] The hypothesis that the opticokinetic response in
man is served by a subcortical reflex arc independent of the
cortical arc[192] is certainly erroneous.

The centers in the *brain stem* mediating the impulses for opticokinetic nystagmus have not been clearly defined. In animals the
superior colliculi are naturally one of the centers,[69] but in man
the counterpart of these visual functions in the lower animals is
to be found in the occipital lobes, and it is likely that the corticofugal fibers for *lateral* movements of the eyes go directly to the
pontine centers without traversing the superior colliculi. The
pontine centers for lateral eye movements have not been identified
in the maze of pontine cells, but it is not impossible that the same
centers are used for vestibular and for opticokinetic impulses.[974, 911]
The occasional *absence of the fast phase* of both the opticokinetic
nystagmus and vestibular nystagmus together[40, 1123, 1113, 318, 795] suggests that opticokinetic and vestibular reflexes have a common
center for the fast phase.

The frequency with which absence of the opticokinetic nystagmus occurs in one direction, associated with an inability to maintain excentric gaze in that direction, also suggests that the pathways and centers serving for the slow phase are identical with
those serving for the maintenance of excentric conjugate gaze.

(b) *Clinical significance of opticokinetic nystagmus.* For clinical
purposes opticokinetic nystagmus is elicited in the horizontal
plane only, and since many of the patients on whom it is desirable

to make a test are confined to bed, it is best to use a simple rotating drum that is portable[965] (Fig. 80). The more elaborate types
of apparatus employing large rotating fields[178] or elaborate recording devices[784, 357, 431, 533, 825, 534] are not necessary for routine
clinical testing. The speed of rotation of the drum is said to be
optimal when there is an angular velocity of approximately 40
degrees per second or less[277] and when the figures on the drum
provide approximately eight contours per second.[882] But the variation among normal subjects is sufficient to make any great amount
of accuracy unprofitable for clinical purposes. Actually one is
interested not in absolute values but in the detection of gross
deficiencies in response or gross differences of the movements of
the patient's eyes on rotating the drum in one direction as compared with those caused by rotating the drum in the other direction.

The opticokinetic response is said not to be present in human
beings at birth. It can be elicited only some time after birth,[145, 771,
772, 555, 671, 717, 410] apparently at a time when the infant first develops
optic fixation.

Opticokinetic nystagmus may be said to be abnormal when it
cannot be elicited on rotating the drum in either direction or
when there is an appreciable difference in response on rotation of
the drum to one side as compared with rotation to the opposite
side. This difference may vary from an easy fatigability to a complete absence of response. Unless response is completely absent,
bilateral reduction in opticokinetic nystagmus is more difficult to
evaluate because of the several extraneous factors such as lack of
attention and uncertainty of fixation which may give falsely positive results.

The relation of disturbances in opticokinetic nystagmus to
cerebral lesions is most important. Here the defect is manifest
by finer excursions, easier fatigability, or absence of the nystagmus
on rotating the drum toward the side of the lesion. On theoretical
grounds one might expect the opticokinetic response to be defective on moving the field toward the side opposite the cerebral
lesion but the reverse is almost invariably the case.[223]

Unfortunately, a confusion has arisen due to the nomenclature
of nystagmus so that one reads in the literature, especially the

German literature, that the nystagmus is defective on the side opposite the lesion. This refers to the fast phase and must not be confused with the fact that the drum is being rotated toward the side of the lesion.

Abnormalities in the opticokinetic response were first noted in patients with hemianopsia,[43] and it was initially assumed that this condition accounted for the defect. In fact, the test was first advanced as an objective means of detecting hemianopsia. Subsequently, it was discovered that some patients with *complete* hemianopsia had normal opticokinetic nystagmus[243, 242, 21, 799, 798] and that many patients without hemianopsia had abnormal opticokinetic nystagmus.[242, 356] It is thus generally agreed that hemianopsia *per se* is not the determining factor in abnormal opticokinetic nystagmus. In fact, opticokinetic nystagmus may be present and essentially normal when only a small portion of the visual field remains.[146, 358, 554] As a rule the opticokinetic response is normal when the hemianopsia is due to a lesion of the optic tract and may or may not be normal when the hemianopsia is due to a cerebral lesion; in other words hemianopsia with abnormalities of the opticokinetic response points to a cerebral lesion, whereas normal opticokinetic response with hemianopsia has no localizing significance.

Lesions in the *middle* or *posterior* half of the cerebral hemisphere, with or without hemianopsia, are especially apt to cause a lasting defect in the opticokinetic nystagmus on rotating the drum to the side of the lesion (Fig. 80). Thus, significant defects have been reported with lesions in the occipital area,[242] in the parietal region[554, 356, 223] (especially about the angular and supramarginal gyri[999, 242, 358, 790]), in the temporal area,[356] and in the internal capsule.[790] Syndromes have been reported in which opticokinetic nystagmus has been found defective with astereognosia[926, 697, 999, 358, 247] and with motor aphasia.[1098, 790, 792] The defect in opticokinetic nystagmus on rotation of the drum to *one* side frequently occurs in patients who have cogwheel eye movements in following an object moved toward *that* side.[242, 247, 554, 555] But not all occipito-parieto-temporary lesions are accompanied by defective opticokinetic nystagmus,[790] and one particularly interesting case has been reported in which the nystagmus was found to be affected only for a short time after an entire occipital lobectomy,[394] suggesting that some compensation takes place.

Lesions in the *anterior* half of the cerebrum are less apt to cause disturbances in the opticokinetic nystagmus,[358, 356, 233] although the same type of disturbance, that is a defect on rotating the drum to the side of the lesion, many occur.[997, 998] Lesions have been reported resulting in motor aphasia with alteration of the opticokinetic nystagmus,[1098, 1099, 790, 792] but the opticokinetic disturbances are not necessarily *always* present with motor aphasia.[697, 241, 358, 1004] With frontal lobe lesions there is fairly rapid compensation for the disturbances in comparison to that with occipital lobe lesions.[1004, 431, 533, 629]

Lesions of the cerebellum and brain stem may produce disturbances of opticokinetic nystagmus on one side, but the defective response is usually bilateral and therefore has little localizing value.[242, 358, 223]

Rarely an inverse or paradoxic type of response may occur wherein the direction of nystagmus is opposite to that usually produced by moving the field; it may even be vertical while the field is rotated horizontally. The most reasonable explanation for this is to assume that there is an underlying occult nystagmus in the observed direction which is held in check by fixation but which may be evoked by the disruption of fixation in the opticokinetic test. Thus the inverse opticokinetic response is seen in persons with congenital nystagmus and the vertical response is seen in patients with brain stem disease.

2. Vestibular Nystagmus

(a) *Characteristics.* Vestibular nystagmus has a jerklike rhythm consisting of a fast component in one direction and a slow component in the other direction; the slow component reflects the effect of impulses derived from the semicircular canals, while the fast component is a corrective movement. The jerky *rhythm* is like that of opticokinetic nystagmus, but unlike the latter, vestibular nystagmus is independent of *visual* stimuli; it is present in the dark or with the lids closed. Vestibular nystagmus may be horizontal, vertical, or rotary; rotary nystagmus is especially characteristic of the vestibular type since it is infrequent with other types.

The direction of the nystagmus is designated, as in the case of the opticokinetic nystagmus, according to the direction of the fast component. This again gives rise to confusion, partly because some of the earlier literature referred the direction of the nystagmus to that of the slow component,[480] but chiefly because the significant or vestibulogenic phase of the nystagmus is the slow component. The vestibular stimulus results in a relatively slow conjugate deviation or torsion of the eyes to the opposite side. There is then a quick compensatory movement (in the direction of the nystagmus) bringing the eyes back to the initial position. The repetition of this cycle makes up the vestibular nystagmus.

The normal or adequate stimulus for the production of vestibular nystagmus is a change in rate of movement of the head, either an acceleration or a deceleration. Movement alone is not sufficient; if there is no change in rate, there is no displacement of the endolymph in the semicircular canals and no nystagmus occurs. The minimum acceleration for the production of eye movements is of the order of 0.2–0.3 degrees/sec./sec.[1037, 1038, 1014, 425, 534]

The semicircular canals provide inertia against any change brought about by movement of the head. Thus, when a person is rotated to the right, there is an opposing increase in extensor tonus of the muscles on the left side of the body, including an increase in tonus of the muscles for conjugate deviation of the eyes to the left (Fig. 84). This deviation of the eyes corresponds to the slow phase of vestibular nystagmus and is always in the direction *opposite* the change in rate of motion; that is, in the direction of greater inertia. Thus, with acceleration of motion the eyes appear to lag, while with deceleration they anticipate the movement. This serves, so far as the eyes are concerned, to stabilize the visual field.[580] When a person's head is rotated in one direction, the eyes remain relatively fixed in their original position in respect to the environment until the rotation of the head causes them to reach the limit of comfortable conjugate gaze; they then make a quick compensatory movement to the primary position, where the new visual field is established, and the cycle is repeated.

Although a part of the vestibular nystagmus the fast phase is not necessarily a function of the vestibular apparatus. It may be selectively absent.[1117, 783, 1113, 318] When the fast phase *is* absent, rotation produces only a maintained conjugate deviation to the side opposite the change of motion.

Changes in the amplitude or direction of nystagmus with different positions of the head is said to be characteristic of vestibular (or cerebellar) disease. This holds for lesions of the end organ[374, 393, 532, 650] or of its connection within the brain stem.[368, 779, 938, 898, 649, 650]

Various means have been employed to elicit vestibular nystagmus, some of which will be discussed with the description of clinical tests. Briefly, the production of vestibular nystagmus depends on displacement of the endolymph in the semicircular canals,[316] either by rotation (adequate stimulus), by caloric irrigation, by compression and suction (inadequate stimuli), or, by galvanic stimulation of the whole end organ and vestibular nerve.

With rotation of the body, vestibular effects and opticokinetic effects serve in common the function of stabilizing the visual field. But with vestibular nystagmus elicited by caloric irrigation or by a sudden stopping of rotation, the opticokinetic and vestibular effects are opposed and optic fixation tends to *inhibit* the vestibular nystagmus.[744, 457] Thus, the vestibular reaction is greatest in the dark[797] or when the eyes are closed;[744] under certain conditions a spontaneous vestibular response is present *only* when illumination is much reduced.[312, 422] To obviate fixation during and after rotation, glasses have been devised that blur the patient's vision[64] or blind him by a light placed close to his eyes;[366] even opaque contact glasses have been used.[577] By these means the sensitivity of the vestibular response is considerably enhanced. By the same token, the vestibular response is much more brisk in blind persons than in normal persons.[529]

For recording eye movements in vestibular nystagmus various types of apparatus have been devised, based on the use of levers,[1136, 784] optical methods,[276, 42, 279, 602] acoustic methods,[72] photography,[687, 1106, 651, 477, 73] and electric methods.[925, 726, 513, 745, 328, 825, 648, 551, 734] These have been reviewed collectively.[699]

Vestibular nystagmus depends ultimately on an asymmetry of the impulses from the semicircular canals of the two labyrinths.

When the eyes are stationary, the innervation from the two sides is equal. Furthermore, if both labyrinths were to be stimulated equally, the eyes would remain stationary. On the other hand, if one labyrinth is stimulated or depressed more than the other, nystagmus results, and the end result is the same whether one labyrinth is stimulated or the opposite labyrinth is depressed. Thus, while stimulation of one labyrinth causes a conjugate deviation of the eyes to the opposite side (with resultant nystagmus to the same side), the same effect is produced by unilateral removal of the opposite labyrinth. This holds true also for torsion; torsion of the eyes to one side is produced by stimulation of the contralateral labyrinth or removal of the homolateral labyrinth.[409] Vertical movements of labyrinthine origin, on the other hand, having no lateralizing component, are, like vertical movements of cerebral origin, not represented simply on one side as are the torsional and horizontal movements. For this reason, vertical nystagmus is not ordinarily produced by stimulation or destruction of one end organ. This fact has considerable diagnostic value, since vertical nystagmus is common with lesions within the brain stem.

While not properly included under the heading of nystagmus, the reactions produced by the otolithic organs are sufficiently related to those produced by the semicircular canals to merit re-emphasis here (see previous discussion on labyrinthine tone p. 21f) and in the subsequent discussion of the end organs. The otolithic reactions of the eyes, the so-called *ophthalmostatic* function, consist of maintained deviations, the stimuli for which are maintained postural or centrifugal forces. Every position of the head in space has a corresponding position of the eyes in the orbit, determined by the degree and character of the otolithic stimulation.[565] Specifically, the eyes tend to assume and maintain a normal orientation to the ground irrespective of the position of the head. This is different from the effect of the semicircular canals, the *ophthalmokinetic* functions, where the eyes respond to acceleration and tend to oppose any change with motion of the body. But like the effects of the semicircular canals, those of the otolithic organs are often inhibited and masked, especially in the higher animals, by optic fixation. Thus, in man it is often impossible to demonstrate the ophthalmostatic reactions unless optic fixation is eliminated by having an optically homogeneous field[929] or by studying it in persons who have a paralysis of their optic fixation functions[887, 994, 352] (Figs. 10 and 60), or by utilizing those ophthalmostatic functions, such as torsion, that play a minor role in optic fixation.

(b) *Origin of vestibular impulses; anatomy of labyrinth.* The labyrinth with which we are concerned consists of a series of interconnecting spaces lodged within the petrous part of the temporal bone. These spaces comprise the bony labyrinth; within the latter are the intercommunicating membranous structures

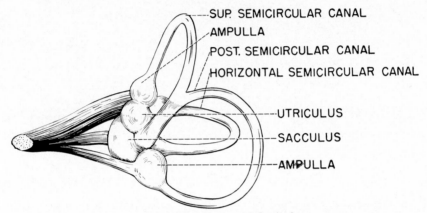

FIG. 81. *Membranous labyrinth*

forming the membranous labyrinth, subdivided into the three semicircular canals, and the subadjacent sacs called the utriculus and sacculus (Fig. 81).

The three semicircular canals are the horizontal, the anterior vertical, and the posterior vertical, each lying in a plane that is approximately at right angles to the others. At one end of each of the canals is a bulbous enlargement, the ampulla, containing a mound of sensory hair cells (the cristae), partially embedded in a gelatinous dome-shaped structure (the cupola). The planes of the semicircular canals and the position of the ampullae are of the utmost importance. The horizontal canal is actually elevated anteriorly but may be placed in the horizontal plane by bending the head 30 degrees forward (or in the vertical plane by bending it 60 degrees backward) (Fig. 82). The vertical canals are situated approximately vertically and at right angles to each other, and each makes an angle of approximately 45 degrees with the anteroposterior axis. The posterior vertical canal lies in a plane that is parallel to that of the anterior vertical canal of the opposite side. The ampullae lie at the anterior extremities of the horizontal canals and at the lateral extremities of the vertical canals. The medial arms of the two vertical canals merge to form a common duct, and all the canals connect freely with the underlying utriculus through their unexpanded portions.

The fluid within the membranous semicircular canals is called

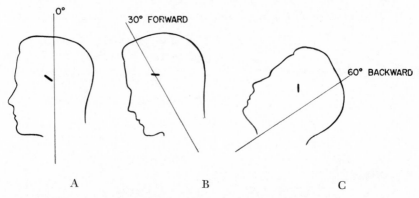

A   B   C

Fig. 82. *Plane of the horizontal semicircular canal with different positions of the head*

In the erect position of the head (A) the horizontal canal is tilted upward approximately 30 degrees but may be made horizontal by tilting the head forward 30 degrees (B) or be made vertical by tilting the head backward 60 degrees (C).

the endolymph. That separating the membranes from the bony wall is called the perilymph.

The utriculus is a sac connecting with the semicircular canals superiorly and with the sacculus inferiorly. The sensory portion of the utriculus is a horizontal plaque of hair cells, the macula, covered by a gelatinous material containing calcareous crystals, the otoliths. The sacculus is a similar sac situated beneath the utriculus and connected with it and with the cochlea. In the sacculus there is also a sensory hair plate called the macula containing otoliths, but unlike that in the utriculus, it is situated vertically.

Vestibular nystagmus arises from asymmetrical disturbances of the semicircular canals or of their pathways in the central nervous system. The classic experiments of Flourens in which the semicircular canals were injured separately[341] still form the basis of our understanding of their physiology and have given rise to the familiar Flouren's law: *Each semicircular canal gives rise to nystagmus in the plane of that canal.*[1011] This is, however, influenced to some extent by the otolithic mechanism (and possibly by the proprioceptive impulses from the neck muscles, for nystagmus induced by rotation may be modified by subsequent tilting of the head into positions different from that during rotation.[578, 354, 581]

The configuration of the canals early gave rise to the concept that the stimulation was brought about by flow of endolymph, but a more exact examination of the canal, especially in squirrels, in which accurate equilibration is a vital necessity,[419] has shown that the diameter of the canals (approximately 0.75 mm.) is scarcely enough to permit flow. Glass models bear this out.[672, 686] As a result, a compromise explanation has come to be accepted whereby no real flow is thought to take place but rather a displacement of the endolymph, resulting in a pressure or tension on the cristae.[712] This mechanical effect on the cristae results in the liberation of a chemical that, after a latent period, gives rise to the nystagmus. That the stimulus is not mediated through the mechanical traction but rather through the generation of a chemical intermediary is suggested by the fact that rotation for as short a period as a fraction of a second can cause, after a latent period, a postrotary nystagmus lasting for twenty seconds. This has been likened to the chemical changes in the visual receptors that are responsible for the continuance of the afterimage on cessation of the stimulus.[686] It accounts for the curious lag between physical acceleration and the subjective illusion of movement of the environment.[421]

The ampulla is the sensory end of the semicircular canal. The rest of the canal apparently provides the necessary momentum to stimulate it or to put traction on it. In the case of the horizontal canals, the stimulus is greatest when the direction of displacement of endolymph is toward the ampulla. Thus, referring to Fig. 83 it is evident that on rotation to the left, the left labyrinth is stimulated maximally during the rotation and the right labyrinth when the rotation is suddenly stopped. The opposite is apparently true for the vertical canals, for stimulation is here greatest when the displacement of endolymph is *away* from the ampullae.[316, 676]

Displacement of the endolymph may be brought about in a variety of ways, and the resultant nystagmus occurs in a manner predictable according to the foregoing considerations. The horizontal canal is the most accessible for analysis. *Rotation* to the right produces a nystagmus with its slow component to the left during the rotation and its slow component to the right after the rotation

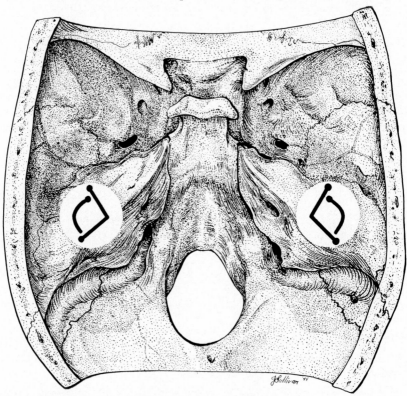

FIG. 83. *Diagrammatic sketch showing the position and arrangement of the semicircular canals and their ampullae in the skull*

is stopped (Fig. 84). The slow component represents, as previously stated, inertia against change, and the stimulus is ultimately derived from the inertia of the endolymph; the slow component of the nystagmus is therefore always in the direction of the displacement of the endolymph. Stimulation of the horizontal canal is of course maximal when rotation is carried out in the plane of the horizontal canal; that is, with the head bowed 30 degrees forward.

Caloric irrigation stimulates the horizontal canal by setting up convection currents. To be maximally effective it must be carried out with the horizontal canal directed vertically; that is, with the head rotated backward 60 degrees. Warm currents then cause a rise

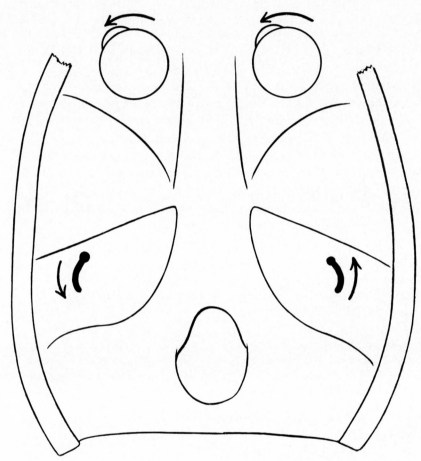

FIG. 84. *Deviation of the eyes and displacement of the endolymph with rotation of the head to the right*

Rotation of the head to the right results in a counter rotation of the endolymph during the rotation and consequent deviation of the eyes (slow phase of vestibular nystagmus) to the left. Since the movement of endolymph is toward the ampulla on the right side and *away* from the ampulla on the left, the right ampulla will be most strongly stimulated during rotation of the head to the right. The reverse occurs with sudden cessation of rotation (postrotary deviation of the eyes and nystagmus).

in fluid toward the ampulla, with consequent deviation of the eyes (slow phase of nystagmus) to the opposite side, whereas cold currents cause a displacement of fluid away from the ampulla, with consequent deviation of the eyes (slow phase) to the ipsilateral side.

In the presence of a fistula, *compression and suction* may be used to elicit a nystagmus, and as might be predicted, compression exerted on the horizontal canal causes a deviation of the eyes to the opposite side (slow phase), while suction causes a deviation of the eyes to the same side.[316, 1036]

Galvanic stimulation need not be discussed here, since it stimulates the entire labyrinth and vestibular nerve and not the semicircular canals individually. But it is noteworthy that the overall stimulation causes a deviation of the eyes to the opposite side (slow phase of the nystagmus). To this extent, stimulation of the horizontal semicircular canal with heat or by compression produces the effect of excitation of the whole labyrinth, whereas cold and suction have an effect analogous to depression of the function of the whole labyrinth.

Since the eye muscles, like the semicircular canals, are arranged in three distinct planes, there have been repeated attempts to demonstrate that their respective planes correspond.[896, 627, 791, 920] No such correspondence has been satisfactorily demonstrated, and other evidence indicates that each semicircular canal is connected with all muscle groups.[571, 324] It cannot be denied, however, that one semicircular canal or group of canals acts most effectively on the eye movements in one particular plane; for example, horizontal canals on lateral eye movements and vertical canals on rotary movements.

The *utriculus and sacculus* are not directly concerned with nystagmus. Cocainization of these sacs does not cause nystagmus, whereas cocainization of the semicircular canal does.[680] Furthermore, nystagmus may be elicited normally even when the otolithic membranes are destroyed by centrifugation so long as the semicircular canals are intact.[1125]

The *utriculus* apparently serves for maintained postural deviation of the eyes (and of the rest of the body). It is the organ of static equilibrium. Cutting the nerves to the utricular maculas abolishes these postural effects.[1054] There is some evidence that while each labyrinth possesses the property of torting the eyes in both directions, this effect is not symmetrical; torsion to one side occurs chiefly with stimulation of the contralateral labyrinth.[404, 414]

The function of the *sacculus* is not so obvious. The fact that the macular membranes in the sacculus are arranged vertically whereas those in the utriculus are arranged horizontally might lead one to suppose that the sacculi act synergistically with the utriculi in maintained postural positions. But this has not been borne out experimentally. No disturbance of posture or equilibration has been found after washing away the saccular otoliths,[618] sectioning the nerves to the saccular membranes,[675] or ablating the sacculi[571, 1054] Indeed, at the present time it cannot be stated whether or not the sacculus has *any* equilibratory function.

(c) **Pathways for the vestibulo-ocular reflexes.** The vestibular nerves have their *peripheral origin* in the sensory epithelium of the semicircular canals (cristae) and otolith sacs (maculas), their *cell bodies* in a ganglion within the internal auditory meatus (the ganglion of Scarpa), and their *central terminations* scattered over a wide area in the vestibular nuclei in the floor of the 4th ventricle.

The vestibular nuclei are made up of multipolar cells occupying a considerable portion of the floor of the 4th ventricle. They are arbitrarily separated into the following four groups (Fig. 85).

1. Superior vestibular nucleus (nucleus of Bechterew; angular nucleus).

2. Medial or principal nucleus (triangular nucleus).

3. Lateral nucleus (nucleus of Deiter).

4. Spinal nucleus (nucleus of Roller).

The anteromedial nuclei (superior vestibular nucleus and medial nucleus) are presumed to be especially and perhaps exclusively concerned with the vestibulo-ocular reflexes. Thus, in man, in whom the increased mobility of the eyes has added to the complexity of the vestibulo-ocular reflexes, there has been a corresponding increase in the proportion of the superior and medial vestibular nuclei,[536, 866, 389] whereas in the owl, which has no ocular muscles, much of this portion of the vestibular nuclei is lacking.[63] There is further some experimental [74, 623, 624] and clinical[696, 840, 996] evidence that the most anterior portion of the nuclei concerned with eye movements mediates vertical eye movements, the most posterior

portion torsional movements, and the in-between portion horizontal movements.[416]

There is still no unanimity regarding the connections, or
the identity[986, 974, 911] of the vestibular nuclei and the so-called
pontine centers for conjugate gaze, but a considerable amount of

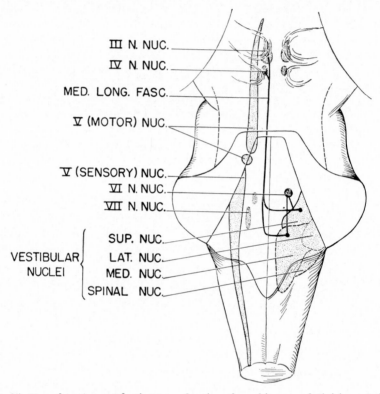

III N. NUC.

IV N. NUC.

MED. LONG. FASC.

V (MOTOR) NUC.

V (SENSORY) NUC.

VI N. NUC.

VII N. NUC.

VESTIBULAR
NUCLEI
{
SUP. NUC.

LAT. NUC.

MED. NUC.

SPINAL NUC.

FIG. 85. *Dorsal surface of brain stem showing the arbitrary subdivision of the
vestibular nucleus and its relation to the ocular motor and other nuclei* (based
on a drawing from Ranson)

experimental and morphologic study has led to the following
conclusions.[1069, 696, 750, 420, 382, 389, 583, 622, 849, 852, 573, 182, 854, 249] The medial vestibular nucleus is connected with the homolateral abducens nucleus
and the contralateral medial rectus nucleus, while the superior
vestibular nucleus is connected with the homolateral medial rectus
(and possibly the contralateral abducens). Furthermore, the fibers
connecting the vestibular nucleus with the medial rectus muscle

course in the medial longitudinal fasciculus on the side of the muscle to be innervated (and possibly in the recticular substance).[660]

Destruction of the medial nuclei in man results in loss of the vestibulo-ocular reflexes,[176] while destruction of the lateral nuclei has no such effect.[1069, 917]

The foregoing represents the neural pathways for the tonic vestibulo-ocular pathways and for the slow phase of vestibular nystagmus. Considerable controversy exists about the origin and pathways for the *fast phase* of vestibular nystagmus. The suggestion that the impulses for the fast phase arise in the orbit[316] or muscle in the manner of a proprioceptive reaction[696, 68, 176, 503] is ruled out on several counts. There is no evidence of typical proprioceptive receptors in the extraocular muscles;[509] anesthetization of the nerves in the orbit[647, 566, 564] or elimination of the trigeminal nerve[599, 600, 479, 564] does not abolish the fast phase selectively; and action potentials from the 6th nerve give no indication of an afferent spike corresponding to the onset of the fast phase.[674] On the other hand, there is considerable evidence that the fast phase is a *compensatory* movement and is not directly dependent on the vestibular stimulus. In some lower animals the fast phase is normally absent despite well developed labyrinths.[57] In the higher species the fast phase is never present without a preceding slow phase, and in certain physiologic and pathologic conditions it may be absent. Normally the fast phase is not present until some time after birth[117, 399] and in sleep or under the influence of a narcotic it disappears sooner than the slow phase. While the fast phase is not influenced by the will, it is influenced by visual stimuli. Thus, with slow rotation in the dark, the fast phase may occur belatedly[280] or not at all.[783] By the same token, the slow phase is especially conspicuous in the blind.[413]

The pathways in the central nervous system mediating the impulses for the fast phase of vestibular nystagmus are not the same as those for the slow phase. Their exact course is disputed. The two schools of thought are represented by those who base their conclusions on animal experimentation, where it is pointed out the slow and fast phase are present if only a small segment of the midbrain is intact, and those who draw their conclusions from clinical observations, where absence of the fast phase occurs with a variety of lesions. The former maintain that the fast phase is a low-order reflex not dependent on centers higher than the vestibular nucleus[74, 567, 566, 564] or reticular substance[660, 979] or other cell complexes between the ocular motor nuclei and the vestibular nuclei.[975] The latter believe that the fast phase is normally mediated through supravestibular centers.[40, 885, 60, 884,24]

Clinically, one obtains the impression that the impulses for the fast phase are mediated through the cerebrum. The difference in opinions may in part be due to a species difference, since it is known that the fast phase is influenced by vision, and vision is represented in the midbrain of animals whereas it is represented in the cerebrum of man. Furthermore, although the fast phase *is* present in animals after decerebration, the nystagmus is nevertheless altered. Hemidecerebration in animals reduces the vestibular nystagmus to the opposite side[174] (or increases it on the same side[870, 773]) and may even eliminate the fast phase altogether.[78] Absence of the fast phase occurs characteristically in man with pseudobulbar palsy, producing the peculiar automatic doll's eye motility (see p. 223). This clinical syndrome, together with the occasional experimental elimination of the fast phase in some animals by combined thalamic and cerebral lesions[1117] suggests that the fast phase is relayed through the basal ganglia.

The *cerebellum* is not essential for vestibular nystagmus. Experimental lesions of the cerebellum or ablation of the entire cerebellum do not prevent the vestibular reaction, nor do they necessarily produce a spontaneous nystagmus.[416] On the other hand, nystagmus is a common symptom of cerebellar disease in man. It is therefore possible that the cerebellar nystagmus is due to secondary pressure effects on the vestibular nuclei in the floor of the 4th ventricle rather than to primary disturbances within the cerebellum.[174]

The *superior colliculi* have little effect on vestibular nystagmus, although lesions in this region have been reported to produce a hyperexcitability of the labyrinth.[777, 983]

(d) **Clinical testing and significance of vestibular nystagmus.** Several techniques are commonly employed in the clinic for producing vestibular nystagmus.

Rotation. The subject is rotated with his eyes closed in a revolving chair at a uniform rate, ten times in twenty seconds. The chair is abruptly stopped, the eyes are opened, and the time is noted, preferably with a stopwatch. After a latent period, which in the normal subject is ten to 15 seconds, nystagmus develops and persists for twenty to 50 seconds. Increased excitability of the labyrinth is manifest by a shorter latent period before the onset of nystagmus and by a longer duration of the nystagmus once it has developed.

To study vestibular reactions in infants, it is more convenient to hold the patient over one's head and pivot about on one's heels, observing the infant's eyes during the rotation rather than watching for postrotary nystagmus.

The plane of the nystagmus is predetermined by having the patient's head in the appropriate position during the rotation. The resultant nystagmus accords with the general rule that the oscillations occur in the plane that was parallel to the ground during the rotation. Thus, horizontal nystagmus is produced by having the head erect during the rotation, rotary nystagmus by having the head bowed forward with chin on chest or with forehead on a rest, and vertical nystagmus by having the head inclined toward the shoulder in the direction of which the patient is being turned. Rotary and vertical nystagmus are less satisfactory to produce than horizontal nystagmus, because they do not last so long and because they are more apt to be accompanied by vertigo and nausea.

A curious response may be seen in patients with marked esotropia when rotated in such a way as would induce rotary nystagmus in the normal subject. Since the obliques act in the vertical plane when the eye is adducted, the esotropic eye shows a vertical nystagmus, while the fixing eye shows a rotary nystagmus.

The direction of the nystagmus, designated by the fast phase, is opposite the movement of the endolymph in the semicircular canals. In the case of postrotary nystagmus, therefore, the nystagmus is in the direction opposite to that in which the head is rotated. The nystagmus also becomes coarser and consequently more striking the more the slow phase is opposed. That is, the nystagmus is maximal on looking in the direction of the rotation.

By rotation, the corresponding semicircular canals of the two labyrinths are not stimulated equally. In the case of the horizontal semicircular canals, the labyrinth that is more strongly stimulated is that in which the movement of the endolymph is *toward* the ampulla. This means that for postrotary nystagmus, the right labyrinth is stimulated most strongly on rotation of the body to the left and, conversely, the left labyrinth is most strongly stimulated by rotation of the body to the right.

Visual fixation reduces the vestibular response. Postrotary nystagmus lasts longer if the eyes are closed during the rotation[744] and if some means is employed to prevent fixation when the eyes are opened after the rotation. For the latter purpose lenses are employed consisting of +20.00 spheres,[64] which serve to blur the patient's vision and at the same time provide magnification for the observer. To these glasses are sometimes added an illumination system that further blinds the subject and yet enhances visibility for the observer.[366] The sensitivity of the vestibular reaction is considerably increased by thus reducing the effect of visual fixation; some investigators have gone so far as to employ opaque contact glasses.[577]

The rotation technique is perhaps the most convenient method of testing vestibular function, but it has the disadvantage that it does not permit the testing of each labyrinth separately as do the other techniques.

Caloric irrigation. According to this method, the external auditory canal is irrigated with either hot or cold water. Usually, 5 to 10 ml. of water at 40 degrees F. (approximately the temperature of ice water) are used, but an alternate procedure of repeatedly filling the canal with 1 ml. of hot or cold water has been successfully used.[493] After a latent period of approximately twenty seconds a nystagmus develops that lasts one to two minutes.

Horizontal nystagmus is best produced by having the patient's head held backward at an angle of 60 degrees during the irrigation, or if he is in bed, by having the head raised about 30 degrees with a pillow. In this position the horizontal semicircular canals are vertical and therefore most suitable for the production of convection currents. Rotary nystagmus to one side may be elicited by irrigating the canal with the head bowed forward, and that to the other side by having the head inclined toward one shoulder. Pure vertical nystagmus cannot be elicited by irrigating the ears.

As in the rotation test, the direction of the nystagmus is opposite the movement of the endolymph, that is, the slow phase is
in the direction of the endolymph. Irrigation with cold water results in a horizontal nystagmus to the opposite side (with respect
to the fast phase), whereas irrigation with hot water results in a
nystagmus to the same side.

Galvanic stimulation. With this method one galvanic electrode
is placed on the mastoid and the indifferent electrode is placed
either on the opposite mastoid or in the patient's hand. A current
of 3 to 5 milliamperes is usually sufficient to elicit a reaction, which
consists of rotary and horizontal nystagmus.[535, 563] Unlike the other
types of stimulation, the position of the head makes no difference
in the plane of the nystagmus produced. Anodal stimulation produces a nystagmus to the opposite side, comparable to depressing
the function of the labyrinth; cathodal stimulation produces a nystagmus to the same side, comparable to excitation.

While the galvanic form of stimulation has been used on occasion, it does not have the general clinical usefulness that rotation and caloric irrigation have, since its stimulation involves the
entire labyrinth.

Compression and suction. When applied over a fistula connecting with the semicircular canals, compression and suction produce nystagmus comparable to stimulation and depression, respectively. This method has obviously little clinical applicability.

Nystagmus may be produced by either rotation or caloric irrigation in all normal mammals. In the human species the vestibular
response is not fully developed until some time after birth. In premature infants the slow phase only may be elicited,[62] and a real
nystagmus may not be elicitable for several months after birth.[1117]
At term only an abortive form of vestibular nystagmus is ordinarily
obtainable. With the development of the vestibular response before the development of visual fixation, the nystagmus is for some
time more evident than it is later when visual fixation develops.

In the normal adult, induced vestibular nystagmus is such a constant and reproducible reaction that when it is diminished or not
elicitable, one may assume there is a lesion in the vestibular end
organ or pathways.

Spontaneous vestibular nystagmus from lesions of the end organ can usually be differentiated from that with lesions of the vestibular nuclei in the central nervous system by the following criteria:

1. Spontaneous *vertical* nystagmus when present is, with rare exceptions,[757, 736] indicative of disease of the central nervous system.[968, 339, 895, 37, 177, 528, 1060, 102] Lesions of the *labyrinth* produce horizontal or rotary nystagmus, and lesions of the *vestibular nuclei* produce horizontal, rotary, or vertical nystagmus. A latent vertical nystagmus with brain stem disease may occasionally be elicited simply by disrupting visual fixation. Thus it sometimes happens that vertical nystagmus is seen when the opticokinetic functions are being tested, even though the field is being rotated horizontally!

2. The *course* of the nystagmus is of significance. Nystagmus from *peripheral* lesions is maximal at the outset and improves in the course of the disease, not lasting more than a few weeks, whereas nystagmus from lesions of the *vestibular nuclei* remains static for considerable lengths of time or increases while under observation.

3. The coexistence of severe *vertigo, tinnitus,* and *deafness* is also indicative of lesions in the end organ or eighth nerve. With lesions of the central nervous system these abnormalities are relatively slight or absent.

The following are some of the more common pathologic states in man accompanied by a nystagmus that is presumably of the vestibular type:

Removal of one labyrinth either by disease or by surgery, results in a nystagmus lasting several days to weeks. The nystagmus is directed to the opposite side (in reference to the fast component) and is predominately horizontal. The slow component of the nystagmus is presumably due to the unopposed action of the remaining labyrinth; removal of both labyrinths simultaneously does not give rise to nystagmus. The nystagmus after unilateral labyrinthectomy gradually disappears; the subject with one remaining labyrinth then responds normally to rotation of the body[426] but the vestibular disturbance may be re-evoked by appropriate narcosis.[877]

If the second labyrinth is removed after compensation has taken place nystagmus develops just as though the first labyrinth were intact. This is called the *compensatory nystagmus of Becht-*

erew.[78] The nature of the compensating mechanism is unknown although it is assumed to be associated with an increased excitability of the vestibular nucleus on the side of the labyrinth that was first destroyed.[976, 973] Such an increased excitability is inferred from the fact that whereas no nystagmus occurs from cerebellar lesions in the presence of intact labyrinths, nystagmus occurs following cerebellar lesions made sometime after a labyrinthectomy.[949] In any case the visual reflexes play an important part in the development of the compensatory mechanism.[283]

Even when the loss of the labyrinth is compensated for so that nystagmus is no longer evident, one may still detect inaccuracies in ocular fixation during movements of the head.[265, 351, 256] With loss of both labyrinths (as from streptomycin) there is a characteristic blurring of vision during movements of the body; such patients complain of being unable to see well while riding on a bicycle or in a car.

Lesions of the labyrinth (labyrinthitis, Ménière's disease) are accompanied by rotary or horizontal nystagmus. They are characterized by precipitous onset with severe vertigo, nausea, and frequently tinnitus. There is also occasionally a vertical divergence of the eyes (skew deviation) with diplopia.[66] Illusory movement of the environment (oculogyral illusion) is a prominent symptom of disease of the semicircular canals whereas maintained disorientation in space (oculogravic illusion) is a symptom of disease of the otoliths.[427]

Involvement of the vestibular nerves or nuclei with consequent nystagmus is frequent in various lesions of the pons, medulla, and midbrain, although it is not always possible to differentiate involvement of the vestibular pathways from that of other pathways for conjugate movements. Spontaneous rotary nystagmus is, however, especially characteristic of lesions of the vestibular nuclei (although a combined horizontal and rotary nystagmus occurs occasionally with cerebral lesions). *Destructive* lesions involving the vestibular nuclei are said to produce a rotary nystagmus that has predominately the same direction of its oscillations irrespective of the direction of gaze and irrespective of vestibular stimulation. This is in contrast to lesions involving the vestibular nuclei by *pressure or traction* on the brain stem, where the direction of the nystagmus varies both with the direction of gaze and with vestibular stimulation.[318]

The lesions of the *central nervous system* that most frequently produce vestibular nystagmus are multiple sclerosis, vascular disease, encephalitis, Wernicke's disease, and lesions secondarily affecting the vestibular nuclei, such as expansive lesions of the cerebellum and of the cerebellopontine angle and compressive lesions such as platybasia and the Arnold-Chiari malformation.

Multiple sclerosis is accompanied by horizontal or rotary nystagmus in a large percentage of patients and less often by vertical nystagmus. The nystagmus is probably due to direct involvement of the vestibular nuclei and is not necessarily a manifestation of intention tremor, as was once asserted and is often reiterated. Illusory movement of the environment which in this connection is called oscillopsia is said to be characteristic of the nystagmus with multiple sclerosis.[158] When the medial longitudinal fasciculus is also involved, there results the highly characteristic syndrome of internuclear ophthalmoplegia (see p. 86f).

Syringobulbia, like multiple sclerosis, generally affects the floor of the 4th ventricle and is then characterized by a predominately rotary nystagmus.[50, 319]

The most frequent vascular lesion involving the vestibular nuclei with nystagmus is *thrombosis of the postero-inferior cerebellar artery* or of its branches. This results in nystagmus (usually rotary), unilateral cerebellar signs, and Horner's syndrome.

Encephalitis may cause horizontal, rotary, or vertical nystagmus. Nystagmus is especially common in the lethargic type of encephalitis but may also occur in the choreiform type.[365] It is frequently the last abnormality to disappear.

Alcoholism frequently causes vertical nystagmus with oscillopsia[102] along with other evidence of Wernicke's disease (6th nerve palsy, horizontal gaze paralysis, ataxia, and Korsakoff's psychosis).[224]

Incidental involvement of the vestibular nuclei is common with *cerebellar and cerebellopontine lesions. Cerebellar tumors and cerebellar abscesses* are especially apt to produce a nystagmus that varies with different positions of the head.[777] This postural nystagmus is said to be present in 80 per cent of tumors of the posterior fossa (cerebellum) and never to be found with tumors in the middle and anterior fossa (cerebrum). The nystagmus may be horizontal, vertical, or rotary. Postural nystagmus is also occasionally found with severe trauma.[936]

Cerebellopontine tumors regularly produce either horizontal or rotary nystagmus and rarely vertical nystagmus. The fast component is toward the side of the lesion.

Herniation of the brain stem through the foramen magnum in the entity of platybasia or in the Arnold-Chiari malformation may cause intermittent compression of the brain stem with consequent vertical nystagmus, palsies of conjugate gaze and hydrocephalus.[220]

With *lesions of the vestibular nerve or nuclei,* there is in addition to the spontaneous nystagmus an absence or reduction in the vestibular response on irrigation of the ears. Thus, vestibular responses are characteristically absent with tumors of the cerebellopontine angle[727] and either absent or impaired with intramedullary lesions of the brain stem.[625] There is also frequently hypesthesia of the cornea on the side of the lesion due to involvement of the mesencephalic root of the trigeminal nerve.[318]

Anomalous vestibular responses such as skew deviation may also occur on caloric irrigation of the ears in patients with brain stem lesions.[711]

Supranuclear lesions have varying effects on vestibular nystagmus. Cerebellar lesions may produce a vestibulbar nystagmus or alter the vestibular reactivity by pressure on the brain stem.[175] This nystagmus changes characteristically with different posture (see p. 203). It may also come and go spontaneously.

The numerous reports of alteration in the vestibular reactions hypoactivity or hyperactivity) by cerebral lesions have not been unanimous.[870, 899, 65, 139, 141, 296, 1124, 51] Especially noteworthy, however, is the occasionally reported absence of the fast phase of induced vestibular nystagmus with unilateral cerebral disease,[46, 884] especially with temporal lobe lesions.[297, 897] The fast phase of vestibular nystagmus and of opticokinetic nystagmus may both be absent.[40,1123]

An especially characteristic disturbance is not infrequently found wherein there is an absence of the fast phase of vestibular nystagmus, together with paralysis of voluntary conjugate gaze in one direction but retention of the slow phase (Roth-Bielschowsky

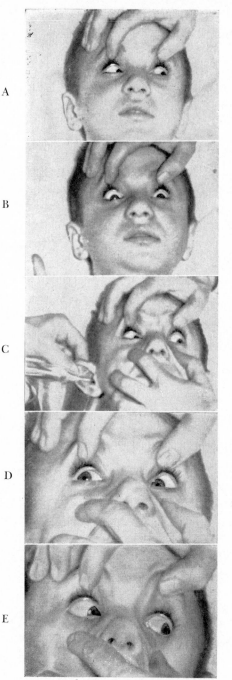

syndrome[887, 124, 994]). Furthermore, the slow phase on stimulation of the labyrinth (e.g., the labyrinth ipsilateral to the paralysis of voluntary conjugate gaze) is compulsory and cannot be voluntarily inhibited resulting in a fixation of gaze.[488] Thus, stimulation of one labyrinth by irrigation of the ear or rotation of the head causes the eyes to turn reflexly in the

← ◁◁◁

Fig. 86. *Patient with supranuclear lesion (pseudo-ophthalmoplegia) manifested by a spontaneous deviation of the eyes to the left at rest (A) and an inability to move the eyes to the right on voluntary effort (B), but on irrigating the ears with cold water (C) a deviation of the eyes to the extreme right after a latent period (D). With similar irrigation of the left ear, the eyes deviate to the extreme left (E) without developing nystagmus.*

The series of events represented in A-D shows that it is possible to have functioning connections between labyrinth and ocular motor nuclei with interruption in the connections between voluntary centers and the ocular motor nuclei. Further, the absence of the fast phase of vestibular nystagmus on irrigating the left ear (E) suggests that the pathways for the fast phase of vestibular nystagmus are associated with or identical with those for voluntary movement.

The site of the lesion was undetermined. The present condition followed a pulmonary lobectomy for bronchiectasis and is believed to have been due to a vascular thrombosis.

direction opposite that of the paralysis. Stimulation of the opposite labyrinth results in a full deviation of the eyes in the direction of the paralysis (Fig. 86). This preservation of ocular gaze on vestibular stimulation with its loss on voluntary and opticokinetic stimuli has been associated with pseudobulbar palsy, whence its name "pseudo-ophthalmoplegia"[1093] and has been likened to the automatic movements of doll's eyes, whence its descriptive name "doll's head" movements[930] (Figs. 10 and 60). It may be present in the horizontal or vertical directions of gaze. Few pathologic studies have been made on patients with this type of disturbance, but those that have been done and the symptoms (athetosis) accompanying others suggest that the responsible lesions are frequently in the basal ganglia or in the centripetal pathways from the cerebrum.

Poisoning with various substances may result in a spontaneous vestibular nystagmus or alter a nystagmus artificially produced. In general, analeptics increase the ease with which vestibular nystagmus may be induced and narcotics decrease it.[1139] The barbiturates are especially noteworthy in producing a *spontaneous* nystagmus of the vestibular type[561, 99, 878] (including vertical nystagmus) and on this account barbiturate poisoning often simulates multiple sclerosis. Dilantin and other anticonvulsants[103] may have similar effects.

3. Nystagmus from Neuromuscular Insufficiency

Nystagmus from neuromuscular insufficiency is a jerk type of nystagmus incorporating a varied group of cases having in common a deficiency in the maintenance of conjugate gaze to one or the other side owing to a defect in the muscle or in the nervous mechanism. The ocular disturbance varies from an inability to maintain conjugate gaze at the extremes (such as is frequently seen in otherwise normal individuals) to a gross paresis of conjugate gaze. When, as a result of the weakness of conjugate gaze, the eyes drift toward the primary position, there is a quick corrective movement bringing the eyes back to the point of fixation, and the repetition of this cycle makes up the nystagmus of neuromuscular insufficiency. The direction of the nystagmus is always toward the side of the gaze. More than any other, this type of nystagmus depends on attention; as soon as the attention is relaxed, the eyes drift away from their excentric position and nystagmus ceases.

This type of nystagmus is frequently present to a slight degree in otherwise normal persons at the limits of conjugate gaze (*Endstellungsnystagmus*), especially after prolonged gaze to the same[1035] or the opposite side.[776] It is increased in neurasthenia, myasthenia, various fatigue states and effort syndromes, and alcohol poisoning.[776] It is then usually present on gaze to either side and is symmetrical. Nystagmus of this type is also present with various cerebral lesions, especially with those of the frontal[769, 65, 776, 358, 407, 777, 1059] and occipital lobes, and with lesions of the subcortical centers for conjugate gaze.

When marked this type of nystagmus is a manifestation of paresis of conjugate gaze.[906] It is therefore found in the recovery states of palsies of conjugate gaze. Unlike nystagmus due to lesions of the vestibular nuclei, which is predominantly rotary, nystagmus of the neuromuscular insufficiency type is always horizontal or vertical, and the fast component is always in the direction of the paresis of conjugate gaze. With pontine lesions and cerebellopontine angle lesions the nystagmus is directed toward the side of the lesion (with reference to the fast component); with cerebral lesions it is to the opposite side, while with cerebellar lesions, especially with lesions of the vermis, the nystagmus is usually bilateral and is especially apt to be vertical.[318]

A peculiar type of eye movement has been described several times in the literature under the name of *nystagmus retractorius*.[582] This consists of irregular jerks of the eye backward into the orbit when the patient attempts to look in one or the other direction. It is usually associated with a paralysis of upward gaze and is caused by lesions in the midbrain, especially by lesions in the vicinity of the aqueduct of Sylvius.[128, 127] It is generally believed that the nuclei and tracts for the extraocular muscles are so compressed that a stimulus going to one portion of the nucleus stimulates all portions of the nucleus at the same time, and it has been suggested that the collective contraction of the recti, which are under voluntary control, elicits a retraction of the globes on any attempt to look upward, while the obliques, which allegedly do not receive voluntary innervation, are not stimulated.[308, 309, 598]

Another, and possibly related, type of movement is a convergence nystagmus. This, as the name implies, consists of a drift apart of the eyes with a quick convergent movement. Its pathogenesis is obscure as no substantial series of cases has been studied. It occurs frequently, however, with lesions in the anterior midbrain so that it is reasonable to assume it involves the convergence centers in the superior colliculi or in Perlia's nucleus. In any case, it is a rare occurrence and, in our present state of knowledge, has little clinical importance.

4. Congenital Nystagmus

Congenital nystagmus of the jerk type is not clearly differentiated from the pendular variety. It consists of a rapid and fine nystagmus the oscillations of which are either pendular or difficult to distinguish from the pendular type in one position of gaze but become converted into the jerk type on deviation to either side. The position of election for the eyes may be the primary position or an excentric position where the eyes show the least nystagmus. To either side of the position of election a relatively coarse nystagmus develops, with the fast phase toward the direction of gaze. The nystagmus is usually much coarser to one side than to the other, and the vision is best when the eyes are in such a position that the nystagmus is least.

Characteristic of this type of nystagmus is a defect in the opticokinetic response and frequently a turning of the head so that the eyes are in the position of least nystagmus. The opticokinetic response may be absent or defective on rotation of the drum to one side only. The vertical opticokinetic responses are normal.

The cause of congenital nystagmus is obscure. In most cases it appears to bear no relation to trauma incident to birth. In some cases it is obviously inherited, being transmitted as a dominant or sex-linked recessive characteristic.[1062, 132] In the majority of cases, however, there is no known history of inheritance. Frequently several siblings are affected without known involvement of the parents, suggesting a recessive type of inheritance. Rarely other types of heredofamilial disease are present within the same family.[1062]

Not infrequently other ocular abnormalities are present in patients with congenital nystagmus. Astigmatism[455] and convergent strabismus[1100] are common. Vestibular responses are frequently anomalous. By the usual methods of testing, the labyrinths are often found to be hypoactive.[455] Rotation to one side often causes a normal response, while rotation to the opposite side causes the nystagmus to cease.

The nystagmus is usually noted during the first few months of life. It is usually horizontal but may be rotary. It is never vertical. It is not usually associated with head nodding but is frequently accompanied by wry positions of the head, hence it is not easily differentiated from spasmus nutans. Unlike the latter, however, congenital nystagmus is present soon after birth, persists throughout life,[248] and affects the two eyes conjugately.

5. Latent Nystagmus

Latent nystagmus is a jerk type of nystagmus that is brought out by covering one eye. When both eyes are open and a clear image is present in both eyes, no nystagmus is present but covering one eye, blurring the image of one eye, or reducing the image brightness in one eye results in a conjugate nystagmus made up of a slow drift of the eyes toward the side of the covered eye, with a fast corrective phase toward the side of the open eye. The nystagmus is least when the gaze is directed toward the side of the covered eye and greatest when the gaze is directed toward the side of the open eye. It is usually present bilaterally, but cases have been reported in which it is elicited on the covering of one eye only.[372, 373, 281]

Contrary to the general impression, it is not the disruption of binocular fixation that gives rise to the nystagmus, since it is frequently seen in patients with strabismus,[475, 474] and a 15 degree prism placed before one eye so as to produce vertical diplopia does not necessarily cause nystagmus.* A $+8.00$ sphere[281] or a graded photometric wedge will, however, bring out the nystagmus, and in the latter case it is at times possible to demonstrate a correspondence between the magnitude of nystagmus and the amount of darkening of the image. Furthermore, the nystagmus may be brought out merely by shining a bright light in one eye,[208] and the resultant nystagmus is in the same direction as though the eye were being covered. Thus, it appears that latent nystagmus is brought about by making the image brightness or distinctness in the two eyes unequal rather than simply by disrupting binocular fixation.

Latent nystagmus is typically horizontal and is usually not accompanied by other abnormalities, although strabismus, monocular amblyopia, and so-called alternating hyperphoria (occlusion

---

* Personal observation; not in accord with the observations of Clarke.[208]

hypertropia) have been reported with it.[1045, 14] The presence of latent nystagmus is frequently unknown to the patient and is first detected by the ophthalmologist in trying to test the vision of each eye separately. The refraction of such patients can be determined only by obstructing macular perception of one eye, as by holding a pencil in front of it, while testing the other eye.[1053] The peripheral vision usually suffices to prevent the latent nystagmus from developing.

Loss of one eye in patients with latent nystagmus results in nystagmus of the other eye[786] either permanent or with periodic spontaneous recurrences.[281]

No satisfactory explanation of all the manifestations of latent nystagmus has been forthcoming.[970] The suggestion that it is due to a bilateral weakness of the lateral recti [323, 1086] is not consistent with the absence of any conspicuous esophoria in these cases. Whatever is the true explanation for latent nystagmus, it is as though the image of each eye in these cases exerted a tonic effect, tending to turn the eyes to the contralateral side. With both eyes open these symmetrical effects balance each other, but occluding one eye or diminishing the image brightness of one eye releases the tonic effect of the other eye, with consequent drifting of the eyes toward the side of the covered eye. When this is followed by the quick corrective component in the opposite direction, the cycle of nystagmus is present. Elaborations of this hypothesis have previously been suggested to account for latent nystagmus.[474, 553, 544]

SUMMARY

At rest, tonic impulses to the eyes arise symmetrically in the two halves of the central nervous system, the two labyrinths, and the two retinas. A unilateral disturbance of these tonic centers results in a conjugate deviation of the eyes in one direction. If, to a continual turning of the eyes in one direction, resulting from an asymmetrical disturbance in tonus, there is added a corrective movement in the opposite direction, the composite cycle makes up the rhythmic oscillations known as *nystagmus*.

An illusion of movement of the environment may or may not occur with nystagmus. Illusory movement of the environment occurs on passive movements of the eyes and with certain low-order reflexes (vestibular reaction) when the cerebral visual centers do not expect displacement of the image on the retina.

Nystagmus is divided into a *pendular* type, in which the oscillations are approximately equal in amplitude in the two directions, and a *jerk* type, in which the excursions in one direction are consistently more rapid than those in the opposite direction.

Pendular nystagmus is associated with loss of central vision. It is believed to be due to the failure of the normal dampening tone that presumably comes from the maculas. In so far as the macular impulses perform for the extraocular muscles the same function as proprioceptive impulses do for other skeletal muscles, pendular nystagmus may be considered a true ataxia of the eyes.

Pendular nystagmus occurs with macular lesions that are congenital (albinism, aniridia, and total color blindness) or are acquired in infancy (bilateral central chorioretinitis), or when the macula although present is not used for long periods (miners' nystagmus). It also occurs with opacities of the media (corneal scars, cataracts) in early life and with other conditions in which the pathogenesis is not known (spasmus nutans and hereditary nystagmus).

Jerk nystagmus is that type of rhythmic oscillations of the eyes in which the movements in one direction are consistently more rapid than those in the opposite direction. It is named according to the direction of the fast component.

Opticokinetic nystagmus is a jerk-type nystagmus that occurs in all normal individuals while looking at a continuously moving panorama. The slow phase is a following reaction mediated through the visual centers. The fast phase is a corrective movement bringing the eyes back to their original position and is presumably mediated through the higher cortical centers.

The opticokinetic response is abnormal when the nystagmus fails to occur on looking at a continuously moving field or when there is considerable asymmetry in the ocular response elicited by moving the field in one direction as compared with that on moving it in the opposite direction. With cerebral lesions, particularly with lesions in the posterior half of the cerebrum, there is absence or easy fatigability of the opticokinetic nystagmus on rotating the drum *toward* the side of the lesion. With brain stem lesions the defect in opticokinetic response is more apt to be bilateral and therefore has less localizing value. In either case the presence or absence of the opticokinetic nystagmus bears no constant relation to hemianopsia.

Vestibular nystagmus has a relatively slow phase in one direction, induced by the labyrinth, and a fast corrective phase in the opposite direction. The direction of the nystagmus may be horizontal, vertical, or rotary. The stimulus for vestibular nystagmus arises in the semicircular canals and is conditioned by change in rate of movement (acceleration or deceleration). The direction of the slow component corresponds to the displacement of the endolymph. The otoliths in the utriculus, but probably not in the sacculus, control static position of the eyes but do not produce nystagmus. The impulses from each labyrinth exert a tonic effect at rest, tending to turn and tort the eyes to the opposite side. Normally, the effects from the two labyrinths balance one another.

The impulses producing the slow phase of vestibular nystagmus are medicated through nuclei in the floor of the 4th ventricle, from whence they go to the ocular motor nuclei. The origin and pathways serving the fast corrective phase of vestibular nystagmus are not known, but presumably they are represented higher in the central nervous system than are those for the slow phase, since the fast phase develops later in the infant and may be selectively abolished in narcosis and in the various supranuclear lesions of the brain.

Vestibular nystagmus may be produced artifically by rotation of the body, caloric irrigation of the ears, compression and suction applied to the semicircular canals through a fistula, and galvanic stimulation of the labyrinth or vestibular nerve. Since vestibular nystagmus is a reliable reflex response, abnormalities of it have considerable localizing significance in labyrinthine and brain stem lesions. With peripheral end organ disease, spontaneous nystagmus occurs in a horizontal and rotary direction, accompanied by considerable vertigo. With brain stem lesions, the spontaneous nystagmus may be not only horizontal and rotary but vertical as well and is usually not accompanied by any marked vertigo. Supranuclear lesions are characterized by selective absence of the fast phase of vestibular nystagmus.

Other types of jerk nystagmus are nystagmus with *neuromuscular insufficiency* due to weakness of the ocular motor mechanism, *congenital* nystagmus, which is frequently familial, and *latent* nystagmus, which is elicited by occluding one eye.

REFERENCES

1. ABDON, N. O., AND HAMMARSKJÖLD, S. O.: Is any free acetylcholine preformed in resting muscles or in heart? *Acta physiol. scandinav., 8:75,* 1944.
2. ADAMS, R. D.: Occlusion of the anterior inferior cerebellar artery. *Arch. Neurol. Psychiat., 49:765,* 1943.
3. ADAMS, R. D., HAKIM, S., AND DREYFUSS, P.: To be published.
4. ADAMSON, J.: A study of the cyclo-rotational powers of the eyes. *Tr. Optical Soc., London, 33:189,* 1932. Abs. *Zentralbl. ges. Ophth., 28:292,* 1933.
5. ADAMÜK, E.: Ueber Innervation der Augenbewegungen. *Centralbl. med. Wissensch., 12:65,* 1870. Abs. *Jahresb. Ophth., 1:158,* 1870.
6. ADIE, W. J.: Argyll-Robertson pupils true and false. *Brit. M. J., 2:136,* 1931.
7. ADIE, W. J.: Tonic pupils and absent tendon reflexes: A benign disorder sui generis; its complete and incomplete forms. *Brain, 55:89,* 1932.
8. ADLER, F. H.: Effect of anoxia on heterophoria and its analogy with convergent concomitant squint. *Arch. Ophth., 34:227,* 1945.
9. ADLER, F. H.: Physiologic factors in differential diagnosis of paralysis of superior rectus and superior oblique muscles. *Arch. Ophth., 36:661,* 1946.
10. ADRIAN, E. D.: Afferent areas in cerebellum connected with limbs. *Brain, 66: 289,* 1943.
11. ALEXANDER: Labyrinthogene Neurasthenie. *München. med. Wchnschr., 29: 1689,* 1910.
12. ALPERS, B. J.: Partial paralysis of upward gaze. *Confinia neurol., 5:1,* 1942.
13. ALPERS, B. J. AND YASKIN, J. C.: Gliomas of the pons, clinical and pathologic characteristics. *Arch. Neurol. & Psychiat., 41:435,* 1939.
14. ANDERSON, J. R.: Latent nystagmus and alternating hyperphoria. *Brit. J. Ophth., 38:217,* 1954.
15. ANDRÉ-THOMAS, AND SCHAEFFER, H.: Syndrome de Parinaud incomplet. Paralysie des inférogyres avec hypertonie du releveur de la paupière supérieure. *Rev. oto-neuro-opht., 10:275,* 1932. Abs. *Zentralbl. ges. Ophth., 28:235,* 1933.
16. ANTON, G.: Beiderseitige Erkrankung der Scheitelgegend des Grosshirns. *Wien. klin. Wchnschr., 48:1899.* Abs. *Jahresb. Ophth., 30:468,* 1899.
17. APTER, J. T.: Projection of retina on superior colliculus of cats. *J. Neurophysiol., 8:123,* 1945.
18. APTER, J. T.: Eye movements following strychninization of the superior colliculi of cats. *J. Neurophysiol., 9:73,* 1946.
19. ARIËNS KAPPERS, C. U.: *Die Vergleichende Anatomie des Nervensystems der Wirbeltiere und des Menschen.* Haarlem, D. E. F. Bohn, 1920, 620 pp.
20. ARING, C. D., AND MERRITT, H. H.: Differential diagnosis between cerebral hemorrhage and cerebral thrombosis; clinical and pathologic study of 245 cases. *Arch. Int. Med., 56:435,* 1935.
21. ARKIN, W.: Ueber den optomotorischen (Eisenbahn-) Nystagmus und seine Anwendung der Neurologie. *Klinika Oczna, 5:191,* 1927. Abs. *Zentralbl. ges. Ophth., 19:862,* 1928.
22. ARKIN, W. AND STERTING, W. Ueber einäugigen Nystagmus. *Neurologia polska, 8:33,* 1925. Abs. *Zetralbl. ges. Ophth., 16:545,* 1926.

23. Asher, H.: Stimulus to convergence in normal and asthenopic subjects. *Brit. J. Ophth., 36:*666, 1952.

24. Asratian, E.: Cited by Graybiel, A., and Niven, J. I., Reference 426.

25. Aubineau, E., and Baron, F.: Le syndrome de Parinaud post-traumatique. *Rev. oto-neuro-opht., 18:*138, 1946.

26. Bach, K.: Die Prüfung des optokinetischen Nystagmus zur Entlarvung einer Scheinblindheit. *Klin. Wchnschr., 2:*1505, 1935.

27. Bach, L.: Experimentelle Untersuchungen und Studien über den Verlauf der Pupillar- und Sehfasern, nebst Eröterungen über die Physiologie und Pathologie der Pupillarbewegung. *Deutsche Ztschr. Nervenh., 17:*428, 1900.

28. Bach, L.: Ueber das Verhalten der motorischen Kerngebiete nach Läsion der peripheren Nerven und über die physiologische Bedeutung der Edinger-Westphalschen Kerne. *Centralbl. Nervenh. u. Psychiat., 29:*140, 1906.

29. Bacq, Z. M., and Weekers, R.: Alterations pupillaires provoquées par la diathermie du corps ciliaire et par l'injection orbitaire d'alcohol. Essais d'interprétation. *Bull. Acad. roy. Méd. Belgique, 14:*379; *14:*489, 1949.

30. Bailey, P., and von Bonin, G.: *The Isocortex of Man.* Urbana, Illinois, Univ. of Illinois Press, 1951.

31. Bakker, A.: Eine fluchtige, doch merkwurdige, Unfallfolge nach einer ortlichen Kontusion des Augapfels. *Ophthalmologica, 101:*364, 1941.

32. Balint, R.: Seelenlähmung des "Schauens," optische Ataxie, räumliche Störung der Aufmerksamkeit. *Monatsschr. Psychiat. u. Neurol., 25:*51, 1909.

33. Ballance, C. A.: *Some Points in the Surgery of the Brain and Its Membranes.* London, Macmillan, 1907, 405 pp.

34. Bárány, R. Augenbewegungen durch Thoraxbewegungen ausgelöst. *Centralbl. Physiol., 20:*298, 1907.

35. Bárány, R.: Latente deviation der Augen und Vorbeizeigen des Kopfes bei Hemiplegie und Epilepsie. *München. med. Wchnschr., 16:*900, 1913.

36. Bárány, R.: Cited by R. Cords. Die Ergebnisse der neueren Nystagmusforschung. *Zentralbl. ges. Ophth., 9:*369, 1923.

37. Bárány, R.: Cited by W. Klestadt. Symptomatologie der Erkrankungen des N. VIII einschliesslich Leitung im Hirnstamm, in *Handbuch der Neurologie,* edited by O. Bumke and O. Forester. Berlin, J. Springer, 1936, vol. 4, p. 359.

38. Bárány, R.: Die Nervösen Störungen des Cochlear- und Vestibularapparates, in *Handbuch der Neurologie,* edited by M. H. Lewandowsky. Berlin, J. Springer, 1910, vol. 1, p. 919.

39. Bárány, R.: Ueber einige Augen- und Halsmuskelreflexe bei Neugeborene. *Acta oto-laryng., 1:*97, 1918.

40. Bárány, R.: Die Untersuchung der reflektorischen vestibulären und optischen Augenbewegungen und ihre Bedeutung für die topische diagnostik der Augenmuskellähmungen. *München. med. Wchnschr., 54:*1072 and 1132, 1907.

41. Bárány, R.: Untersuchungen über die Funktion des Flocculus am Kaninchen. *Jahrb. Psychiat. u. Neurol., 36:*631, 1914.

42. Bárány, R.: Verbesserter Apparat zur Untersuchung der Gegenrollung der Augen und des Nystagmus. *Acta oto-laryng., 8:*25, 1925. *Zentralbl. ges. Ophth., 16:*478, 1926.

43. Bárány, R.: Zur Klinik und Theorie des Eisenbahnystagmus. *Acta oto-laryng., 3:*260, 1920.

44. BÁRÁNY, R., VOGT, C., AND VOGT, O.: Zur reizphysiologischen Analyse der corticalen Augenbewegungen. *J. Psychol. u. Neurol., 30:*87, 1923, Abs. *Zentralbl. ges. Ophth., 12:*397, 1924.

45. BARD, L.: De l'origine sensorielle de la déviation conjugée des yeux avec rotation de la tête chez les hémiplégiques. *Semaine méd., 24:*9, 1904. Abs. *Jahresb. Ophth., 35:*438, 1904.

46. BARD, L.: Du nystagmus artificiel chez les hémiplégiques le nystagmus à rebours. *Rev. Neurol., 36* (1):179, 1929.

47. BARDRAM, M. T.: Oculomotor pareses and nonparetic diplopia in pituitary adenomata. *Acta ophth., 27:*225, 1949.

48. BARKAN, O.: Pupillometer and keratometer cards. *Am. J. Ophth., 32:*267, 1947.

49. BARON AND SOUDET: Scoliose d'origine oculaire. *Rev. oto-neuro-opht., 24:*181, 1952.

50. BARRÉ, J. A.: Essai sur les syndromes topographiques des voies vestibulaires centrales de l'homme. *Rev. oto-neuro-opht., 15:*353, 1937.

51. BARRÉ, J. A.: Les troubles vestibulaires dans l'hypertension cranienne. II. *Rev. oto-neuro-ocul., 4:*241, 1926. Abs. *Zentralbl. ges. Ophth., 17:*678, 1927.

52: Barris, R. W.: A pupillo-constrictor area in the cerebral cortex of the cat and its relationship to the pretectal area. *J. Comp. Neurol., 63:*353, 1936.

53. BARRIS, R. W., INGRAM, W. R., AND RANSON, S. W.: Optic connections of the diencephalon and midbrain of the cat. *J. Comp. Neurol., 62:*117, 1935.

54. BARTELS, M.: Aufgaben der vergleichenden Physiologie der Augenbewegungen. *Arch. f. Ophth., 101:*299, 1920.

55. BARTELS, M.: Auge und Ohr (Die Ohr-Augen-Bewegungen.), in *Kurzes Handbuch der Ophthalmologie,* edited by F. Schieck and A. Brückner. Berlin, J. Springer, 1930, vol. 3, p. 652.

56. BARTELS, M.: Augenerscheinungen bei der sog. Encephalitis lethargica. *Klin. Monatsbl. Augenh., 65:*64, 1920(2).

57. BARTELS, M.: Beobachtungen an Wirbeltieren und Menschen über unwillkürliche Augenbewegungen bei Störungen des Sehens. *Klin. Monastbl. Augenh., 78:*478, 1927(1).

58. BARTELS, M.: Beobachtungen an Wirbeltieren und Menschen über unwillkürliche Augenbewegungen bei Störungen des Sehens. Mitteilung 2: *Beobachtungen an Menschen. Klin. Monatsbl. Augenh., 80:*145, 1928(1).

59. BARTELS, M.: Ophthalmostatik und Ophthalmokinetik. *Arch. f. Ophth., 118:* 270, 1927.

60. BARTELS, M.: Die Reflexbahnen für die Ohr- Augenbewegungen. *Arch. f. Ophth., 117:*538, 1926.

61. BARTELS, [M.]: Sehnervendurchschneidung und Dunkelzittern. *Ber. ü. d.* 44 *Zusammenkunft deutsch. ophth. Gesellsch., Heidelberg, 44:*21, 1924.

62. BARTELS, [M.]: Ueber Augenbewegungen bei Neugeborenen. *Deutsche med. Wchnschr., 58:*1477, 1932(2).

63. BARTELS, M.: Ueber die Gegend des Deiters- und Bechterew-Kernes bei Vögeln. *Ztschr. ges. Anat.,* pt. 1, *Ztschr. Anat. u. Entwicklungsgesch., 77:*726, 1925.

64. BARTELS, M.: Ueber Drehnystagmus mit und Ohne Fixation. *Arch. f. Ophth., 110:*426, 1922.

65. BARTELS, M.: Ueber kortikale Augenabweichungen und Nystagmus sowie über das motorische Rindenfeld für die Augen- und Halswender. *Klin. Monatsbl. Augenh., 62:*673, 1919(1).

66. BARTELS, M.: Ueber Regulierung der Augenstellung durch den Ohrapparat. II. (Weitere Mitteilung.) Schielen und Ohrapparat. *Arch. f. Ophth., 77:*531, 1910.

67. BARTELS, M.: Ueber Regulierung der Augenstellung durch den Ohrapparat. Mitteilung III. Kurven des Spannungszustandes einzelner Augenmuskeln durch Ohrrreflexe. *Arch. f. Ophth., 78:*129, 1911.

68. BARTELS, M.: Ueber willkürliche und unwillkürliche Augenbewegungen. (Nystagmus der Blinden, Proprioreflexe, Blickbewegungen der Tiere.) *Klin. Monatsbl. Augenh., 53:*358, 1914(2).

69. BARTELS, M.: Vergleichendes über Augenbewegungen, in *Handbuch der normalen und pathologischen Physiologie,* edited by A. Bethe, G. v. Bergmann, G. Embden, and A. Ellinger. Berlin, J. Springer, 1931, vol. 12, pt. 2, p. 1113.

70. BARTELS, M.: Zur Lage de Seitenwenderbahnen in der Brücke. *Klin. Monatsbl. Augenh., 75:*61, 1925(2).

71. VON BASEDOW, C.: Exophthalmus durch Hypertrophie des Zellgewebes in der Augenhöhle. *Wchnschr. ges. Heilk., 6:*197, 1840.

72. BASSENGE, W. L.: Ein Verfahren zur akustischen Registrierung des Nystagmus. *Klin. Monatsbl. Augenh., 113:*173, 1948.

73. BAUDOUIN, A., FISCHGOLD, H., CAUSSE, R., AND LERIQUE, J.: Une vielle notion trop oubliée: La différence de potentiel rétino-cornéenne. Son intérét théorique et pratique. *Bull. Acad. méd., 121:*688, 1939.

74. BAUER, J., AND LEIDLER, R.: Ueber den Einfluss der Ausschaltung verschiedener Hirnabschnitte auf die vestibulären Augenreflexe. *Arb. neurol. Inst. Wien. Univ., 19:*155, 1911-1912.

75. BEATTIE, J., BROW, G. R., AND LONG, C. N. H.: Physiological and anatomical evidence for the existence of nerve tracts connecting the hypothalmus with spinal sympathetic centers. *Proc. Roy. Soc., s. B., London, 106:*253, 1930.

76. BEATTIE, J., DUEL, A. B., AND BALLANCE, C.: The effects of stimulation of the hypothalamic pupillo-dilator center after successful anastomoses between the cervical sympathetic and certain motor nerves. *J. Anat., 66:*283, 1932.

77. VON BECHTEREW, W.: Cited by H. Oloff and H. Korbsch. Ueber das Hertwig-Magendiesche Phänomenon (Vertikaldivergenz der Augen). *Klin. Monatsbl. Augenh., 77:*618, 1926(2).

78. VON BECHTEREW, W.: Durchschneidung des nervus acusticus. *Arch. ges. Physiol., 30:*312, 1883.

79. VON BECHTEREW, W.: *Les Fonctions Nerveuses. Les Fonctions Bulbo-medullaires.* I. Paris, O. Dion, 1909, 372 pp.

80. VON BECHTEREW, W.: Die *Funktionen der Nervencentra.* Vol. 2. Mittelhirn, Zwischenhirn und subkortikale Ganglien. Jena, G. Fischer, 1909, [373] pp.

81. VON BECHTEREW, W.: Ueber das corticale Sehcentrum. *Monatsschr. Psychiat. u. Neurol., 10:*432, 1901.

82. VON BECHTEREW, W.: Ueber die Lage der motorischen Centra in der Hirnrinde des Menschen, auf Grund der Resultate der Reizung desselben vermittelst des faradischen Stromes bei Reizung am Gehirn. Neurolog. Westnik., VII 3. p. 1. Abs. *Jahresb. Ophth., 31:*443, 1900.

83. BEEVOR, C. E., AND HORSLEY, V.: A further minute analysis by electrical stimulation of the so-called motor region of the cortex cerebri in the monkey. *Phil. Tr. Roy. Soc., London, 179:*205, 1888.

84. BEEVOR, C. E., AND HORSLEY, V.: On the pallio-tectal or cortico-mesencephalic system of fibres. *Brain, 25:*436, 1902.

85. BEEVOR, C. E., AND HORSLEY, V.: A record of the results obtained by electrical stimulation of the so-called motor cortex and internal capsule in the Orang-Outang (Simia Satyrus). *Phil. Tr. Roy. Soc., s. B., London, 181:*129, 1890.

86. BEHR, C.: Die Erkrankungen der Augennerven, in Kurzes *Handbuch der Ophthalmologie,* edited by F. Schieck and A. Brückner. Berlin J. Springer, 1931, vol. 6, p. 156.

87. BEHR, C.: Hemianopische Pupillenstarre ohne homonyme Hemianopsie. *Ztschr. Augenh., 58:*398, 1926.

88. BEHR, C.: *Die Lehre von den Pupillenbewegungen.* Berlin, J. Springer, 1924, 225 pp. Abs. *Zentralbl. ges. Ophth., 13:*225, 1925.

89. BEHR, C.: Zur Diagnose und Symptomatologie der Erkrankungen in der Gegend der Fissura orbitalis superior und des Sinus cavernosus. *Klin. Monatsbl. Augenh., 71:*81, 1923(2).

90. BEHR, C.: Zur topischen Diagnose der Hemianopsie. *Arch. f. Ophth., 70:*340, 1909.

91. BEHR, K.: Die bedeutung der Pupillenströungen für die Herddiagnose der homonymen Hemianopsie und ihre Beziehungen zur Theorie der Pupillen-bewegung. *Deutsche Ztschr. Nervenh., 46:*88, 1912-1913.

92. BEHR, W.: Die Diphtherie. Bibliographie und neue Ergebnisse der Klinik und Forschung. *Ergebn. inn. Med. u. Kinderh., 52:*160, 1937.

93. BELINOFF, S.: Eine neue Methode der klinischen Anwendung des auropalpe-bralen Reflexes. *Monatsschr. Ohrenh., 52:*423, 1918.

94. BELLECCI, P.: Il nistagmo ottocinetico nella practica medico-legale. Ann. Med. Navale e Coloniale, *54:*450, 1949. Abs. Ophthamology Sect. XII, *Excerpta Medica, 4:*1207, 1950.

95. BENDER, M. B.: Contractions in denervated muscles induced by fright as evidence of secretion of a parasympathetic hormone. *J. Mt. Sinai Hosp., 5:*411, 1938.

96. BENDER, M. B.: Eyelid closure reaction. *Arch. Ophth., 29:*435, 1943.

97. BENDER, M. B.: The nerve supply to the orbicularis muscle and the physiology of movements of the upper eyelid; with particular reference to the pseudo-Graefe phenomenon. *Arch. Ophth., 15:*21, 1936.

98. BENDER, M. B.: Synkinetic pupillary phenomena and the Argyll-Robertson pupil. *Arch. Neurol. & Psychiat., 53:*418, 1945.

99. BENDER, M. B.: Effects of barbiturates on ocular movements (nystagmus). *Confinia neurol., 7:*144, 1946.

100. BENDER, M. B., AND ALPERT, S.: Abnormal ocular and pupillary movements following oculomotor paralysis; report of a case. *Arch. Ophth., 18:*411, 1937.

101. BENDER, M. B., AND FULTON J. F.: Functional recovery in ocular muscles of a chimpanzee after section of the oculomotor nerve. *J. Neurophysiol., 1:*144, 1938.

102. BENDER, M. B., AND GORMAN, W. F.: Vertical nystagmus on direct forward gaze with vertical oscillopsia. *Am. J. Ophth., 32:*967, 1949.

103. BENDER, M. B., NATHANSON, M., AND GREEN, M.: Effects of intravenous tolserol on normal and abnormal ocular movements (nystagmus). *Am. J. Ophth., 34:*579, 1951.

104. BENDER, M. B., AND SAVITSKY, N.: Paralysis of divergence. *Arch. Ophth., 23:*1046, 1940.

105. BENDER, M. B., AND WEINSTEIN, E. A.: Effects of stimulation and lesion of

median longitudinal fasciculus in the monkey. *Arch. Neurol. & Psychiat., 52:*106, 1944.

106. BENDER, M. B., AND WEINSTEIN, E. A.: Functional representation in oculomotor and trochlear nuclei. *Arch. Neurol. & Psychiat., 49:*98, 1943.

107. BENJAMIN, J. W.: The nucleus of the oculomotor nerve with special reference to innervation of pupil and fibers from the pretectal region. *J. Nerv. & Ment. Dis., 89:*294, 1939.

108. BENNETT, A. E.: Clinical investigations with curare in organic neurologic disorders. *Am. J. M. Sc., 202:*102, 1941.

109. BERGER, H.: Experimentelle Untersuchungen über die von der Sehsphäre aus ausgelöstern Augenbewegungen. *Monatsschr. Phychiat. u. Neurol. 9:*185, 1901.

110. BERL.: Einiges über die Beziehungen der Sehbahnen zu dem vorderen Zweihügel des Kaninchens. *Arb. neurol. Inst. Wien. Univ., 8:*308, 1902.

111. BERNHEIMER, S.: Experimentelle Studien zur Kenntnis der Bahnen der synergischen Augenbewegungen beim Affen und der Beziehungen der Vierhügel zu denselben. *Sitzungsb. Akad. Wissensch. Math.-naturw. Cl., 108:*229, 1899. Abs. *Jahresb. Ophth., 30:*6, 1899.

112. BERNHEIMER, S.: Experimentelle Studien zur Kenntnis der Innervation der inneren und Ausseren vom Oculomotorius versorgten Muskeln des Auges. *Arch. f. Ophth., 44:*481, 1897.

113. BERNHEIMER, S.: Weitere experimentelle Studien zur Kenntnis der Lage des Sphinkter- un der Levatorkerns. *Arch. f. Ophth., 70:*539, 1909.

114. BERNHEIMER, S.: Die Wurzelgebiete der Augennerven, ihre Verbindungen und ihr Anschluss an die Gehirnrinde. Graefe-Saemisch *Handbuch der Augenheilkunde,* 2 ed. Leipzig, W. Engelmann, 1900, pt. 1, vol. 1, chapter VI, p. 1.

115. BERRY, G. A.: Habit; as exemplified in the functional activity in the eye muscle. *Edinburgh M. J., 9:*399, 1912.

116. BERTELSEN, E., AND RÖNNE, H.: Ein Fall von Polioencephalitis mit assoziierter Blicklähmung supranuklearen Ursprunges. *Monatsschr. Psychiat u. Neurol., 25:*148, 1909.

117. BEST, F.: Die Augenveränderungen bei den organischen nichtenzündlichen Erkrankungen des Zentralnervensystems, in *Kurzes Handbuch der Ophthalmologie,* edited by F. Schieck and A. Brückner. Berlin, J. Springer, 1931, vol. 6. p. 531.

118. BEST, F.: Hemianopsie und Seelenblindheit bei Hirnverletzungen. *Arch. f. Ophth., 93:*49, 1917.

119. BEST, F.: Die vom Grosshirn ausgelösten gleichsinnigen Blickbewegungen. *Arch. f. Ophth., 144:*25, 1941.

120. BIANCHI, L.: The functions of the frontal lobes. *Brain, 18:*497, 1895.

121. BIANCHI, L.: *The Mechanism of the Brain and the Function of the Frontal Lobes.* New York, W. Wood, 1922, 348 pp.

122. BIELSCHOWSKY, A.: Discussion (p. 299) in N. P. Scala and E. A. Spiegel, The mechanism of optokinetic nystagmus. *Tr. Am. Acad. Ophth. 43:*277, 1938.

123. BIELSCHOWSKY, A.: Die einseitigen und gegensinnigen ("'dissoziierten") Vertikalbewegungen der Augen. *Arch. f. Ophth., 125:*493, 1930.

124. BIELSCHOWSKY, A.: Das klinische Bild der assoziierten Blicklähmung und

seine Bedeutung für die topische Diagnostik. *München. med. Wchnschr.,* 50:1666, 1903.

125. BIELSCHOWSKY, A.: Mitbewegungsphänomene bei Augenmuskellähmungen. *Deutsche med. Wchnschr., 36*:1348, 1910.

126. BIELSCHOWSKY, A.: Ueber einseitige bzw. nichtassoziierte Innervationen der Augenmuskeln. *Arch. ges. Physiol., 136*:658, 1910.

127. BIELSCHOWSKY, A.: Symptomatologie der Störungen im Augenbewegungsapparat, in *Handbuch der Neurologie,* edited by O. Bumke and O. Foerster. Berlin, J. Springer, 1936, vol. 4, p. 173.

128. BIELSCHOWSKY, A.: Ueber Retraktionbewegungen und andere ungewöhnliche Bewegungsphänomene der Augen. *Klin. Monatsbl. Augenh., 73*:577, 1924 (2).

129. BIELSCHOWSKY, A.: Ueber totale Rindenblindheit. *München. med Wchnschr.,* p. 2308, 1911(2). Abs. *Jahresb. Ophth., 42*:484, 1911.

130. BIEMOND, A.: Experimentellanatomische Untersuchungen über die corticofugalen optischen Verbindungen bei Kaninchen und Affen. *Ztschr. ges. Neurol. u. Psychiat., 129*:65, 1930.

131. BIETTI, G. B., and GIARDINI, A.: Influence of anoxia on ocular movements. II Comparison between the action of anoxia and of alcohol on the ocular muscular equilibrium. *Riv. med. aeronaut., 12*:198, 1949. Abs. Ophthalmology Sect. XII, *Excerpta Medica, 4*:887, 1950.

132. BILLINGS, M. L.: Nystagmus through 4 generations. *J. Hered., 34*:457, 1943.

133. BING, R.: *Gehirn und Auge. Kurzgefasste Darstellung der physiopathologischen Zusammenhange zwischen beiden Organen, sowie der Augensymptome bei Gehirnkrankheiten,* ed. 2. Munich, J. F. Bergmann, 1923, 88 pp. Abs. *Zentralbl. ges. Ophth., 11*:163, 1924.

134. BIRUKOW, G.: Untersuchungen über den optischen Drehnystagmus und über die Sehschärfe des Grasfrosches (Rana temporaria). *Ztschr. vergl. Physiol., 25*:92, 1937. Abs. *Zentralbl. ges. Ophth., 40*:461, 1938.

135. BISHOP, G. H., AND HEINBECKER, P.: A functional analysis of the cervical sympathetic nerve supply to the eye. *Am. J. Physiol., 100*:519, 1932.

136. BJÖRK, A., AND KUGELBERG, E.: The electrical activity of the muscles of the eye and eyelids in various positions and during movement. *Electroencephalog. & Clin. Neurophysiol., 5*:595, 1953.

137. BJÖRK, A., AND KUGELBERG, E.: Motor unit activity in the human extraocular muscles. *Ibid., 5*:271, 1953.

138. BLALOCK, A.: Thymectomy in treatment of myasthenia gravis. *J. Thoracic Surg., 13*:316, 1944.

139. BLOHMKE, A.: Beitrag zur Frage des Vorbeizeigens und seiner cerebralen Auslösung. *Ztschr. Hals-, Nasen- u. Ohrenh., 4*:366, 1922-23.

140. BLOHMKE, [A.]: Ueber das Verhalten des Dunkelnystagmus beim Hunde nach zentraler Vestibularausschaltung. Ber. ü. d. 46 *Zusammenkunft deutsch. ophth. Gesellsch., Heidelberg, 46*:444, 1927.

141. BLOHMKE, A.: Zur Diagnose von Hirntumoren. *Ztschr. Hals-, Nasen- u. Ohrenh., 6*:340, 1923.

142. BOEKE, J.: Die morphologische Grundlage der sympathischen Innervation der quergestreiften Muskelfasern. *Ztschr. mikr.-anat. Forsch., 8*:561, 1927.

143. VAN BOGAERT, L.: Sur des modalités exceptionnelles des crises oculogyres. 1. Crises de convergence au cours d'une forme myasthénique chez l'enfant. 2. Crises du regard direct avec rétropulsion et attitude décérébrée d'un

membre et syndrome d'obsessions sexuelles. 3. Crises oculogyres vers le bas seulement au cours d'une hémiplégie encéphalitique. *J. neurol. et psychiat., 28:*379, 1928. Abs. *Zentralbl. ges. Ophth., 20:*543, 1929.

144. BOLK, L.: *Das Cerebellum der Säugetiere; eine vergleichend anatomische Untersuchung.* Jena, G. Fischer, 1906, 338 pp.

145. BORRIES, G. V. T.: *Fixation und Nystagmus. Klinische, experimentelle und theoretische Studien.* Copenhagen, T. Linds, and Leipzig, K. F. Koehler, 1926, 112 pp. Abs. *Zentralbl. ges. Ophth., 17:*147, 1927.

146. BORRIES, G. V. T.: Fortgesetzte Untersuchungen über experimentellen optischen Nystagmus. *Hospitalstid., 66:*201, 1923. Abs. *Zentralbl ges. Ophth., 10:*298, 1923.

147. BORRIES, G. V. T.: Konvergenzspasmus und Labyrinthleiden. *Monatssch. Ohrenh., 60:*736, 1926. Abs. *Zentralbl. ges. Ophth., 17:*912, 1927.

148. BORS, E.: Ueber das Zahlenverhaltnis zwischen Nerven- und Muskelfasern. *Anat. Anz., 60:*415, 1925/26.

149. BORSOTTI, L.: Considerazioni sulla paralisi dell'abducente da puntura lombare. (A proposita di un insorto in seguito a puntura lombar in un malato di meningite cerebrospinale.) *Riv. otol. ecc., 15:*205, 1938. Abs. *Zentralbl. ges. Ophth., 42:*193, 1939.

150. BORSOTTI: Cited by Marrucci, L. La restituzione psichica del riflesso pupillare affaticato alla luce studiata col metado pupillografice di Lowenstein e Borsotti. *Ann. ottal. e clin. ocul., 72:*502, 1946.

151. BRAMWELL, E.: Etiology of recurrent ocular paralysis, including periodic ocular paralysis and ophthalmoplegic migraine. *Tr. Med. Chir. Soc. Edinburgh,* pp. 209, 1932/33: in *Edinburgh M. J.,* 1933.

152. BRAUN, G.: Ein neues Hemikinesimeter. *Klin. Monatsbl. Augenh., 87:*441, 1931(2).

153. BRAUN, G.: Ein neues Hemikinesimeter. *Klin. Monatsbl. Augenh., 88:*61, 1932(1).

154. BRECHER, G. A.: Optisch ausgelöste Augen- und Körperreflexe am Kaninchen. *Ztschr. vergl. Physiol., 23:*374, 1936. Abs. *Zentralbl. ges. Ophth., 37:*230, 1937.

155. BRECHER, G. A.: Die optokinetische Auslösung von Augenrollung und rotatorischem Nystagmus. *Arch. ges. Physiol., 234:*13, 1934.

156. BREMER, F.: Activité électrique du cortex cérébral dans les états de sommeil et de veille chez le chat. *Compt. rend. Soc. biol., 122:*464, 1936.

157. BREMER, L.: Ueber die Endigungen der markhaltigen und marklosen Nerven im quergestreiften Muskel. *Arch. mikr. Anat., 21:*165, 1882.

158. BRICKNER, R. M.: Oscillopsia; a new symptom commonly occurring in multiple sclerosis. *Arch. Neurol. & Psychiat., 36:*586, 1936.

159. BRISCOE, G.: Antagonism between curarine and prostigmine in myasthenia gravis. *Lancet, 1:*470, 1936.

160. BRISCOE, G.: Antagonism between curarine and acetylcholine. *J. Physiol., 87:* 425, 1936.

161. BROCA, A.: Un pupillometre. Abs. *Zentralbl. ges. Ophth., 14:*907, 1925.

162. BROUWER, B.: Klinisch-anatomische Untersuchung über den Oculomotoriuskern. *Ztschr. ges. Neurol. u. Psychiat., 40:*152, 1918.

163. BROUWER, B., and Zeeman, W. P. C.: The projection of the retina in the primary optic neuron in monkeys. *Brain, 49:*1, 1926.

164. BROWN, G. L., and Feldberg, W.: Action of potassium on superior cervical ganglion of cat. *J. Physiol., 86:*290, 1936.

165. BROWN, G. L., and HARVEY, A. M.: Neuro-muscular transmission in the extrinsic muscles of the eye. *J. Physiol., 99:*379, 1941.

166. BROWN, G. L., AND HARVEY, A. M.: Reactions of avian muscle to acetylcholine and eserine. J. Physiol., *94:*101, 1938.

167. BROWN, H. W.: Congenital paralysis of inferior oblique. *J. Michigan M. Soc., 50:*509, 549, 1951.

168. BROWN, [T.] GRAHAM: Die Grosshirnhemispheres, in *Handbuch der Normalen und Pathologischen Physiologie,* edited by A. Bethe, G. v. Bergmann, G. Embden, and A. Ellinger. Berlin, J. Springer, 1927, vol. 10, p. 418.

169. BROWN, T. GRAHAM: Reflex orientation of the optical axes and the influence upon it of the cerebral cortex. *Arch. néerl. physiol., 7:*571, 1922. Abs. *Zentralbl. ges. Ophth., 9:*159, 1923.

170. BROWNE, R. C.: Experimental nystagmus. *Lancet, 13:*721, 1951.

171. BRUCE, G. M.: Ocular divergence: its physiology and pathology. *Arch. Ophth., 13:*639, 1935.

172 BRÜCKNER, A.: Zur Kenntnis des sogenannten willkürlichen Nystagmus. *Ztschr. Augenh., 37:*184, 1917.

173. VON BRUNN, M.: Die Lumbalanästhesie. *Neue Deutsche Chirurgie, 29:*1, 1922.

174. BRUNNER, H.: Beiträge zur otologischen Diagnostik der Hirntumoren. XV. Ueber den Einfluss der corticalen Innervation auf den labyrinthären Nystagmus. *Monatsschr. Ohrenh., 70:*40, 1936. Abs. *Zentralbl. ges. Ophth., 36:*207, 1936.

175. BRUNNER, H.: Beiträge zur otologischen Diagnostik der Hirntumoren. XVI. Ergebnisse der calorischen Prüfung des labyrinthes bei Hirntumoren. *Monatsschr. Ohrenh., 70:*206, 1936. Abs. *Zentralbl. ges. Ophth., 37:*232, 1937.

176. BRUNNER, H.: Bemerkungen zum zentralen Mechanismus des vestibulären Nystagmus. *Monatsschr. Ohrenh., 53:*1, 1919.

177. BRUNNER, H.: Cited by W. Klestadt, Symptomatologie der Erkrankungen des N. VIII einschliesslich Leitung im Hirnstamm, in *Handbuch der Neurologie,* edited by O. Bumke and O. Foerster. Berlin, J. Springer, 1936, vol. 4, p. 359.

178. BRUNNER, H.: Demonstration des Drehschirmes zur Prüfung des experimentellen "optischen Nystagmus" und eines Patienten mit Inversion des "optischen" Nystagmus. *Monatsschr. Ohrenh., 56:*318, 1922.

179. BRUNNER, H.: Ueber die Inversion des experimentellen optischen Nystagmus. *Monatsschr. Ohrenh., 55:*574, 1921.

180. BRYCE-SMITH, R., AND MACINTOSH, R. R.: Sixth-nerve palsy after lumbar puncture and spinal analgesia. *Brit. M. J., 4701:*275, 1951.

181. BUCCIANTE, L.: Modalita delle inserzioni dei muscoli sul bulbo oculare nell uoma (ricerche statistiche). *Monitore zool. ital., 44:*Suppl., 246, 1933. Abs. *Zentralbl. ges. Ophth., 31:*735, 1934.

182. BUCHANAN, A. R.: Nystagmus and eye deviations in guinea pigs with lesions in the brain stem. *Laryngoscope, 50:*1002, 1940.

183. BUCHTHAL, F., AND LINDHARD, J.: Elektrostatische Messungen an einzelnen, motorischen Endplatten und Muskelfasern; Änderung der Potentialdifferenz bei Erregung und Kontraktion. *Skandinav. Arch. Physiol., 77:*224, 1937.

184. BUCKLEY, R. C.: Pontile gliomas; a pathologic study and classification of 25 cases. *Arch. Path., 9:*779, 1930.

185. BUCY, P. C., AND WEAVER, T. A., Jr.: Paralysis of conjugate lateral movement of the eyes in association with cerebellar abscess. *Arch. Surg., 42:*839, 1941.

186. BUMKE, O. C.: *Die Pupillenstörungen bei Geistes- und Nervenkrankheiten,* ed. 2. Jena, G. Fischer, 1911, 262 pp.

187. BURIAN, H. M., AND CAHILL, J. E.: Congenital paralysis of medical rectus muscle with unusual synergism of the horizontal muscles. *Tr. Am. Ophth. Soc., 50:*87, 1953.

188. BUTLER, T. H., AND WILSON, A. J.: Ocular paralyses following mumps. *Brit. M. J., 1:*752, 1937.

189. BUYS, E.: Un cas de nystagmus spontané dirigé aternativement vers la droite et vers la gauche. *J. neurol. et psychiat., 32:*715, 1932.

190. BYRNE, J. G.: *Studies on the Physiology of the Eye; Still Reaction, Sleep, Dreams, Hibernation, Repression, Hypnosis, Narcosis, Coma, and Allied Conditions.* London, H. K. Lewis, 1933, 428 pp.

191. CANNON, W. B., AND ROSENBLUETH, A.: *Autonomic Neuro-Effector Systems.* New York, Macmillan, 1937.

192. CARMICHAEL, E. A., DIX, M. A., AND HALLPIKE, C. S.: Lesions of the cerebral hemispheres and their effects upon optokinetic and caloric nystagmus. *Brain, 77:*345, 1954.

193. CARREA, R. M. E.: Physiologic effects of bilateral cerebellar removals in the primate. *Federation Proc., 5:*15, 1946.

194. Case Records of the Massachusetts General Hospital, Case 39451. *New England J. Med., 249:*776, 1953.

195. Case Records of the Massachusetts General Hospital, Case 37451. *New England J. Med., 245:*736, 1951.

196. CASTALDI, L.: Contributo allo studio dei nuclei degli oculomotori e dei tubercoli quadrigenelli. Nota prelim. *Boll. ocul., 1:*470, 1922. Abs. *Zentralbl. ges. Ophth., 9:*274, 1923.

197. CASTEN, V. G.: Isolated congenital absence of the inferior rectus muscle; report of two cases in which operation was performed. *Arch. Ophth., 24:*55, 55, 1940.

198. CHAMLIN, M., AND DAVIDOFF, L. M.: Divergence paralysis with increased intracranial pressure. Further observations. *Arch. Ophth., 46:*145, 1951.

199. CHARNWOOD: Effect of posture on involuntary eye movements. *Nature, 166:* 348, 1950.

200. CHODERA, J., AND SABATA, C. A.: Contribution to pupillometric methods. *Čas. Lek Čes., 98:*977, 1950. Abs., Ophthalmology Sect. XII, *Excerpta Medica 5:*725, 1951.

201. CILIMBARIS, P.: Histologische Untersuchungen über die Muskelspindeln der Augenmuskeln. *Arch. mikr. Anat., 75:*692, 1910. Abs. *Jahresb. Ophth., 41:*32, 1910.

202. CLAES, E.: Contribution à l'étude physiologique de la fonction visuelle. II. Étude des centres oculomoteurs corticaux chez le chat non anesthésie. *Arch. internat. physiol., 48:*238, 1939.

203. CLAES, E.: Contribution à l'étude physiologique de la fonction visuelle. III. Activités pupilo-motrices du diencéphale et du mésencéphale chez le chat non anesthésie. *Arch. internat. physiol., 48:*261, 1939.

204. CLAES, E.: Étude des relations fonctionnelles des cortex sensitifs visuel et auditif avec les regions oculomotrices corticales. *Compt. rend. Soc. biol., 127:*1116, 1938.

205. CLARK, G., AND LASHLEY, K. S.: Visual disturbances following frontal ablations in the monkey. *Anat. Rec., 97:*381, 1947.

206. CLARK, W. E. L.: A morphological study of the lateral geniculate body. *Brit. J. Ophth., 16:*264, 1932.

207. CLARK, W. E. L.: The visual centers of the brain and their connections. *Physiol. Rev., 22:*205, 1942.

208. CLARKE, E.: A rare form of nystagmus. *Tr. Ophth. Soc. U. Kingdom, 16:*327, 1896.

209. CLARKE, R. H.: Experimental stimulation of the cerebellum. *Brain, 49:*557, 1926.

210. COBB, S., AND SCARLETT, H. W.: A report of eleven cases of cervical sympathetic injury, causing the oculopupillary syndrome. *Arch. Neurol. & Psychiat., 3:*636, 1920.

211. COGAN, D. G.: Accommodation and the autonomic nervous system. *Tr. Sect. Ophth., A. M. A., 88:*189, 1937.

212. COGAN, D. G.: Unpublished.

213. COGAN, D. G.: The waltzing (circling) phenomenon in rabbits. *J. Comp. Psychol., 35:*111, 1943.

214. COGAN, D. G.: Waltzing guinea pigs with particular reference to ocular movements and righting reflexes. *Arch. Ophth., 24:*78, 1940.

215. COGAN, D. G.: A simplified entoptic pupillometer. *Am. J. Ophth., 24:*1431, 1941.

216. COGAN, D. G.: Neurologic significance of lateral conjugate deviation of the eyes on forced closure of the lids. *Arch. Ophth., 39:*37, 1948.

217. COGAN, D. G.: A type of congenital ocular motor apraxia presenting jerky head movements. *Tr. Am. Acad. Ophth., 56:*853, 1952.

218. COGAN, D. G.: Ocular dysmetria, flutter-like oscillations of the eyes, and opsoconus. *Arch. Ophth., 51:*318, 1954.

219. COGAN, D. G., AND ADAMS, R. D.: A type of paralysis of conjugate gaze (ocular motor apraxia.) *Arch. Ophth., 50:*434, 1953.

220. COGAN, D. G., AND BARROWS, L. J.: Platybasia and the Arnold-Chiari malformation. *Arch. Ophth., 52:*13, 1954.

221. COGAN, D. G., AND FREESE, C. G.: Spasm of the near reflex. *Arch. Ophth., 54:*752, 1955.

222. COGAN, D. G., KUBIK, C. S., AND SMITH, W. L.: Unilateral internuclear ophthalmoplegia: report of eight clinical cases with one post-mortem study. *Arch. Ophth., 44:*783, 1950.

223. COGAN, D. G., AND LOEB, D. R.: Optokinetic response and intracranial lesions. *Arch. Neurol. & Psychiat., 61:*183, 1949.

224. COGAN, D. G., AND VICTOR, M.: Ocular signs of Wernicke's disease. *Arch. Ophth., 51:*204, 1954.

225. COLLIER, J.: Nuclear ophthalmoplegia, with especial reference to retraction of the lids and ptosis and to lesions of the posterior commissure. *Brain, 50:*448, 1927.

226. COLLINS, E. T.: Hereditary ocular degenerations—"Ophthalmic Abiotrophies." *Internat. Cong. Ophthal.* (Washington, D.C.), p. 103, 1922.

227. COLSON, Z. W.: The effect of alcohol on vision. An experimental investigation. *J.A.M.A., 115:*1525, 1940.

228. COMBES, X.: Myosis et paralysis alterne. Paris thesis, 1903, 57 pp., No. 499.

229. CONSTANT, G. A., PORTER, E. L., ANDRONIS, A., AND RIDER, J. A.: The effect of thymus extracts on neuromuscular response. *Texas Rep. Biol. & Med., 7:*350, 1949.

230. CONTINO, F.: A new method for measuring the diameter of the pupil. *Rass. ital. ottal., 15:*450, 1946. Abs., Ophthalmology Sect. XII, *Excerpta Medica, 1:*904, 1947.

231. COOPER, S., AND DANIEL, P. M.: Muscle spindles in human extrinsic eye muscles. *Brain, 72:*1, 1949.

232. COOPER, S., DANIEL, P., AND WHITTERIDGE, D.: Cells of origin of proprioceptive fibers from eye muscles. *J. Physiol., 111:*25 (p), 1950.

233. COOPER, S., DANIEL, P., AND WHITTERIDGE, D.: Nerve impulses in the brain stem of the goat. Short latency responses obtained by stretching the extrinsic eye muscles and the jaw muscles. *J. Physiol., 120:*471, 1953.

234. COOPER, S., DANIEL, P., AND WHITTERIDGE, D.: Nerve impulse in the brain stem and cortex of the goat. Spontaneous discharges and responses to visual and other afferent stimuli. *J. Physiol., 120:*514, 1953.

235. COOPER, S., AND ECCLES, J. C.: Isometric responses of mammalian muscles. *J. Physiol., 69:*377, 1930.

236. COOPER, S., DANIEL, P., AND WHITTERIDGE, D.: Afferent impulses in the oculomotor nerve, from the extrinsic eye muscles. *J. Physiol., 113:*463, 1951.

237. COPPERS, A. C.: *An Introduction to Clinical Orbitonometry.* Leiden, H. E. Stenfert, 1948.

238. COPPOLA, L.: Paralisi del retto estérno sinistro consecutiva a rachianestesia, in soggetto con sfondo climaterico. *Riv. oto-neuro-oftal., 16:*448, 1939.

239. CORBIN, K. B., AND HARRISON, F.: Further attempts to trace origin of afferent nerves to extrinsic eye muscles. *J. Comp. Neurol., 77:*187, 1942.

240. CORBIN, K. B., AND OLIVER, R. K.: Origin of fibres to the grape-like endings in insertion third of the extraocular muscles. *J. Comp. Neurol., 77:*171, 1942.

241. CORDS, R.: Die Bedeutung des optomotorischen Nystagmus für die neurologische Diagnostik. *Deutsche Ztschr. Nervenh., 84:*152, 1925.

242. CORDS, R.: Optisch-motorisches Feld und optisch-motorische Bahn. Ein Beitrag zur Physiologie und Pathologie der Rindeninnervation der Augenmuskeln. *Arch. f. Ophth., 117:*58, 1926.

243. CORDS, R.: Optomotorischer Nystagmus und Gesichtsfeld. *Klin. Monatsbl. Augenh., 73:*513, 1924(2).

244. CORDS, R.: Die Pathologie der Augenbewegungen, in Kurzes *Handbuch der Ophthalmologie,* edited by F. Schieck and A. Brückner. Berlin, J. Springer, 1930, vol. 3, p. 491.

245. CORDS, R.: Physiologie und Pathologie des Bewegungsapparates. Augenmuskelspasmen and Nystagmus. *Uebersichtsreferet. Jahresb. ges. Ophth., 48:*348, 1921.

246. CORDS, R.: Zur Pathologie der Führungsbewegungen. *Arch. f. Ophth., 123:* 173, 1929.

247. CORDS, R., AND NOLZEN, L.: Weitere Untersuchungen über den optokinestischen (optomotorischen) Nystagmus. *Arch. f. Ophth., 120:*506, 1928.

248. Cox, R. A.: Congenital head-nodding and nystagmus; report of a case. *Arch. Ophth., 15:*1032, 1936.

249. Cranmer, R.: Nystagmus related to lesion of the central vestibular apparatus and the cerebellum. *Ann. Otol. Rhin. & Laryng., 60:*186, 1951.

250. Crevatin, F.: Sull'unione di cellule nervose. Mem. d. r. Accad. d. sc. d. Ist. di Bologna *8:*503, 1900.

251. Critchley, A. M.: Ocular manifestations following encephalitis lethargica. Bristol med.-chir. J. *45:*113, 1928. Abs. Zentralbl. f. d. ges. Ophth. *20:*683, 1929.

252. Crosby, E. C.: The application of neuro-anatomical data to the diagnosis of selected neurosurgical and neurological cases. *J. Neurosurg., 7:*566, 1950.

253. Crosby, E. C.: Relations of brain centers to normal and abnormal eye movements in the horizontal plane. *J. Comp. Neurol., 99:*437, 1953.

254. Crosby, E. C., and Henderson, J. W.: Mammalian midbrain and isthmus regions; fiber connections of superior colliculus; pathways concerned in automatic eye movements. *J. Comp. Neurol., 88:*53, 1948.

255. Crosby, E. C., Yoss, R. E., and Henderson, J. W.: Mammalian midbrain and isthmus regions; fiber connections; pattern for eye movements on frontal eye field and discharge of specific portions of this field to and through midbrain levels. *J. Comp. Neurol., 97:*357, 1952.

256. Crowe, S. J.: Ménière's disease; study based on examinations made before and after intracranial division of vestibular nerve. *Medicine, 17:*1, 1939.

257. Cummins, J. D.: Note on Wernicke's pupillary reaction. *Brit. J. Ophth., 7:*421, 1923.

258. Cuppers, C.: Eine neue Methode zur stetigen Registrierung der konsensuellen Pupillenreaktion. *Klin. Monatsbl. Augenh., 119:*411, 1951.

259. Cuppers, C., and Graff, T.: Ueber ein neues Gerät zur stetigen Beobachtung und Aufzeichnung des normalen und pathologischen Pupillarreflexes. (Ein Beitrag zur Frage der objektiven Perimetrie.) *Klin. Monätsbl. Augenh., 119:*189, 1951.

260. Curschmann, H.: Ueber Convergenzkrämpfe bei Tabes Dorsalis. *Neurol. Centralbl., 24:*10, 1905.

261. Cushing, H.: Experiences with the cerebellar astrocytomas. A critical review of seventy-six cases. *Surg., Gynec. & Obst., 52:*129, 1931.

262. Cushing, H.: Strangulation of the nervi abducentes by lateral branches of the basilar artery in cases of brain tumour. *Brain, 33:*204, 1910-1911.

263. Dale, H. H.: The action of certain esters and ethers of choline, and their relation to muscarine. *J. Pharmacol. & Exper. Therap., 6:*147, 1914.

264. Dale, H. H., Feldberg, W., and Vogt, M.: Release of acetylcholine at voluntary motor nerve endings. *J. Physiol., 86:*353, 1936.

265. Dandy, W. E.: Ménière's disease; symptoms, objective findings and treatment in 42 cases. *Arch. Otolaryng., 20:*1, 1934.

266. Daniel, P.: Spiral nerve endings in the extrinsic eye muscles of man. *J. Anat., 80:*189, 1946.

267. Danis, P. C.: The functional organization of the third-nerve nucleus in the cat. *Am. J. Ophth., 31:*1122, 1948.

267a. Danis, P. C., and Brihaye-van Geertruyden, M.: Nouvelle observation de paralysie oculo-faciale congenitale. *Bull. Soc. Belg. Opht., No. 102:*624-633, 1952.

268. DÉJERINE, [J.], GAUCKLER, [E.], AND ROUSSY, [G.]: Un cas de ptosis congénital de la paupière droite avec déficit cellulaire dans le noyau de la 3e paire. *Rev. Neurol., 12:*1243, 1904.

269. DÉJERINE, J., AND ROUSSY, G.: Un cas d'hémiplégie avec déviation conjugée de la tête et des yeux chez une aveugle de naissance. *Rev. Neurol., 13:*161, 1905.

270. DEJONG, R. N.: Horner's syndrome; report of 10 cases. *Arch. Neurol. & Psychiat., 34:*734, 1935.

271. DEJONG, R. N.: Nystagmus; an appraisal and a classification. *Arch. Neurol. & Psychiat. 55:*43, 1946.

272. DEUSCH, G.: Zur Symptomotologie und Etiologie der Myelitis (Encephalomyelitis) disseminata acuta. *Deutsche Ztchr. Nervenh., 80:*211, 1923.

273. DIMMER, F.: Zur Lehre von der Sehnervenbahnen. *Arch. f. Ophth., 48:*473, 1899.

274. DITTLER, R.: Ueber die Raumfunktion der Netzhaut in ihrer Abhängigkeit von Lagegefühl der Augen und vom Labyrinth. *Ztschr. Psychol. u. Physiol. Sinnesorg., 52:(2):*274, 1921. Abs. *Zentralbl. ges. Ophth., 6:*493, 1922.

275. DODGE, R.: Five types of eye movements in the horizontal meridian plane of the field of regard. *Am. J. Physiol., 8:*307, 1903.

276. DODGE, R.: A mirror-recorder for photographing the compensatory movements of closed eyes. *J. Exper. Psychol., 4:*165, 1921. Abs. *Zentralbl. ges. Ophth., 7:*236, 1922.

277. DODGE, R., TRAVIS, R. C., AND FOX, J. C., JR.: Optic nystagmus. III. Characteristics of the slow phase. *Arch. Neurol. & Psychiat., 24:*21, 1930.

278. DOGIEL, A. S.: Die Endigungen der sensiblen Nerven in den Augenmuskeln und deren Sehnen beim Menschen und den Säugetieren. *Arch. mikr. Anat., 68:*501, 1906. Abs. *Jahresb. Ophth., 37:*24, 1906.

279. DOHLMAN, [G.]: Demonstration eines Apparates zur optischen Registrierung der vestibulären Augenbewegen. *Ber. ü. d. 47 Zusammenkunft d. deutsch. ophth. Gesellsch., Heidelberg, 47:*459, 1928.

280. DOHLMAN, G.: Physikalische und physiologische Studien zur Theorie des Kalorischen Nystagmus. *Acta oto-laryng.,* Suppl. 5, 1925.

281. DORFF, H.: Ueber latenten Nystagmus. *Klin. Monatsbl. Augenh., 53:*503, 1914(1).

282. DÖRING, G. K., AND SCHÄFFERS, E.: Ueber die Tagesrhythmik der Pupillenweite beim Menschen. *Pfluger's Arch. ges. Physiol., 252:*537, 1950.

283. DOW, R. S.: The effects of unilateral and bilateral labyrinthectomy in monkey, baboon and chimpanzee. *Am. J. Physiol., 121:*392, 1938.

284. DOW, R. S. The relation of the paraflocculus to the movements of the eyes. *Am. J. Physiol., 113:*296, 1935.

285. DOW, R. S.: Cerebellar action potentials in response to stimulation of the cerebral cortex in monkeys and cats. *J. Neurophysiol., 5:*121, 1942.

286. DUANE, A.: The monocular movements. *Arch. Ophth., 8:*530, 1932.

287. DUBOIS-RAYMOND, R., AND SILEX, P.: Ueber corticale Reizung der Augenmuskeln. *Arch. Anat. u. Physiol.,* p. 174, 1899.

288. DUGUET, J.: Syndrome de Parinaud congenital. *Bull. Soc. opht., Paris, 6:* 424, 1937.

289. DUGUET, J.: Etude des effects de l'anoxemie sur les heterophories. *Bull. Soc. opht. Paris, 26:*12, 1947.

290. DUKE-ELDER, W. S.: New observations on the physiology of the extraocular muscles. *Tr. Ophth. Soc. U. Kingdom, 50:*181, 1930.

291. DUKE-ELDER, W. S., AND DUKE-ELDER, P. M.: Contraction of the extrinsic muscles of the eye by choline and nicotine. *Proc. Roy. Soc., London,* s. B. *170:*332, 1930.

292. DUNNINGTON, J. H., AND BERKE, R. N.: Exophthalmos due to chronic orbital myositis. *Arch. Ophth., 30:*446, 1943.

293. DUSSER DE BARENNE, J. G.: Die Funktionen des Kleinhirns; Physiologie und allgemeine Neuropathologie, in *Handbuch der Neurologie des Ohres,* edited by G. Alexander and O. Marburg. Berlin, Urban & Schwarzenberg, 1924, vol. 1, p. 589.

294. DUSSER DE BARENNE, J. G., AND McCULLOCH, W. S.: Functional organization in sensory cortex of monkey (Macaca mulatta). *J. Neurophysiol., 1:*69, 1938.

295. DUVAL, AND LABORDE, J. V.: De l'innervation des mouvements associés des globes oculaires. *J. anat. et physiol.,* p. 56, 1880. Abs. *Jahresb. Ophth., 11:* 37, 1880.

296. EAGLETON, W. P.: Clinical studies of vestibular and auditory tests in intracranial surgery. *Laryngoscope, 33:*483, 1923.

297. EAGLETON, W. P.: Discussion, in J. G. Wilson, The relation of otology to neurology. *Laryngoscope, 34:*573, 1924.

298. EARECKSON, V. O., AND MILLER, J. M.: Third-nerve palsy with sparing of pupil in diabetes mellitus. A subsequent identical lesion of the opposite eye. *Arch. Ophth., 47:*607, 1952.

299. EATON, L. M.: Diagnostic tests for myasthenia gravis with prostigmine and quinine. *Proc. Staff Meet., Mayo Clin., 18:*230, 1943.

300. ECCLES, J. C., KATZ, B., AND KUFFLER, S. W.: Effect of eserine on neuromuscular transmission. *J. Neurophysiol., 5:*211, 1942.

301. ECCLES, J. C.: Electrical hypothesis of synaptic and neuromuscular transmission. *Nature* (London), *156:*680, 1945.

302. ECKHARD, C.: Der auf Lichtreiz erfolgende Lidreflex. *Centralbl. Physiol., 9:* 353, 1895. Abs. *Jahresb. Ophth., 26:*60, 1895.

303. ECKHARD, C.: Das sogennante Rindenfeld des Facialis in seiner Beziehung zu den Blinzelbewegungen. *Centralbl. Physiol., 12:*1, 1898. Abs. *Jahresb. Ophth., 29:*107, 1898.

304. VON ECONOMO, C., AND KOSKINAS, G. N.: *Die cytoarchitektonik der Hirnrinde des erwachsenen Menschen.* Revised by J. Wagner. Vienna, J. Springer, 1925, 810 pp.

305. EDGEWORTH, F. H.: The development of some of the cranial muscles of ganoid fishes. *Phil. Tr. Roy. Soc., London,* s. B. *217:*39, 1928.

306. EDINGER, L.: Ueber den Verlauf centralen Hirnnervenbahnen mit Demonstration von Präpareten. *Arch. Psychiat., 16:*858, 1885.

307. EDINGER, L., AND FISCHER, B.: Ein Mensch ohne Grosshirn. *Arch. ges. Physiol., 152:*535, 1913.

308. ELSCHNIG, A.: Nystagmus retractorius ein zerebralis Herdsymptom. *Med. Klin.,* p. 8, 1913. Abs. *Jahresb. Ophth., 44:*580, 1913.

309. ELSCHNIG, A.: Oberlidretraktion als Herdsymptom. *Med. Klin., 20:*75, 1924.

310. ELSCHNIG, A.: Zur Anatomie des menschlichen Albinoauges. *Arch. f. Ophth., 84:*401, 1913.

311. van Emde Boas, C.: Abducensparese nach Lumbalpunktion. *Nederl. tijdschr. geneesk., p.* 36, 1937. Abs. *Zentralbl. ges. Ophth., 38:*224, 1937.

312. Engelbrecht: Ueber ein bisher noch nicht beschriebenes Augensymptom bei Encephalitis lethargica. *Klin. Monatsbl. Augenh., 77:*413, 1926(2).

313. Engelking, E.: Ueber den Nystagmus bei der angeborenen totalen Farbenblindheit. *Arch. ges. Physiol., 201:*220, 1923. Abs. *Zentralbl. ges. Ophth., 11:*458, 1924.

314. Van Essen, J.: Bewegung Bereitschaft und Netzhautbeleuchtung. *Ztschr. Sinnesphysiol., 66:*146, 1935.

315. Estable, C., and Baldomir, J. M.: Untersuchung der thalamischen Zentren in ihrer Beziehung zu Auge und Gehör durch permanente Elektroden. I. *An. otorino-laring. Uruguay, 3:*37, 1933. Abs. *Zentralbl. ges. Ophth., 30,* 167, 1934.

316. Ewald, J. R.: *Physiologische Untersuchungen über das Endorgan des Nervus octavus.* Wiesbaden, J. F. Bergmann, 1892, 324 pp.

317. Exner, S., and Paneth, J.: Das Rindenfeld des Facialis und seine Verbindungen bei Hund und Kaninchen. *Arch. ges. Physiol., 41:*349, 1887.

318. Falkenberg, K.: Zur lokaldiagnostischen Bedeutung der Nystagmusbeobachtung bei Prozessen der hinteren Schädelgrube. *Arch. Ohren-, Nasen- u. Kehlkopfh., 151:*134, 1942.

319. Falkenberg, K.: Zur Lokalisation des Nystagmus. *Deutsche Ztschr. Nervenh., 153:*40, 1941.

320. Falls, H. F., Kruse, W. T., and Cotterman, C. W.: Three cases of Marcus Gunn phenomenon in two generations. *Am. J. Ophth., 32:*53, 1949.

321. Falta, M.: Bemerkungen zum Artikel "Der akustische Blinzelreflex in der militärärztlichen Konstatierungspraxis" von Dr. Cemah. *Wien. med. Wchnschr., 68:*2194, 1918.

322. Falta, M.: Zur Auslösung des cochlearen Lidreflexes. *Monatsschr. Augenh. 55:*319, 1921. Abs. *Zentralbl. ges. Ophth., 6:*313, 1922.

323. Faucon, A.: Nystagmus par insuffisance des droits externes. *J. opht., 1:*223, 1872. Abs. *Jahresb. Ophth., 3:*466, 1872.

324. Favill, J.: The Relationship of Eye Muscles to Semicircular Canal Currents in Rotationally Induced Nystagmus in the Cerebellum; An Investigation of Recent Advances. Baltimore, Williams & Wilkins, 1929, vol. 6, of a series of research publications published by Assoc. for Research in Nerv. and Ment. Dis., p. 530.

325. Feigenbaum, A., and Kornbleuth, W.: Paralysis of convergence with bilateral ring scotoma following injury to occipital region; report of a case. *Arch. Ophth., 35:*218, 1946.

326. Feldberg, W.: Present views on mode of action of acetylcholine in central nervous system. *Physiol. Rev., 25:*596, 1945.

327. Feng, T. P., and Li, T.: Studies on the neuro-muscular junction. XVI. Acetylcholine sensitivity of a muscle and its aptitude to give contracture of the eserine type. *Chinese J. Physiol., 15:*197, 1940.

328. Fenn, W. O., and Hursh, J. B.: Movements of the eyes when the lids are closed. *Am. J. Physiol., 118:*8, 1937.

329. Ferrier, [D.]: The Croonian lectures on cerebral localization. *Lancet, 1:*1225, 1287, 1343, and 1409, 1890.

330. FERRIER, D.: Experimental researches in cerebral physiology and pathology. *West Riding Lunatic Asylum Med. Rep., 3:*1, 1873.

331. FERRIER, D.: Experiments on the brain of the monkey. *Proc. Roy. Soc., London, 23:*409, 1875.

332. FERRIER, D.: *Functions of the Brain,* ed. 2. London, Smith, Elder & Co., 1886, 498 pp.

333. FERRIER, D.: The localization of function in the brain. *Proc. Roy. Soc. London, 22:*229, 1874.

334. FERRIER, D., AND TURNER, W. A.: Experimental lesion of the corpora quadrigemina in monkeys. *Brain, 24:*27, 1901.

335. FINK, W. H.: A study of the anatomical variations in the attachment of the oblique muscles of the eyeball. *Tr. Am. Acad. Ophth., 51:*500, 1947.

336. FINK, W. H.: Etiologic considerations of vertical muscle defects. *Tr. Am. Ophth. Soc., 50:*135, 1953.

337. FISCHER, M. H.: In Sachen des Drehnystagmus. *Acta oto-laryng., 8:*495, 1926. Abs. *Zentralbl. ges. Ophth., 17:*267, 1927.

338. FISHER, J. H.: Presidential address. The personal equation. *Tr. Ophth. Soc. U. Kingdom, 61:*1, 1921.

339. FISHER, L., AND GLASER, M. A.: New vestibular complexes for localization of lesions of the brain. An analysis of one hundred and thirty-nine verified lesions. *Arch. Neurol. & Psychiat., 21:*876, 1929.

340. FLECHSIG, P. E.: *Anatomie des menschlichen Gehirns und Rückenmarks auf myelogenetischer Grundlage.* Leipzig, G. Thieme, 1920, 68 pp.

341. FLOURENS, P.: *Recherches Expérimentales sur les Propriétés et les Fonctions du Système Nerveux dans les Animaux Vertébrés,* ed. 2. Paris, J. B. Baillière, 1842, 516 pp.

342. FOCOSI, M., AND TOSELLI, C.: Sulla comparasa di una divergenza verticale da eccitamento labirintico e in assenza del processo di fusione. *Boll. ocul., 32:*3, 1953.

343. FOERSTER: Reference in Morone, G. and Andreani, F. Il comportamento della pupilla dopo resezione del simpatico cervicale sotto l'azione di alcuni medicamenti. *Riv. oto-neuro-oftal., 23:*250, 1948.

344. FOERSTER, O.: Cerebral cortex in man. *Lancet, 2:*309, 1931.

345. FOERSTER, O.: The motor cortex in man in the light of Hughlings Jackson's doctrines. *Brain, 59:*135, 1936.

346. FOERSTER, O.: Die Topik der Hirnrinde in ihrer Bedeutung für Motilität. *Deutsche Ztschr. Nervenh., 77:*124, 1924.

347. FOERSTER, O.: Zur Pupillarinnervation. *Deutsche Ztschr. Nervenh., 106:*311, 1928.

348. FOERSTER, O., AND GAGEL, O.: Die Vorderseitenstrandurchschneidung beim Menschen. Eine klinisch-patho-physiologisch-anatomische Studie. *Ztschr. ges. Neurol. u. Psychiat., 138:*1, 1932.

349. FOERSTER, O., GAGEL, O., AND MAHONEY, W.: Ueber die Anatomie, Physiologie und Pathologie der Pupillarinnervation. *Verhandl. deutsch. Gesellsch. inn. Med., 48:*386, 1936. Abs. *Zentralbl. ges. Ophth., 37:*615, 1937.

350. FOIX, C.: Syndrome de la paroi externe du sinus caverneux. (Ophthalmoplégie unilatérale à marche rapidement progressive. Algie du territoire de l'ophtalmique.) Amélioration considérable par le traitement radiothérapique. *Rev. neurol., 29:*827, 1922.

351. FORD, F. R., AND WALSH, F. B.: Clinical observations upon the importance of the vestibular reflexes in ocular movements. The effects of section of one or both vestibular nerves. *Bull. Johns Hopkins Hosp., 58:*80, 1936.

352. FORD, F. R., AND WALSH, F. B.: Tonic deviations of eyes produced by movements of head with special reference to otolith reflexes; clinical observations. *Arch. Ophth., 23:*1274, 1940.

353. FORD, F. R., WALSH, F. B., AND KING, A.: Clinical observations on the pupillary phenomena resulting from regeneration of the third nerve with especial reference to the Argyll-Robertson pupil. *Bull. Johns Hopkins Hosp., 68:*309, 1941.

354. FORSTER, G.: Der Augennachnystagmus bei Stellungsänderungen des Kopfes. *Helvet. physiol. et pharmacol. acta, 7:*382, 1949.

355. FOVILLE, [A.]:Note sur un paralysie peu connue des certains muscles de l'oeil, et sa liaison avec quelques points de l'anatomie et la physiologie de la protubérance annulaire. *Bull. Soc. anat. Paris, 33:*393, 1858.

356. FOX, J. C., JR.: Disorders of optic nystagmus due to cerebral tumors. *Arch. Neurol. & Psychiat., 28:*1007, 1932.

357. FOX, J. C. JR., AND DODGE, R.: Optic nystagmus. II. Variations in nystagmographic records of eye movement. *Arch. Neurol. & Psychiat., 22:*55, 1929.

358. FOX, J. C., AND HOLMES, G.: Optic nystagmus and its value in the localization of cerebral lesions. *Brain, 49:*333, 1926.

359. FRANCESCHETTI, A., AND BISCHLER, V.: Some pharmacodynamic effects upon pupillotonia and accomodotonia in Adie's syndrome. *Rev. Bulgar. opht.,* 9 (anniv. edit.): 85, 1943. Abs., Ophthalmology Sect. XII, *Excrepta Medica;* 2:1072, 1948.

360. FRANCIS, J.: Zone ophthalmique et paralysies ocularies. *J. belge neurol. et psychiat., 36:*8, 1936. Abs. *Zentralbl. ges. Ophth., 36:*447, 1936.

361. FRANK, C.: Ueber die Lokalisation in den Augenmuskelnervenkern und zwei noch unbekannte Kerne im Mittelhirn des Menschen. Pathologisch-anatomische Untersuchungen. *J. Psychol. u. Neurol., 26:*200, 1921.

362. FRANK, E., NORTHMANN, M., AND HIRSCH-KAUFFMANN, H.: Ueber die Tonische Kontraktion des quergestreiften Säugetieremuskeln nach Ausschaltung des motorischen Nerven. *Arch. ges. Physiol., 197:*270, 1922.

363. FREEMAN, W., AMMERMAN, H. H., AND STANLEY, M.: Syndromes of the pontile tegmentum; Foville's syndrome: report of three cases. *Arch. Neurol. & Psychiat., 50:*462, 1943.

364. FREEMAN, W., AND JAFFE, O.: Occlusion of the superior cerebellar artery; report of a case with neecropsy. *Arch. Neurol. & Psychiat., 46:*115, 1941.

365. FREMEL, F.: Der Vestibularapparat bei Grippe-Encephalitis. *Acta oto-laryng., 4:*471, 1922.

366. FRENZEL, H.: Nystagmusbeobachtung während der Drehung. *Ztschr. Hals-, Nasen- u. Ohrenh.,* 12 Kongressber. pt. 2, p. 637 and 653, 1925. Abs. *Zentralbl. ges Ophth., 16:*177, 1926.

367. FRENZEL, H.: Rücknystagmus als Halsreflex und Schlagfeldverlagerung des labyrinthären Drehynstagmus durch Halsreflexe. *Ztschr. Hals-, Nasen- u. Ohrenh., 21:*177, 1928.

368. FRENZEL, H.: Das Fahnden nach Spontannystagmus der wichtigste Teil der vestibularisuntersuchung in der Praxis. *Ztschr. Hals-Nasen-u Ohrenh., 44:*347, 1938.

369. FRIEDGOOD, H. B., CATTELL, R. B., AND BEETHAM, W. P.: Cited by J. F. Fulton, *Physiology of the Nervous System.* London, Oxford, 1938, 644 pp.

370. FRITSCH: Vergleichende Untersuchungen der Fovea Centralis des Menschen. *Anat. Anz. 30:*462, 1907. Abs. *Jahresb. Ophth., 38:*8, 1907.

371. FROHSE, F.: Ueber die Verzweigung der Nerven zu und in den menschlichen Muskeln. *Anat. Anaz., 41:*321, 1897/98.

372. FROMAGET, C., AND FROMAGET, H.: Nystagmus latent (nystagmus et strabisme). *Ann. ocul., 147:*344, 1912.

373. FROMAGET, H.: Nystagmus latent. *Ann. ocul., 149:*241, 1913.

374. FROMM, B., AND NYLEN, C. O.: Contribution to symptomatology of transplanted brain tumors in rats with and without labyrinths. *Acta oto-laryng., 23:*1, 1935.

375. FRONINOPOULOS, J.: Ein Beitrag zur Frage der Aetiologie der sogenannten rheumatischen Abduzensparese. *Klin. Monatsbl. Augenh., 101:*253, 1938(2).

376. FUCHS, E.: Ueber isolierte doppelseitige Ptosis. *Arch. f. Ophth., 36:*234, 1890.

377. FUCHS, E.: Association von Lidbewegungen mit seitlichen Bewegungen des Auges. *Beitr. Augenh., 2:*12, 1895.

378. FULTON, J. E.: *Muscular Contraction and the Reflex Control of Movement.* Baltimore, Williams & Wilkins, 1926, 644 pp.

379. FULTON, J. F., AND DOW, R. S.: The cerebellum; a summary of functional localization. *Yale J. Biol. & Med., 10:*89, 1937.

380. FULTON, J. F.: Neurophysiology. 1942-48. *New England J. Med., 240:*920, 1949.

381. FULTON, J. F.: *Physiology of the Nervous System.* New York, Oxford, 1949.

382. FUSE: Cited by M. Bartels. Auge und Ohr (Die Ohr-Augenbewegungen.), in *Kurzes Handbuch der Ophthalmologie,* edited by F. Schieck and A. Brückner. Berlin, J. Springer, 1930, vol. 3, p. 652.

383. GAGEL, O.: Ein Pons oblongata-astrocytom mit ungewöhnlichem Verlauf. *Nervenarzt, 14:*343, 1941.

384. GALANT, S.: Reflexus cochleopalpebralis und Ohr-Lidschlagreflex. *Arch. ges. Physiol., 176:*221, 1919.

385. VAN GANNEYT, M.: Zona ophthalmique avec paralysis isolée du nerf VI. *Bull. soc. belge opht., 83:*81, 1946.

386. GARCIN, R., AND KIPFER, M.: Syndrome de Claude Bernard. Horner homolatéral dans certaines lésions experimentales du thalamus optique; contribution à l'étude des centres et voies oculosympathiques du diencéphale. *Compt. rend. Soc. biol., 126:*864, 1937.

387. GAREL, J.: Nouveau fait de paralysie de la sixième paire avec déviation conjuguée dans un cas d'hémiplégie alterne. *Rev. med., Paris, 7:*1882. Abs. *Jahresb. Ophth., 13:*318, 1882.

388. GARVEN, H. S. D.: Cited by M. Hines. Studies on the innervation of skeletal muscle. III. Innervation of the extrinsic eye muscles of the rabbit. *Am. J. Anat., 47:*1, 1931.

389. VAN GEHUCHTEN, P.: Un cas de paralysie latérale du regard par lésion protubérantielle. Contribution a l'étude des voies oculogyres. *Rev. oto-neuro-opht., 8:*701, 1930. Abs. *Zentralbl. ges. Ophth., 25:*270, 1931.

390. VAN GEHUCHTEN, P.: Syndrome de Parinaud. Étude anatomique. *J. belge neurol. et psychiat., 40:*126, 1940.

391. van Gehuchten, P.: Les voies nerveuses du nystagmus. *Rev. neurol., 35*(2):849, 1928. Abs. *Zentralbl. ges. Ophth., 21:*841, 1929.

392. van Gehuchten, P.: Les mouvements conjugues des yeux et le système vestibulaire. *Bull. schweiz. Akad. med. Wissensch., 3:*333, 1948.

393. Gerlings, P. G.: Peripheral positional nystagmus. *J. Laryng. & Otol., 62:*147, 1948.

394. German, W. J., and Fox, J. C., Jr.: Observations following unilateral lobectomies. *A. Res. Nerv. & Ment. Dis., Proc., 13:*378, 1932.

395. Gifford, S. R.: Paradoxic elevation of the lid. *Arch. Ophth., 22:*252, 1939.

396. Gilbert, W.: Ueber Pigmentanomalien des Auges. *Arch. Augenh., 88:*143, 1921.

397. Gillan, R. U.: Report on a case of Parkinson's syndrome with oculogyric crises. *Tr. Ophth. Soc. U. Kingdom, 57:*577, 1938.

398. di Giorgio, A. M.: Sur l'activité des muscles oculaires dans le nystagmus de differente origine. *Acta oto-laryng., 43:*300, 1953.

399. di Giorgio, A. M., and Castelli-Borgiotti, G.: Sul graduale instaurarsi nell'uomo della corrispondeza fra il piano dell'orbita in cui si manifesta il nistagmo oculare da eccitamento rotatorio del labirinto ed il piano di rotazione. *Arch. fisiol., 38:*117, 1938-1939. Abs. *Zentralbl. ges. Ophth., 41:*681, 1938.

400. Givner, I., and Jaffe, N. S.: Myokymia of the eyelids. *Am. J. Ophth., 32:*51, 1949.

401. Godlowski, W.: Les centres sous-corticaux du regard et des mouvements associés des globes oculaires. *Trav. clin. Mal. Nerv. Univ. Cracovia*, 1936.

402. Goinard, P., Larmande, A., and Descuns, P.: Réhabilitation de la mydriase unilatéral en traumatologie cranienne. *Presse med., 55:*281, 1947.

403. Goldberg, F. R., and Kisin, P. E.: Pathogenesis of paralysis of the ocular muscles after spinal anaesthesia and lumbar puncture. *Vestn. oftal., 32:*31, 1953. Abs., Ophthalmology Sect. XII, *Excerpta Medica, 8:*1284, 1954.

404. Goldflam, S.: Beitrag zur Symptomatologie des Schläfenlappenabscesses. *Deutsch Ztschr. Nervenh., 90:*38, 1926.

405. Goldman, H.: Objektive Sehschärfenbestimmung. *Ophthalmologica, 105:*240, 1943.

406. Goldstein, A., Krayer, O., Root, M. A., Acheson, G. H., and Doherty, M. E.: Plasma neostigmine levels and cholinesterase inhibition in dogs and myasthenic patients. *J. Pharmacol. & Exper. Therap., 96:*56, 1949.

407. Goldstein, K.: Das Kleinhirn, in *Handbuch der Normalen und Pathologischen Physiologie*, edited by A. Bethe, G. v. Bergmann, G. Embden, and A. Ellinger. Berlin, J. Springer, 1927, vol. 10, p. 222.

408. Goldstein, K.: Ueber induzierte Veränderungen des Tonus (Halsreflex, Labyrinthreflex und ähnliche Erscheinungen). *Acta oto-laryng., 7:*13, 1924.

409. Gollas, E.: Untersuchung der Raddrehung der Augen bei einseitigem Labyrinthausfall. *Arch. Ohren-, Nasen-, u. Kehlkopfh., 140:*340, 1936. Abs. *Zentralbl. ges. Ophth., 36:*669, 1936.

410. Gorman, J. J.: Unpublished.

411. Gordon, G.: Observations upon the movements of the eyelids. *Brit. J. Ophth., 35:*339, 1951.

412. Gorman, W. F., and Brock, S.: Periodic alternating nystagmus in Friedreich's ataxia. *Am. J. Ophth., 33:*860, 1950.

413. Göthlin, G. F.: Die Bewegungen und die Physiologischen Konsequenzen der Bewegungen eines Zentralen Optischen Nachbildes in Dunklem Blickfield bei Postrotatorische und Kalorischer Reizung des Vestibularapparates. Uppsala, Almquist & Wiksell, 1927, 69 pp. Abs. *Zentralbl. ges. Ophth., 19:* 289, 1928.

414. Grahe, K.: Raddrehung der Augen und Otolithenstellung beim Menschen. *Acta oto-laryng., 26:*268, 1938. Abs. *Zentralbl. ges. Ophth., 42:*69, 1940.

415. Grahe, K.: Ueber Halsreflexe und Vestibularreaktion beim Menschen. *Ztschr. Hals-, Nasen- u. Ohrenh., 3:*550, 1922.

416. Grahe, K.: Das Verhalten der Haltungs- und Bewegungsreaktionen (der Vestibularapparte) bei zentralen Erkrankungen (Medulla oblongata, Kleinhirn usw.), in *Handbuch der Normalen und Pathologischen Physiologie,* edited by A. Bethe, G. v. Bergmann, G. Embden, and A. Ellinger. Berlin, J. Springer, 1930, vol. 15, pt. 1, p. 411.

417. Grant, F. C.: The Marcus Gunn phenomena. Report of a case with suggestions as to relief. *Arch. Neurol. & Psychiat., 35:*487, 1936.

418. Grasset, J., and Gaussel, A.: Paralysie des deux hémioculomoteurs (abolition des mouvements de latéralité à droit et à gauche): tubercule de la protubérance. *Rev. neurol.,* No. 2, 1905. Abs. *Jahresb. Ophth., 36:*434, 1905.

419. Gray, A. A.: *The Labyrinth of Animals, Including Mammals, Birds, Reptiles, and Amphibians.* London, J. & A. Churchill, 1907-1908, 2 vols.

420. Gray, L. P.: Connections of the vestibular mechanism in the cat. *J. Comp. Neurol., 41:*319, 1926.

421. Graybiel, A., and Brown, R. H.: The delay in visual reorientation following exposure to a change in direction of resultant force on a human centrifuge. *J. Gen. Psychol., 45:*143, 1951.

422. Graybiel, A., and Clark, B.: Autokinetic illusion and its significance in night flying. *J. Aviation Med., 16:*111, 1945.

423. Graybiel, A., and Clark, B.: Duration of oculogyral illusion as a function of the interval between angular acceleration and deceleration. Its significance in terms of dynamics of semicircular canals in man. *J. Appl. Physiol., 5:*147, 1952.

424. Graybiel, A., and Hupp, D.: The oculo-gyral illusion: a form of apparent motion which may be observed following stimulation of the semicircular canals. *J. Aviation Med., 17:*3, 1946.

425. Graybiel, A., Kerr, W. A., and Bartley, S. H.: Stimulus thresholds of the semicircular canals as a function of angular acceleration. *Am. J. Psychol., 61:*21, 1948.

426. Graybiel, A., and Niven, J. I.: The absence of residual effects attributable to the otolith organs following unilateral labyrinthectomy in man. *Laryngoscope, 63:*18, 1953.

427. Graybiel, A., Niven, J. I., and Walsh, T. E.: The differentiation between symptoms referable to the otolith organs and semicircular canals in patients with nonsuppurative labyrinthitis. *Laryngoscope, 62:*924, 1952.

428. Grinker, R. R., and Bucy, P. C.: *Neurology.* Springfield, Thomas, 1949.

429. Grünbaum, A. S. F., and Sherrington, C. S.: A discussion of the motor cortex exemplified in the anthropoid apes. *Brit. M. J., 2:*784, 1902.

430. Grundfest, H.: Bioelectric potentials in the nervous system and in muscle. *Ann. Rev. Physiol., 9:*477, 1947.

431. GRÜTTNER, R.: Experimentelle Untersuchungen über den optokinetischen Nystagmus. *Ztschr. Sinnesphysiol., 68:*1, 1939.

432. GUNN, M.: Congenital ptosis. *Lancet, 2:*104, 1883.

433. GÜTTICH, A.: Ueber den Antagonismus der Hals- und Bogengangsreflexe bei der Bewegung des menschlichen Auges. *Arch. Ohren-, Nasen- u. Kehlkopfh., 147:*1, 1940.

434. HALPERN, L., AND LANDAU, J.: Head posture and visual functions. *Monatsschr. Psychiat. u. Neurol., 125:*148, 1953.

435. HAMPEL, C. W.: Effect of denervation on sensitivity to adrenine of smooth muscle in nictiating membrane of the cat. *Am. J. Physiol., 111:*611, 1935.

436. HAMPSON, J. L., HARRISON, C. R., AND WOOLSEY, C. N.: Somatotopic localization in anterior lobe and lobulus simplex of cerebellum in cat and dog. *Federation Proc. 4:*31, 1945.

437. HAMPSON, J. L., HARRISON, C. R., AND WOOLSEY, C. N.: Somatotopic localization in the cerebellum. *Federation Proc., 5:*41, 1946.

438. HAMPSON, J. L., HARRISON, C. R., AND WOOLSEY, C. N.: Cerebro-cerebellar projections and the somatotopic localization of motor function in the cerebellum. *A. Res. Nerv. & Ment. Dis., Proc., 30:*299, 1950.

439. HARE, W. K., MAGOUN, H. W., AND RANSON, S. W.: Localization within the cerebellum of reactions to faradic cerebellar stimulation. *J. Comp. Neurol., 67:*145, 1937.

440. HARE, W. K., MAGOUN, H. W., AND RANSON, S. W.: Pathways for pupillary constriction; location of synapses in the path for the pupillary light reflex and of the constrictor fibers of cortical origin. *Arch. Neurol. & Psychiat., 34:*1188, 1935.

441. HARMS, H.: Grundlagen: Methodik und Bedeutung der Pupillenperimetrie für die Physiologie und Pathologie des Sehorgans. *von Graefe's Arch. Ophth., 149:*1, 1949.

442. HARMS, H.: Hemianopische Pupillenstarre. *Klin. Monatsbl. Augenh., 118:*133, 1951.

443. HARRINGTON, D. O., AND FLOCKS, M.: Ophthalmoplegic migraine. A discussion of its pathogenesis with a report of the pathologic findings in a case of recurrent oculomotor palsy. *Tr. Am. Acad. Ophth., 57:*517, 1953.

444. HARRIS, A. J., HODES, R., AND MAGOUN, H. W.: The afferent path of the pupillodilator reflex in the cat. *J. Neurophysiol., 7:*231, 1944.

445. HARRIS, W.: Ataxic nystagmus: A pathognomonic sign in disseminated sclerosis. *Brit. J. Ophth., 28:*40, 1944.

446. HARVEY, A. M.: Some preliminary observations on the clinical course of myasthenia gravis before and after thymectomy. *Bull. New York Acad. Med., 24:*505, 1948.

447. HARVEY, A. M., AND LILENTHAL, J. L., JR.: Observations on nature of myasthenia gravis; intra-arterial injection of acetylcholine, prostigmine and adrenaline. *Bull. Johns Hopkins Hosp., 69:*566, 1941.

448. HARVEY, A. M., AND WHITEHILL, M. R.: Quinine as an adjuvant to prostigmine in the diagnosis of myasthenia gravis. Preliminary report. *Bull. Johns Hopkins Hosp., 61:*216, 1937.

449. HAYNE, H. W.: Report of a case of paralysis of convergence without impairment of associated movements. *Arch. Ophth., 25:*329, 1896.

450. HECAEN, H., AJURIAGUERRA, J., ROUQUES, L., DAVID, M., AND DELL, M. B.: Para-

lysie psychique du regard de balint au cours de l'evolution d'une leuco-encephalite type balo. *Rev. neurol., 83:*81, 1950.

451. HACAEN, H., AND AJURIAGUERRA, J. DE: Balint's syndrome (psychic paralysis of visual fixation) and its minor forms. *Brain, 77:*373, 1954.

452. HEDDÄEUS, E.: *Klinische Studien über die Beziehungen zwischen Pupillareaction und Sehvermögen.* Halle a. S., Plötz, 1880, 65 pp.

453. HELMHOLTZ, H. VON: *Hb. der Physiologischen Optik.* Vol. III, 3rd ed. Hamburg and Leipzig, Voss, 1910.

454. HELSPER, R.: Ueber Parkinsonismus bei luetischen Hirnerkrankungen. *Monatsschr. Psychiat. u. Neurol., 83:*286, 1932. Abs. *Zentralbl. ges. Ophth., 28:*412, 1933.

455. HEMMES, G. D.: *Ueber Hereditären Nystagmus.* Wageningen, H. Veenman, 1924, 105 pp. Abs. *Zentralbl. ges. Ophth., 13:*262, 1925.

456. HEMMES, G. D.: Zur Analyse der Augenbewegungen bei Nystagmus latens. *Arch. Augenh., 103:*246, 1930.

457. HENDERSON, J. W.: Optokinetic and other factors modifying vestibular nystagmus. *Arch. Ophth., 37:*459, 1947.

458. HENDERSON, J. W., AND CROSBY, E. C.: An experimental study of optokinetic responses. *Arch. Ophth., 47:*43, 1952.

459. HENSEN, V., AND VÖLCKERS, C.: Ueber den Ursprung der Accommodationsnerven, nebst Bemerkungen über die Function der Wurzeln des Nervus oculomotorius. Physiologische Untersuchung. *Arch. f. Ophth., 24(1):*1, 1878.

460. HERTWIG: Cited by H. Oloff and H. Korbsch. Ueber das Hertwig-Magendiesche Phänomenon (Vertikaldivergenz der Augen). *Klin. Monatsbl. Augenh., 77:* 618, 1926 (2).

461. HERTZ, M.: Zur Physiologie des Formen- und Bewegungssehens. II. Auflösungsvermögen des Bienenauges und Optomotorische Reaktion. *Ztschr. vergl. Physiol., 21:*579, 1934. Abs. *Zentralbl. ges. Ophth., 33:*322, 1935.

462. HERTZ, M.: Zur Physiologie des Formen- und Bewegungssehens. III. Figurale Unterscheidung und reziproke Dressuren bei der Biene. *Ztschr. vergl. Physiol., 21:*604, 1934. Abs. *Zentralbl. ges. Ophth., 33:*323, 1935.

463. HESS, C.: Untersuchungen zur Physiologie und Pathologie des Pupillenspieles. *Arch. Augenh., 60:*327, 1908.

464. HESS, W. R.: Pupille und Zwischenhirn. *Klin. Monatsbl. Augenh., 103:*407, 1939 (2).

465. HICKS, A. M.: Congenital paralysis of lateral rotators of eyes with paralysis of muscles of face. *Arch. Ophth., 30:*38, 1943.

466. HICKS, A. M., AND HOSFORD, G. N.: Cyclic paralysis of the oculomotor nerve. *Arch. Ophth., 17:*213, 1937.

467. HINES, M.: Nerve and muscle. *Quart. Rev. Biol., 2:*149, 1927.

468. HINES, M.: Studies on the innervation of skeletal muscle. III. Innervation of the extrinsic eye muscles of the rabbit. *Am. J. Anat., 47:*1, 1931.

469. HIRANO, N.: Histologische Untersuchungen über die nervösen Innervation der menschlichen äusseren Augenmuskeln. *Arch. f. Ophth., 142:*560, 1941.

470. HIRASAWA, K., AND KATO, K.: Ueber die Fasern, insbesondere die corticalen extrapyramidalen aus den areae 8 (α, β, γ, δ) und 9 (c, d) der Grosshirnrinde beim Affen. *Folia anat. japon., 13:*189, 1935.

471. HITZIG, E.: *Physiologische und klinische Untersuchungen über das Gehirn. Gesammelte Abhandlungen.* Part I. Untersuchungen über das Gehirn.

Part II. Alte und neue Untersuchungen über das Gehirn. Berlin, R. Hirschwald, 1904, 618 pp.

472. HITZIG, E.: *Untersuchungen über das Gehirn.* Berlin, A. Hirschwald, 1874, 276 pp.

473. HODES, R., AND MAGOUN, H. W.: Autonomic responses to electrical stimulation of the forebrain and midbrain with special reference to the pupil. *J. Comp. Neurol., 72:*169, 1942.

474. VAN DER HOEVE, J.: Latent Nystagmus. *Nederl. tijdschr. geneesk.,* p. 790, 1918 (1).

475. VAN DER HOEVE, J.: Nystagmus latent. *Ann. ocul., 154:*738, 1917.

476. VOM HOFF, K.: Untersuchungen über das Verhalten eines centralen optischen Nachbildes bei und nach unwillkürlichen Bewegungen sowie mechanischen Verlagerung des Auges. *Arch. f. Ophth., 144:*164, 1941.

477. HOFFMAN, A. C., WELLMAN, B., AND CARMICHAEL, L.: A quantitative comparison of the electrical and photographic techniques of eye-movement recording. *J. Exper. Psychol., 24:*40, 1939.

478. HOFFMAN, M. [P]: Ueber die Atkionsströme der Augenmuskeln bei Ruhe des Tieres und beim Nystagmus. *Arch. Anat. u. Physiol.,* (Physiol. Sec.) p. 23, 1913, and (*Physik-med. ges. Würzburg*) *Med. Klin.,* p. 560, 1913. Abs. *Jahresb. Ophth., 44:*88, 1913.

479. HÖGYES, A.: Ueber den Nervenmechanismus der associerten Augenbewegungen. *Monatsschr. Ohrenh., 46:*685 and 809, 1912. Abs. *Jahresb. Ophth., 43:* 119, 1912.

480. HÖGYES, A.: Ueber die wahren Ursachen der Schwindelerscheinungen bei der Drucksteigerung in der Paukenhöhle. *Arch. ges. Physiol., 26:*558, 1881. Abs. *Jahresb. Ophth., 12:*153, 1881.

481. HOHMAN, L. B.: Forced conjugate upward movements of the eyes in post-encephalitis Parkinson's syndrome. *J.A.M.A., 84:*1489, 1925.

482. HOLMES, G.: Cerebral integration of ocular movements. *Brit. M. J., 2:*107, 1938.

483. HOLMES, G.: Discussion of Symposium on the cerebellum. *Brain, 50:*275, 1927.

484. HOLMES, G.: Disturbances of vision by cerebral lesions. *Brit. J. Ophth., 2:*353, 1918.

485. HOLMES, G.: Observations on ocular palsies. *Brit. M. J., 2:*1165, 1931.

486. HOLMES, G.: Palsies of the conjugate ocular movements. *Brit. J. Ophth., 5:* 241, 1921.

487. HOLMES, G.: Partial iridoplegia associated with symptoms of other diseases of the nervous system. *Tr. Ophth. Soc. U. Kingdom, 51:*209, 1931.

488. HOLMES, G.: Spasm of fixation. *Tr. Ophth. Soc. U. Kingdom, 50:*253, 1930.

489. HOLMES, G.: Symptoms of acute cerebellar injury due to gun shot injuries. *Brain, 40:*461, 1917.

490. HOLT, H.: Convergent spasm. *Am. J. Ophth., 26:*865, 1943.

491. HOORENS, A. J. F.: Studies on the pharmacological action of ephedrine on the pupil. *Kon. Vlaamse Acad. Geneesk. Belgi* (Verhand), *12:*277, 1950. Abs., Ophthalmology Sect. XII, *Excerpta Medica, 6:*333, 1952.

492. HOORENS, A., AND PHILIPS, A.: Contribution à l'étude de l'action du chlorure de tétraethylammonium sur la pupille. *Bull. Soc. belge. opht., 96:*603, 1950.

493. HOPMANN, E.: Quantitative calorische Prüfung am Normalen mittels Wasser-

füllung des Gehörgangs. *Arch. Ohren-, Nasen- u. Kehlkopfh., 141:*155, 1936. Abs. *Zentralbl. ges. Ophth., 37:*295, 1937.

494. HORRAX, G., AND BUCKLEY, R. C.: Clinical study of differentiation of certain pontile tumors from acoustic tumors. *Arch. Neurol. & Psychiat., 24:*1217, 1930.

495. HORSLEY, V., AND CLARKE, R. H.: The structure and functions of the cerebellum examined by a new method. *Brain 31:*45, 1908.

496. HORSLEY, [V.], AND SCHÄFFER, [E. A.]: A record of experiments upon the functions of the cerebral cortex. *Phil. Tr. Roy. Soc. Lond.,* s. B. *179:*1, 1888.

497. HOSHINO, T.: Beiträge zur Funktion des Kleinhirnwurmes beim Kaninchen. *Acta oto-laryng.,* Suppl. 2, 1921.

498. HOWE, H. A., TOWER, S. S., AND DUEL, A. B.: Facial tic in relation to injury of the facial nerve. An experimental study. *Arch. Neurol. & Psychiat., 38:* 1190, 1937.

499. HUBER, G. C.: A note on the sensory nerve endings in the extrinsic eye muscles of the rabbit. *Anat. Anz., 15:*335, 1899.

500. HUET, W. G.: Zwischenhirn und Halssympathicus. *Arch. ges. Physiol., 137:* 627, 1911.

501. HUGGER, H.: Beitrag zur objektiven Sehschärfenbestimmung nach dem Ohmschen Prinzip. *Klin. Monatsbl. Augenh., 116:*651, 1950.

502. HUNNIUS, H.: Zur Symptomatologie der Brückenerkrankungen und über die conjugierte Deviation der Augen bei Hirnkrankheiten, Bonn. Abs. *Jahresb. Ophth., 12:*310, 1881.

503. HYNDMAN, O. R.: Physiology of the vestibular labyrinth. *Arch. Otolaryng., 29:*759, 1939.

504. INGRAHAM, F. D., AND CAMPBELL, J. B.: Marcus Gunn phenomenon. *Arch. Neurol. & Psychiat., 46:*127, 1941.

505. INGRAM, W. R., RANSON, S. W., AND HANNETT, F. I.: Pupillary dilatation produced by direct stimulation of the tegmentum of the brain stem. *Am. J. Physiol., 98:*687, 1931.

506. INGRAM, W. R., AND OTHERS: Results of stimulation of tegmentum with Horsley-Clarke stereotaxic apparatus. *Arch. Neurol. & Psychiat., 28:*513, 1932.

507. INGVAR, S.: On pathogenesis of Argyll-Robertson phenomenon. *Bull. Johns Hopkins Hosp., 43:*363, 1928.

508. IGERSHEIMER, J.: Visual changes in progressive exophthalmos. *Arch. Ophth., 53:*94, 1955.

509. IRVINE, S. R.: Histology of the extra-ocular muscles. *Arch. Ophth., 15:*847, 1936.

510. IRVINE, S. R., AND LUDVIGH, E. J.: Is ocular proprioceptive sense concerned in vision? *Arch. Ophth., 15:*1037, 1936.

511. IVY, A. C.: The physiology of vestibular nystagmus. *Arch. Otolaryng., 9:*123, 1929.

512. JACKSON, J. H.: Cited by O. Foerster. The motor cortex in man in the light of Hughlings Jackson's doctrines. *Brain, 59:*135, 1936.

513. JACOBSON, E.: Electrical measurements of neuromuscular states during mental activities; visual imagination and recollection. *Am. J. Physiol., 95:*694, 1930.

514. JAEGER, R.: Aneurism of the intracranial carotid artery: syndrome of frontal headache with oculomotor nerve paralysis. *J.A.M.A., 142:*304, 1950.

515. JAFFE, N. S.: Practical application of the denervated iris. *Arch. Ophth., 40:* 317, 1948.

516. JAFFE, N. S.: True psychosensory dilation and delayed psychosensory dilation of the pupil. *Am. J. Ophth., 32:*1681, 1949.

517. JAFFE, N. S.: Localization of lesions causing Horner's syndrome. *Arch. Ophth., 44:*710, 1950.

518. JAKOB AND BOEDEKER: Cited by C. Frank. Ueber die Lokalisation in den Augenmuskelnervenkernen und zwei noch unbekannte Kerne im Mittelhirn des Menschen. *J. Psychol. u. Neurol., 26:*200, 1920.

519. JAENSCH, P. A.: Atypischer torticollis ocularis durch Fehlen des geradem Senkers. *Klin. Monatsbl. Augenh., 104:*733, 1940.

520. JAENSCH, P. A.: Zur Klinik der supranuclearen Medialisparese und internuclearen Ophthalmoplegie. *Arch. f. Ophth., 125:*592, 1930.

521. JANISCHEWSKY, A.: Un cas de maladie de Parkinson avec syndrome pseudobulbaire et pseudo-ophthalmoplégique. *Rev. Neurol., 17:*823, 1909.

522. JAVAL, E.: In *Traité des Maladies de Yeux* by L. Wecker, Paris, Delahaye, 1866, vol. 2, p. 815.

523. JEFFERSON, G.: On saccular aneurysms of internal carotid artery in cavernous sinus. *Brit. J. Surg., 26:*267, 1938.

524. JEFFERSON, G.: Isolated oculomotor palsy caused by intracranial aneurysm. *Proc. Rev. Soc. Med., 40:*419, 1947.

525. JESS, A.: Hemikinesimeter. *Klin. Monatsbl. Augenh., 52:*147, 1914 (1).

526. JESS, A.: Ueber die hemianopische Pupillenstarre und das hemiopische Prismenphänomen. *Arch. Augenh., 71:*66, 1912.

527. JOHNSON, L. V.: Adherence syndrome: pseudoparalysis of the lateral or superior rectus muscles. *Arch. Ophth., 44:*870, 1950.

528. JONES: Cited by W. Klestadt. Symptomatologie der Erkrankungen des N. VIII einschliesslich Leitung im Hirnstamm, in *Handbuch der Neurologie,* edited by O. Bumke and O. Foerster. Berlin, J. Springer, 1936, vol. 4, p. 359.

529. JONES, I. H.: *Equilibrium and Vertigo.* Philadelphia, J. B. Lippincott, 1918, 444 pp.

530. JONES, I. H., AND SPILLER, W. G.: The central tracts of the nervus vestibularis. *Tr. Am. Neurol. A., [51]:*181, 1925.

531. JONES, M. S., AND STADIE, W. C.: Cholinesterase content of the muscle of myasthenia gravis and of serum of four other groups of clinical conditions. *Quart. J. Exper. Physiol., 29:*63, 1939.

532. JONGKEES, L. B.: Positional nystagmus of peripheral origin. *J. Physiol., 110:* 447, 1949.

533. JUNG, R., AND MITTERMAIER, R.: Zur objektiven Registrierung und Analyse verschiedener Nystagmusformen; vestibulärer, optokinetischer und spontaner Nystagmus in ihren Wechselbeziehungen. *Arch. Ohren-, Nasen- u. Kehlkopfh., 146:*410, 1939. Abs. *Ztschr. Hals-, Nasen- u. Ohrenh., 46:*320, 1939.

534. JUNG, R., AND TÖNNIES, J. F.: Die Registrierung und Auswertung des Drehnystagmus beim Menschen. *München. med. Wchnschr., 33:*513, 1948.

535. JUNGER, I.: Methodik und klinische Bedeutung der galvanischen Prüfung des Labyrinthes. *Monatsschr. Ohrenh., 56:*451, 1922. Abs. *Zentralbl. ges. Ophth., 9:*43, 1923.

536. KAPLAN, M.: Die spinale Acusticuswurzel und die in ihr eingelagerten

Zellsysteme. Nucleus Deiters.—Nucleus Bechterew. *Arb. neurol. Inst. Wien. Univ., 20:*375, 1913.

537. KARPLUS, J. P., AND KREIDL, A.: Gehirn und Sympathicus. I. Zwischenhirnbasis und Halssympathicus. *Arch. ges. Physiol., 129:*138, 1909.

538. KARPLUS, J. P., AND KREIDL, A.: Gehirn und Sympathicus. II. Ein Sympathicuszentrum im Zwischenhirn. *Arch. ges. Physiol., 135:*401, 1910.

539. KARPLUS, J. P., AND KREIDL, A.: Gehirn und Sympathicus. III. Sympathicusleitung im Gehirn und Halsmark. *Arch. ges. Physiol., 143:*109, 1911-1912.

540. KARPLUS, J. P., AND KREIDL, A.: Ueber die Bahn des Pupillarreflexes. *Arch. ges. Physiol., 149:*115, 1912.

541. KÄSLIN, W.: *Postencephalitische und Sonstige Parkinsonismen nach Trauma* (an Hand der in den Jahren 1930-1934 bei der Suva angemeldeten Fälle). Basel Diss. 1935, 29 pp. Abs. *Zentralbl. ges. Ophth., 36:*447, 1936.

542. KATO, T.: Ueber histologische Untersuchungen der Augenmuskeln von Menschen und Säugetieren. *Okajimas Folia anat. japon., 16:*131, 1938. Abs. *Zentralbl. Ophth., 42:*28, 1939.

543. KEHRER, F.: *Die Kuppelungen von Pupillenstörungen mit Aufheben der Sehnenreflexe.* Stuttgart, Thieme, 1937.

544. KEINER, G. B. J., AND ROELOFS, C. O.: Nystagmus latens in monocular patients. Abs. from Program of International Congress Ophth., 1954.

545. KELLER, A. D.: Autonomic discharges elicited by physiological stimuli in midbrain preparations. *Am. J. Physiol., 100:*576, 1932.

546. KELLER, A. D.: An intense and enduring miosis following transection of the brain stem, caudal to the level of exit of the oculomotor nerves. *Federation Proc., 3:*23, 1944.

547. KELLER, A. D., AND STEWART, L.: The superior colliculi and the pupillary light reflex in the cat. *Am. J. Physiol., 101:*64, 1932.

548. KENNARD, M. A.: Alterations in response to visual stimuli following lesions of the frontal lobe in monkeys. *Arch. Neurol. & Psychiat., 41:*1153, 1939.

549. KENNARD, M. A.: Experimental analysis of the functions of the basal ganglia in monkeys and chimpanzees. *J. Neurophysiol., 7:*127, 1944.

550. KENNARD, M. A., AND ECTORS, L.: Forced circling in monkeys following lesions of the frontal lobes. *J. Neurophysiol., 1:*45, 1938.

551. KESER, H. :Variationen des Drehnystagmus beim Gesunden nach der Amplitudenauswertung. *Ber. Kongres. Neurol. u. Psychiat.,* Tübingen 1947.

522. KESTENBAUM, A.: Der Mechanismus des Nystagmus. *Arch. f. Ophth., 105:*799, 1921.

553. Kestenbaum, A.: Ueber latenten Nystagmus und seine Beziehungen zur Fixation. *Klin. Monatsbl. Augenh., 65:*426, 1920 (2).

554. KESTENBAUM, A.: Zur Klinik des optokinetischen Nystagmus. *Arch. f. Ophth., 124:*339, 1930.

555. KESTENBAUM, A.: Zur Entwicklung der Augenbewegungen und des optokinetischen Nystagmus. *Arch. f. Ophth., 124:*113, 1930.

556. KESTENBAUM, A.: Periodisch umschlagender Nystagmus. *Klin. Monatsbl. Augenh., 84:*552, 1930.

557. KESTENBAUM, A.: *Clinical Methods of Neuro-ophthalmologic Examination.* New York, Grune & Stratton, 1946.

558. KEYNES, G.: Results of thymectomy in myasthenia gravis. *Brit. M. J., 2:*611, 1949.

559. KILOH, L. G., AND NEVIN, S.: Progressive dystrophy of the external ocular muscles (ocular myopathy.) *Brain, 74:*115, 1951.

560. KINDT, P., AND KNUDTZON, K.: Eye symptoms in poliomyelitis. *Nord. med., 34:* 1422, 1947. Abs., Ophthalmology Sect. XII, *Excerpta Medica, 2:*495, 1948.

561. KISCH, B.: New method (of using pentobarbital sodium) to produce nystagmus. *Exper. Med. & Surg., 1:*169, 1943.

562. KLEIST, K.: Gehirn-Pathologie, vornehmlich auf Grund der Kriegserfahrungen, in *Handbuch der ärztlichen Erfahrungen im Weltkriege.* Leipzig, Barth, 1934, vol. 4, pt. 2, p. 343.

563. KLESTADT, W.: Symptomatologie der Erkrankungen des N. VIII einschliesslich Leitung im Hirnstamm, in *Handbuch der Neurologie,* edited by O. Bumke and O. Foerster. Berlin, J. Springer, 1936, vol. 4, p. 359.

564. de Kleyn, A.: Some remarks on vestibular nystagmus. *Confinia Neurol., 2:*257, 1939.

565. DE KLEYN, A.: Tonische Labyrinth- und Halsreflexe auf die Augen. *Arch. ges. Physiol., 186:*82, 1921.

566. DE KLEYN, A.: Ueber vestibulare Augenreflexe. IV. Experimentelle Untersuchungen über die schnelle Phase des vestibulären Nystagmus beim Kaninchen. *Arch. f. Ophth., 107:*480, 1922.

567. DE KLEYN, A., AND MAGNUS, R.: Ueber die Unabhängigkeit der Labyrinthreflexe vom Kleinhirn und über die Lage der Zentren für die Labyrinth reflexe im Hirnstamm. *Arch. ges. Physiol., 178:*124, 1920. Abs. *Zentralbl. ges. Ophth., 3:* 26, 1920.

568. DE KLEYN, A., AND STENVERS, H.: Tonische labyrinthreflexen op de oogen bij menschen. *Nederl. tijdschr. geneesk., 1:*486, 1922.

569. DE KLEYN, A., AND VERSTEEGH, C.: Experimentelle Untersuchungen über den sogenannten Lagenystagmus während akuten Alkoholvergiftung beim Kaninchen. *Acta oto-laryng., 14:*356, 1930.

570. DE KLEYN, A., AND VERSTEEGH, C.: Schwindelanfälle und Nystagmus bei einer bestimmten Lage des Kopfes. *Acta oto-laryng., 7:*422, 1925.

571. DE KLEYN, A., AND VERSTEEGH, C.: Some remarks upon the present position of the physiology of the labyrinth. *J. Laryng. & Otol., 42:*649, 1927.

572. DE KLEYN, A., AND VERSTEEGH, C.: Ueber die Unabhängigkeit des Dunkelnystagmus der Hunde vom Labyrinth. *Arch. f. Ophth., 101:*228, 1920.

573. KLOSSOWSKY, B., AND LEVIKOWA, A. M.: Der Mechanismus der vestibularen Nystagmus. (Ueber die homonyme keineswegs cruciate Innervation der Musculi recti interni von dem Oculomotoriuskern beim Nystagmus.) *Arch. ges. Physiol., 228:*198, 1931.

574. KNOLL, P.: Beiträge zur Physiologie der Vierhügel. *Beitr. Anat. u. Physiol., 4:* 109, 1869.

575. KNOLLER, G.: Zur Spasmus nutans- und Nystagmusforschung. Versuch einer aktiven Therapie. *Monatsschr. Kinderh., 37:*21, 1927.

576. KOBRAK, F.: Zur Wirkungsweise des kalorischen Schwachreizes. *Beitr. Anat., Physiol., Path. u. Therap. Ohres, 18:*351, 1922.

577. KOBRAK, H.: Zur Ausschaltung der Fixation bei der Nystagmusbeobachtung. *Ztschr. Laryng., Rhin., Otol., 22:*426, 1932. Abs. *Zentralbl. ges. Ophth., 28:* 613, 1933.

578. KOELLA, W.: Experimentell-physiologischer Beitrag zum Nystagmusproblem. *Helvet. physiol. et pharmacol. acta, 5:*430, 1947.

579. KOELLA, W.: Die Beeinflussbarkeit des postrotatorischen Augennystagmus durch propriozeptive Halsreflexe beim Kaninchen. *Helvet. physiol. et pharmacol. acta, 5:*430, 1947.

580. KOELLA, W.: Das Verhalten des perrotatorischen Augennystagmus beim Kaninchen bei Drehungen um nicht latrechte Achsen. *Helvet. Physiol. et pharmacol. acta, 6:*280, 1948.

581. KOELLA, W.: The labyrinthine system and system of the eye muscles in the light of the coordination theory. *Vischr. nature. Ges., Zurich, 95* (suppl. 1), 1950. Abs., Ophthalmology Sect. XII, *Excerpta Medica, 5:*1682, 1951.

582. KOERBER, [H.]: Trois observations de mouvements de rétraction de bulbe (Nystagmus retractorius). *Clinique Ophth., p.* 147. Abs. *Jahresb. Ophth., 34:*683, 1903.

583. KOHNSTAMM: Cited by M. Bartels. Auge und Ohr (Die Ohr-Augen-Bewegungen.), in *Kurzes Handbuch der Ophthalmologie,* edited by F. Schieck and A. Brückner. Berlin, J. Springer, 1930, vol. 3, p. 652.

584. KÖLLNER, H.: Scheinbewegungen beim Nystagmus und ihr diagnostischer Wert. *Arch. Augenh., 93:*130, 1923.

585. KÖLLNER, H.: Ueber den Wilbrandschen Prismenversuch bei der Hemianopsie. *Ztschr. Augenh., 24:*9, 1910.

586. KÖLLNER, H., AND HOFFMAN, P.: Der Einfluss des Vestibularapparates auf die Innervation der Augenmuskeln. *Arch. Augenh., 90:*170, 1922.

587. KOMPANEJETZ, S.: Investigation on the counterrolling of the eyes in optimum head-positions. *Acta oto-laryng., 12:*332, 1928.

588. KÖNIG, A.: Bemerkungen über angeborene totale Farbenblindheit. *Ztschr. Psychol. u. Physiol. Sinnesorg., 20:*425, 1899.

589. KOOMEN, M., TOUSEY, R., AND KNOLL, H. A.: An infra-red pupillometer. *J. Optic. Soc. Am., 38:*719, 1948.

590. [VON] KORNILOW, [A.]: Zur Frage der Associationslähmungen der Augen. *Deutsche Ztschr. Nervenh., 23:*417, 1903. Abs. *Jahresb. Ophth., 34:*466, 1903.

591. KORNMÜLLER, A. E.: Eine experimentelle Anästhesie der äusseren Augenmuskeln am Menschen und ihre Auswirkungen. *J. Psychol. u. Neurol., 41:*354, 1931. Abs. *Zentralbl. ges. Ophth., 25:*267, 1931.

592. KRABBE, K. H.: Crises oculogyres et Parkinsonisme dans la syphilis cérébrospinale. *Acta psychiat. et neurol.. 6:*457, 1931. Abs. *Zentralbl. ges. Ophth., 26:*400, 1932.

593. KRAMER, V., AND BLAGOVEŠCENSKIJ, M.: Zur Ätiologie des Konvergenzspasmus. *Vestnik oftal., 4:*161, 1934. Abs. *Zentralbl. ges. Ophth., 32:*537, 1935.

593a. KRAUSE, F.: Die Sehbahn im chirurgischen Beziehung und die faradische Reizung des Sehzentrums. *Klin. Wchnschr., 3:*1260, 1924.

594. KRIES, J. VON: Wettstreit der Sehrichtungen bei Divergengschielen. *Arch. f. Ophth., 4:*117, 1878.

595. KRUSIUS, F. F.: Klinische Beiträge zur Frage des topischen Werthes des hemianopischen Prismenphänomens und der Hemikinesie bei hemianopischen Störungen. *Arch. Augenh., 65:*383, 1910.

596. KUBIK, C. S., AND ADAMS, R. D.: Subdural empyema. *Brain, 66:*18, 1943.

597. KUBIK, C. S., AND ADAMS, R. D.: Occlusion of the basilar artery—a clinical and pathological study. *Brain, 69:*73, 1946.

598. KUBIK, J.: Retraktionsbewegungen des Bulbus als zerebrales Herdsymptom. *Klin. Monatsbl. Augenh., 86:*251. 1931 (1).

599. KUBO, [I.]: Ueber die vom nervus acusticus ausgelösten Augenbewegungen (besonders bei thermischen Reizungen). *Arch. ges. Physiol., 114:*143, 1906.

600. KUBO, [I.]: Ueber die vom nervus acusticus ausgelösten Augenbewegungen (besonders bei thermischen Reizungen). Part II. *Arch. ges. Physiol., 115:*457, 1906.

601. KUFFLER, S. W.: Specific excitability of endplate region in normal and denervated muscle. *J. Neurophysiol., 6:*99, 1943.

602. KUILMAN, J.: Nystagmographie während der Drehung. *Ztschr. Hals-, Nasenu. Ohrenh., 35:*85, 1933. Abs. *Zentralbl. ges. Ophth., 31:*308, 1934.

603. KULCHITSKY, N.: Nerve endings in the muscles of the frog. *J. Anat., 49:*1, 1924.

604. KUNTZ, A., AND RICHINS, C. A.: Reflex pupillodilator mechanisms. An experimental analysis. *J. Neurophysiol., 9:*1, 1946.

605. KURÉ, K., SUSUKI, T., KANEKO, Y., AND OKINAKA, S.: Histologische Studien über die extrapyramidalen Bahnen; die Kerne der extrapyramidalen Fasern für die Augenmuskeln. *Ztschr. Zellsforsch. u. mikr. Anat., 17:*453, 1933.

606. KYRIELEIS, W.: Beobachtungen bei Pupillotonie. *Deutsche Ophth. Gesell., 57:* 59, 1951.

607. LABORD: Cited by H. Oloff and H. Korbsch. Ueber das Hertwig-Magendiesche Phänomenon (Vertikaldivergenz der Augen). *Klin. Monatsbl. Augenh., 77:* 618, 1926 (2).

608. LABRANCHE, H. G., AND JEFFERSON, R. N.: Congenital myasthenia gravis. *Pediatrics, 4:*16, 1949.

609. LAFON, C.: La vision des nystagmiques. *Ann. ocul., 151:*4, 1914.

610. LAIGNEL-LAVASTINE, M. M., AND BERNAL, P.: Encéphalite aiguë avec syndrome de Parinaud précoce, compliqué et transitoire (Présentation de la malade). *Rev. neurol., 1:*479, 1929.

611. LANGE, F.: Ueber die Pupillomotorik im Alter. *Klin. Monatsbl. Augenh., 124:* 76, 1954.

612. LANGLEY, J. N.: Several communications. *J. Physiol., 36:*347, 1907; *37:*165, 1908; *39:*235, 1909; *47:*159, 1913; *48:*73, 1914.

613. LANGWORTHY, O. R., AND KOLB, L. C.: Cited by O. R. Langworthy and E. S. Tauber. The control of the pupillary reaction by the central nervous system; a review. *J. Nerv. & Ment. Dis., 86:*462, 1937.

614. LARSELL, O.: The development of the cerebellum in man in relation to its comparative anatomy. *J. Comp. Neurol., 87:*85, 1947.

615. LASHLEY, K. S.: The mechanism of vision; cerebral areas necessary for pattern vision in rat. *J. Comp. Neurol., 53:*419, 1931.

616. LASHLEY, K. S.: The mechanism of vision; projection of retina upon primary optic centers in rat. *J. Comp. Neurol., 59:*341, 1934.

617. LAST, S. L., AND VOGELSANG, K.: Gutachten über einen Fall von psychogener Blindheit. (Mit Berücksichtigung des optokinetischen Nystagmus.) *Nervenarzt, 4:*645, 1931.

618. LAUDENBACH, J.: Zur Otolithen-Frage. *Arch. ges. Physiol., 77:*311, 1899.

619. LAUGHLIN, R. C.: Hereditary paralysis of the abducens nerve. Report of a case. *Am. J. Ophth., 20:*396, 1937.

620. LAURENS, H.: Studies on the relative physiological value of spectral lights. III. The pupillomotor effects of wave-lengths of equal energy content. *Am. J. Physiol., 64:*97, 1923.

621. LE CONTE, J.: On some phenomena of binocular vision. *Am. J. Sc. & Arts, 47:* 1872. Abs. *Jahresb. Ophth., 3:*128, 1872.

622. LEIDLER, R.: Cited by M. Bartels. Auge und Ohr (Die Ohr-Augen-Bewegungen.), in *Kurzes Handbuch der Ophthalmologie*, edited by F. Schieck and R. Brückner. Berlin, J. Springer, 1930, vol. 3, p. 652.

623. LEIDLER, R.: Experimentelle Untersuchungen über das Endigungsgebiet des Nervus vestibularis. 1. Mitteilung. *Arb. neurol. Inst. Wien. Univ., 20:*256, 1912-1913.

624. LEIDLER, R.: Experimentelle Untersuchungen über das Endigungsgebiet des Nervus vestibularis. 2. Mitteilung. *Arb. neurol. ist. Wien. Univ., 21:*151, 1916.

625. LEIDLER, R.: Fragen der Lokalisation innerhalb des zentralen Vestibularsystems. I. Die entzündlichen, nichteitrigen Erkrankungen des Hirnstammes (Encephalitis). *Monatsschr. Ohrenh., 70:*176, 267, 472, 544, 725, and 801, 1936. Abs. *Zentralbl. ges. Ophth., 38:*692, 1937.

626. LEINFELDER, P. J., AND BLACK, N. M., JR.: Experimental transposition of the extraocular muscles in monkeys. Preliminary report. Am. J. Ophth. *24:*1115, 1941.

627. LEMERE, [H. B.]: Oculomotor reaction to labyrinthine stimulation. *J.A.M.A., 71:*901, 1918.

628. LEMMEN, L. J.: Anatomical and experimental study of temporal and occipital association areas. *J. Comp. Neurol., 95:*521, 1951.

629. LENZ: Das Verhalten des optokinetic Nystagmus bie einigen Fällen von Lappenresektionen. *Nervenarzt, 14:*124, 1941.

630. LEVINSOHN, G.: *Auge und Nervensystem. Die Beziehungen des Auges zum normalen und kranken Cerebrospinalnervensystem.* Munich, J. F. Bergmann, 1920, 91 pp. Abs. *Zentralbl. ges. Ophth., 5:*265, 1921.

631. LEVINSOHN, G.: Beiträge zur Physiologie des Pupillenreflexes. II. *Arch. f. Ophth., 59* (3):436, 1904.

632. LEVINSOHN, G.: Doppelte Kreuzung der zentripetalen Pupill- und Lidbahnen. *Verhandl. Berlin. Physiol. Gesellsch., 26*(2):568, 1904.

633. LEVINSOHN, G.: Der optische Blinzelreflex. *Ztschr. ges. Neurol. u. Psychiat., 20:* 377, 1913.

634. LEVINSOHN, [G.]: Ueber die Beziehung der Grosshirnrinde beim Affen zu den Bewegungen des Auges. *Arch. f. Ophth., 71:*313, 1909.

635. LEVINSOHN, G.: Zur Kenntnis der Physiologie und Pathologie der Pupillenbahnen. *Deutsche Ztschr. Nervenh., 56:*300, 1917. Abs. *Jahresb. Ophth., 45*(3):492, 1916-1917.

636. LEVINSOHN, G., AND LIEPMANN: Cited by G. Levinsohn. Der optische Blinzelreflex. *Ztschr. f. d. ges. Neurol. u. Psychiat., 20:*377, 1913.

637. LEVIT, L., AND GIQUEAUX, R.: Oftalmoplejias supranucleares. *An. argent. oftal., 7:*75, 1946.

638. LEWANDOWSKY, M.: *Handbuch der Neurologie.* Berlin, Springer, 1910, vol. I, pt. 2, p. 734.

639. LEWANDOWSKY, M., AND SIMON, A.: Zur Physiologie der vorderen und der hinteren Zentralwindung. *Arch. ges. Physiol., 129:*240, 1909.

640. LEWY, F. H.: Reizversuche zur zentralen Pupilleninnervation. *Deutsche Ztschr. Nervenh., 102:*89, 1928.

641. LEWY, F. H., GROFF, R. A., AND GRANT, F. C.: Autonomic innervation of the eye-

lids and the Marcus Gunn phenomenon. An experimental study. *Arch. Neurol. & Psychiat., 37:*1289, 1937.

642. LEYDHECKER, W.: Divergenzlähmung. *Klin. Monatsbl. Augenh., 123:*83, 1953.

643. LEYSER, E.: Ein Angiom der Brücke. *Monatschr. Psychiat. u. Neurol., 51:*83, 1922.

644. LEYTON, A. S. F., AND SHERRINGTON, C. S.: Observations on the excitable cortex of the chimpanzee, orangutan and gorilla. *Quart. J. Exper. Physiol., 11:*135, 1917.

645. LHERMITTE, J.: L'encéphalite léthargique. Anatomie et physiologie pathologiques; pathologie expérimentale, microbiologie. *Arch. ophth., 38:*11, 1921.

646. LHERMITTE, J., AND KRAUS, W.: Note sur les lésions anatomiques du syndrome de Parinaud. *Bull. Soc. ophth. Paris,* p. 220, 1924.

647. LILJESTRAND, G., AND MAGNUS, R.: Ueber die Wirkung des Novokains auf den normalen und den tetanusstarren Skelettmuskel und über die die Enstehung der lokalen Muskelstarre beim Wundstarrkrampf. *Arch. ges. Physiol., 176:*168, 1919.

648. LINDSLEY, D. B., AND HUNTER, W. S.: A note on the polarity potentials from the human eye. *Proc. Nat. Acad. Sc., 25:*180, 1939.

649. LINDSAY, J. R.: Significance of positional nystagmus in otoneurological diagnosis. *Laryngoscope, 55:*527, 1945.

650. LINDSAY, J. R.: Postural vertigo and positional nystagmus. *Ann. Otol., Rhin. & Laryng., 60:*1134, 1951.

651. LINTHICUM, F. H.: Nystagmography; a method for graphic recording of nystagmus during and after turning and of caloric nystagmus. *Arch. Otolaryng., 32:*464, 1940.

652. LIPPMANN, O.: Paralysis of divergence due to cerebellar tumor. *Arch. Ophth., 31:*299, 1944.

653. LIPSCHITZ: Beitrag zur Lehre von der Facialslähmung nebst Bemerkungen zur Frage der Nervenregeneration. *Monatssch. Psychiat. u. Neurol., 20:*84, 1906.

654. LISMAN, J. B.: Rheumatoid involvement of the extraocular muscles. Case report. *Arch. Ophth., 38:*547, 1947.

655. LISMAN, J. V.: Ocular myasthenia gravis. *Am. J. Ophth., 32:*565, 1949.

656. LISMAN, J. V.: Rheumatoid involvement of the extraocular muscles. *Arch. Ophth., 42:*410, 1949.

657. LOEWI, O.: Ueber humorale Übertragbarkeit der Herznervenwirkung. I. Mitteilung. *Arch. ges. Physiol. 189:*239, 1921.

658. LORD, M. P.: Effect of a posture change on head and monocular fixation eye movements. *Nature (London), 166:*349, 1950.

659. LORENTE DE NÓ, R.: Ausgewählte Kapitel aus der vergleichenden Physiologie des Labyrinthes. Die Augenmuskelreflexe beim Kaninchen und ihre Grundlagen. *Ergebn. Physiol., 32:*73, 1931. Abs. *Zentralbl. ges. Ophth., 26:*835, 1932.

660. LORENTE DE NÓ, R.: Ueber den Nervenmechanismus der vestibulären Augenbewegungen. *Acta oto-laryng., 12:*243, 1928.

661. LORENTE DE NÓ, R.: Untersuchungen über die Anatomie und die Physiologie des Nervus octavus und des Ohrlabyrinths. Part IV. Die Drehreflexe auf die Augenmuskeln. *Arch. Ohren-, Nasen- u. Kehlkorpfh., 118:*241, 1928.

662. LÖWENSTEIN, K., AND BORCHARDT, M.: Symptomatologie und elektrische Reizung bei einer Schussverletzung des Hinterhauptlappens. *Deutsche Ztschr. Nervenh., 58:*264, 1918.

663. LOWENSTEIN, O., AND FRIEDMAN, E. D.: Pupillographic studies. I. Recent

state of pupillography; its method and diagnostic method. *Arch. Ophth.,* 27:969, 1942.

664. LOWENSTEIN, O., AND FRIEDMAN, E. D.: Adie's syndrome (pupillotonic pseudotabes.) *Arch. Ophth., 28:*1042, 1942.

665. LOWENSTEIN, O., AND LOEWENFELD, I. E.: Mutual role of sympathetic and parasympathetic in shaping of the pupillary reflex to light. *Arch. Neurol. & Psychiat., 64:*341, 1950.

666. LUCIANI, L.: *Il Cervelletto. Nuovi Studi di Fisiologia Normale e Pathologica.* Firenze, successori Le Monnier, 1891, 320 pp.

667. LUDVIGH, E.: Possible role of proprioception in the extraocular muscles. *Arch. Ophth., 48:*436, 1952.

668. LUDVIGH, E.: Control of ocular movements and visual interpretation of environment. *Arch. Ophth., 48:*442, 1952.

669. LUFT, R.: Meningealblutungen, entstanden durch Aneurysmenruptur der basalen Hirnarterien. *Hygiea, 100:*177, 1938. Abs. *Zentralbl. ges. Ophth., 41:* 671, 1938.

670. LUTZ, A.: Ueber die Bahnen der Blickwendung und deren Dissoziierung. (Nebst Mitteilung eines Falles von Ophthalmoplegia internuclearis anterior in Verbindung mit Dissoziierung der Bogengänge.) *Klin. Monatsbl. Augenh., 70:*213, 1923.

671. McGINNIS, J. M.: Eye-movements and optic nystagmus in early infancy. *Genet. Psychol. Monogr., 8:*321, 1930.

672. MACH, E.: Physikalische Versuche über den Gleichgewichtssinn des Menschen. *Sitzungsb. Akad. Wissensch. Math.-naturw. Cl., 68:*124, 1873.

673. McINTYRE, A. K.: Physiology of nerve endings in extrinsic ocular muscles. *Tr. Ophth. Soc. Australia* (1941), *3:*99, 1942.

674. McINTYRE, A. K.: Quick component of nystagmus. *J. Physiol., 97:*8, 1939.

675. McNALLY, W. J., AND TAIT, J.: Ablation experiments on labyrinth of frog. *Am. J. Physiol., 75:*155, 1925.

676. MAGENDIE: Cited by H. Oloff and H. Korbsch. Ueber das Hertwig-Magendiesche Phänomen (Vertikaldivergenz der Augen). *Klin. Monatsbl. Augenh., 77:*618, 1926(2).

677. MAGNUS, R.: *Körperstellung.* Monograph. Berlin, Springer, 1924.

678. MAGNUS, R.: Cameron prize lectures on some results of studies in the physiology of posture. Part I. *Lancet, 2:*531, 1926. Part II. *Lancet, 2:*585, 1926.

679. MAGNUS, R.: Welche Teile des Zentralnervensystems müssen für das Zustandekommen der tonischen Hals- und Labyrinthreflexe auf die Körpermuskulatur vorhanden sein? *Arch. ges. Physiol., 159:*224, 1914.

680. MAGNUS, R., AND DE KLEYN, A.: Cited by O. R. Hyndman. Physiology of the vestibular labyrinth. *Arch. Otolaryng., 29:*759, 1939.

681. MAGNUS, R., AND DE KLEYN, A.: Experimentelle Physiologie des Vestibularapparates bei Säugetieren mit Ausschluss des Menschen, in *Handbuch der Neurologie des Ohres,* edited by G. Alexander and O. Marburg. Berlin, & Schwarzenberg, 1924, vol. 1, p. 465.

682. MAGOUN, H. W.: Maintenance of light reflex after destruction of superior colliculus in cat. *Am. J. Physiol., 111:*91, 1935.

683. MAGOUN, H. W.: ATLAS, D., HARE, W. K., AND RANSON, S. W.: Afferent path of pupillary light reflex in monkey. *Brain, 59:*234, 1936.

684. MAGOUN, H. W., HARE, W. K., AND RANSON, S. W.: Electrical stimulation of interior of cerebellum in monkey. *Am. J. Physiol., 112:*329, 1935.

685. MAGOUN, H. W., AND RANSON, S. W.: The central path of the light reflex; a study of the effect of lesions. *Arch. Ophth., 13:*791, 1935.

686. MAIER, M., AND LION, H.: Ueber den experimentellen Nachweis der Endolymphbewegung in Bogengangsapparat des Ohrlabyrinthes bei adaquäter und kalorischer Reizung. Physiologische Erklärung der Auslösung des Nystagmus durch Endolymphbewegung. *Arch. ges. Physiol., 187:*47, 1921.

687. MAJEWSKI, K.: Eine neue Methode der klinischen Nystagmographie. *Arch f. Ophth., 96:*140, 1918.

688. MALBRAN, J.: Paralisis del musculo recto inferior. *Arch. oftal. Buenos Aires, 17:*311, 1942.

689. MALTESOS, C.: Eine Methode zur fortlaufenden Registrierung der Pupillenweite. *Arch. ges. Physiol., 241:*129, 1938.

690. MANCALL, I.: Opticociliary neuritis. *Arch. Ophth., 54:*436-437, 1955.

691. MANN, C. W.: The effects of auditory-vestibular nerve pathology on space perception. The Bureau of Medicine and Surgery Project No. 001063, 01. 22, 1951.

692. MANN: Ueber die galvanische Vestibularreaktion. *Neurol. Centralbl., 31:*1356, 1912.

693. MANN, I. C.: Developing third nerve nucleus in human embroys. *J. Anat., 61:*424, 1927.

694. MARBURG, O.: Probleme der vertikalen Blickbewegung. *Ztschr. Augenh., 58:*253, 1926.

695. MARBURG, O.: Ueber die neueren Fortschritte in der topischen Diagnostik des Pons und der Oblongata. *Deutsche Ztschr. Nervenh., 41:*41, 1911.

696. MARBURG, O.: Zur Lokalisation des Nystagmus. (Zystizerkus am Boden des 4. Ventrikels). *Neurol. Centralbl., 31:*1366, 1912.

697. MARCUS, A.: *Untersuchungen über den Ausfall der Optomotorischen Nystagmusreaktion bei Nervenerkrankungen.* Diss. Cologne, 1923 (1924).

698. MARCUS, H., SAHLGREN, E., AND BJERLÖV, H.: Métastases carcinomateuses du cerveau avec syndrome de Charcot-Adams-Stokes et crises oculogyres. *Acta med. scandinav., 98:*58, 1938.

699. MARG, E.: Development of electro-oculography; standing potential of the eye in registration of eye movement. *Arch. Ophth., 45:*169, 1951.

700. MARGULIS, M. S., AND MODEL, M. M.: Zur Pathologie der assoziierten Bewegungen der Augenmuskeln in Zusammenhang mit vestibulärem Symptomenkomplex bei Encephalitis. *Deutsche Ztschr. f. Nervenh., 93:*80, 1926.

701. MARINA, [A.]: Das Neuron des Ganglion ciliare und die Centra der Pupillenbewegungen. Eine experimentelle Studie. *Deutsche Ztschr. Nervenh., 14:*356, 1899.

702. MARINA, [A.]: Die Relationen des Paläencephalons (Edinger) sind nicht fixiert. *Neurol. Centralbl., 34:*338, 1915.

703. MARQUEZ, M.: Explicacion fisologica de la ley de Hering en conexion con la doble inervacion del musculo recto interno del ojo. *An. Soc. Mexico oftal., 21:*3, 1947.

704. MARQUIS, D. G.: Effects of removal of the visual cortex in mammals, with observations on the retention of light discrimination in dogs. *A. Res. Nerv. & Ment. Dis., Proc., 13:*558, 1932.

705. MARQUIS, D. G.: Phylogenetic interpretation of the functions of the visual cortex. *Arch. Neurol. & Psychiat., 33:*807, 1935.

706. MARQUIS, D. G., AND HILGARD, E. R.: Conditional lid responses to light in dogs after removal of visual cortex. *J. Comp. Psychol., 22:*157, 1936.

707. MARQUIS, D. G., AND HILGARD, E. R.: Conditioned responses to light in monkeys after removal of the occipital lobes. *Brain, 60:*1, 1937.

708. MATTEUCCI, P.: Sulla presenza di particolari fibre pupillari nel nerve ottico. *Oto-rino-laring. ital., 17:*441, 1948.

709. MATTHES, K.: Ueber die Registrierung von Bewegungsvorgängen mit dem lichtelektrischen Reflexionsmesser. *Klin. Wchnschr., 20:*295, 1941.

710. MATTIS, R. D.: Ocular manifestations in myasthenia gravis. *Arch. Ophth., 26:*969, 1941.

711. MAUTHNER, O.: Zur Kenntnis nur scheinbar otogener zerebraler Komplikationen bei akuten Infektionskrankheiten. *Monatsschr. Ohrenh., 59:*272, 1925.

712. MAXWELL, S. S.: Labyrinth and Equilibrium. II. The mechanism of the dynamic functions of the labyrinth. *J. Gen. Physiol., 2:*349, 1920.

713. MAXWELL, S. S., AND HUDDLESTON, O. L.: Relations of individual ampullae of semicircular canals to individual eye muscles; horizontal canals. *J. Gen. Physiol., 8:*441, 1926.

714. MAYER, O.: Die Pyramidenzelleneiterungen. *Ztschr. Hals.-, Nasen- u. Ohrenh., 42:*87, 1937.

715. McCULLOCH, W. S.: *Corticocortical connections.* Chap. VIII of *Precentral Motor Cortex.* Illinois Monogr. in Med. Sc., 1948.

716. McEACHERN, D.: The thymus in relation to myasthenia gravis. *Medicine, 20:*1, 1943.

717. McGINNIS, J. M.: Eye-movements and optic nystagmus in early infancy. *Genet. Psychol. Monogr., 8:*321, 1930.

718. McGOUGH, G. P., AND ADLER, F. H.: Extraocular reflexes. *Am. J. Physiol., 100:*78, 1932.

719. McKEEVER, G. E.: Myasthenia gravis in mother and her newborn son. *J.A.M.A., 147:*320-322, 1951.

720. MERRILLEES, N. C. R., SUNDERLAND, S., AND HAYHEW, W.: Neuromuscular spindles in the extraocular muscles in man. *Anat. Rec., 108:*23-30, 1950.

721. MERRITT, H. H., AND FINLAND, M.: Vascular lesions of hindbrain (lateral medullary syndrome). *Brain, 53:*290, 1930.

722. MERRITT, H. H., AND MOORE, M.: The Argyll-Robertson pupil. An anatomic physiologic explanation of the phenomenon, with a survey of its occurrence in neurosyphilis. *Arch. Neurol. & Psychiat., 30:*357, 1933.

723. METTLER, F. A.: Corticofugal fiber connections of the cortex of Macaca mulatta. The frontal region. *J. Comp. Neurol., 61:*221, 1935.

724. METZGER, E.: Tonusänderungen auf optische Reize. *Deutsche. Ophth. Gesellsch,. Heidelberg, 45:*278, 1925.

725. MEYER, I. L.: Conjugate deviation of the head and eyes. Its value in the diagnosis and localization of abscess of the brain. *Arch. Otolaryng., 13:*683, 1931.

726. MEYERS, I. L.: Electronystagmography; a graphic study of the action currents in nystagmus. *Arch. Neurol. & Psychiat., 21:*901, 1929.

727. MICHEL, V.: *Beiträge zur Frage der Kleinhirnbrückenwinkeltumoren.* Diss., Frankfort, 1936, 24 pp. Abs. *Zentralbl. ges. Ophth., 41:*301, 1936.

728. MIKLOS, A.: Ueber einen Fall von willkürlichen Nystagmus. *Klin. Monatsbl. Augenh., 100:*186, 1938(1).

729. MILLIKAN, C. H., AND HAINES, S. F.: The thyroid in relation to neuromuscular disease. *Arch. Int. Med., 92:*5, 1953.

730. MINKOWSKI, M.: Zur Physiologie der Sehsphäre. *Arch. ges. Physiol., 141:*171, 1911.

731. MOHNEY, J. B., MORGAN, M. W., JR., OLMSTED, J. M. D., AND WAGMAN, I. H.: The pathway of sympathetic nerves to the ciliary muscles in the eye. *Am. J. Physiol., 135:*759, 1942.

732. VON MONAKOW, C.: *Gehirnpathologie,* ed. 2, 2 Parts. Vienna, Hölder, 1905, 1319 pp.

733. VON MONAKOW, C.: *Die Lokalisation im Grosshirn und der Abbau der Funktion durch Kortikale Herde.* Wiesbaden, J. F. Bergmann, 1914, 1033 pp.

734. MONNIER, M., AND RUHSCHMID, H. J.: Das Elektro-Oculogramm (EOG) und Elektro-nystagmogram (ENG) beim Menschen. *Helvet. physiol. et pharmacol. acta, 9:*348, 1951.

735. MONNIER, M. AND SIGWALD, J.: L'influence de la fonction optique sur le tonus musculaire (contribution à l'étude pathogénique du torticolis spasmodique). *Ann. méd., 42:*138, 1937.

736. MONTANDON, A.: Nystagmus vertical spontane d'origine peripherique (polyny-stagmus a composante verticale predominante, dans une labyrinthite circonscrite interessant le canal vertical anterieur). *Rev. oto-neuro-opht., 18:* 449, 1946.

737. MORAN, P. V.: Les paralyses des mouvements associés des yeux; étude clinique et physiopathologique. *Ann ocul., 176:*337, 1939.

738. MORGAN, L. O.: Corpus striatum; study of secondary degenerations following lesions in man and of symptoms and acute degenerations following experimental lesions in cats. *Arch. Neurol. & Psychiat., 18:*495, 1927.

739. MORGAN, M. W., JR., OLMSTED, J. M. D., AND WATROUS, W. G.: Sympathetic action in accommodation for far vision. *Am. J. Physiol., 128:*588, 1940.

740. DE MORSIER, G., AND BALAVOINE, C.: Spasmes de la convergence. *Ophthalmologica, 116:*248, 1948.

741. MORSON, S. M.: The anatomy of the "sensory" ending in extrinsic ocular muscles. *Tr. Ophth. Soc. Australia* (1941), *3:*91, 1942.

742. MOTT, [F. W.], AND SCHÄFER, [E. A.]: On associated eye movements produced by cortical faradisation of the monkey's brain. *Brain, 13:*165, 1890.

743. MOWRER, O. H.: A comparison of the reaction mechanisms mediating optokinetic nystagmus in human beings and in pigeons. *Psychol. Monogr., 47:*294, 1936.

744. MOWRER, O. H.: The influence of vision during bodily rotation upon the duration of post-rotational vestibular nystagmus. *Acta oto-laryng., 25:*351, 1937.

745. MOWRER, O. H., RUCH, T. C., AND MILLER, N. E.: Corneo-retinal potential difference as the basis of the galvanometric method of recording eye movements. *Am. J. Physiol., 114:*423, 1936.

746. MÜLLER, H. K., AND MANI, P.: Ueber die isolierte, einseitige, supranucleare Medialislähmung. *Klin. Monatsbl. Augenh., 97:*685. 1936. Abs. *Zentralbl. ges. Ophth., 38:*161, 1937.

747. MUNK, H.: Ueber die centralen Organe für das Sehen und das Hören bei den Wirbeltieren. *Sitzungsb. preuss. Akad. Wissensch., 30:*615, 1889. Abs. *Jahresb. Ophth., 20:*41, 1889.

748. MUNK, H.: *Ueber die Functionen der Grosshirnrinde; gesammelte Mittheilungen mit Anmerkungen,* ed. 2. Berlin, A. Hirschwalt, 1890, 320 pp.

749. MUNRO, D., AND SISSON, W.: Hernia through the incisura of the tentorium cerebelli in connection with craniocerebral trauma. *New England J. Med., 247:*699, 1952.

750. MUSKENS, L. J. J.: An anatomico-physiological study of the posterior longitudinal bundle in its relation to forced movements. *Brain, 36:*352, 1914.

751. MUSKENS, L. J. J.: The central connections of the vestibular nuclei with the corpus striatum, and their significance for ocular movements and for locomotion. *Brain, 45:*454, 1922.

752. MUSKENS, L. J. J.: Cortical innervation of ocular movements in the horizontal plane. *Arch. Ophth., 18:*527, 1937.

753. MUSKENS, L. J. J.: On tracts and centers involved in upward and downward associated movements of eyes after experiments in birds. *J. Comp. Neurol., 50:*289, 1930.

754. MUSSEN, A. T.: Experimental investigations on the cerebellum. *Brain, 50:*313, 1927.

755. MUTCH, J. R.: Pupil after cervico-thoracic sympathetic ganglionectomy; photographic observations in man. *Edinburgh M. J., 43:*743, 1936.

756. MYERSON, A.: Tap and thrust responses in Parkinson's disease. *Arch. Neurol. & Psychiat., 51:*480, 1944.

757. MYGIND, S. H.: Ueber vertikalen Nystagmus. *Arch. Ohren-, Nasen- u. Kehlkopfh., 128:*69, 1931.

758. NACHMANSOHN, D.: *Currents in Biochemical Research.* New York, Interscience, 1946.

759. NAFFZIGER, H. C.: Exophthalmos. Some principles of surgical management from the neurosurgical aspect. *Am. J. Surg., 75:*25, 1948.

760. NATHANSON, M., BERGMAN, P. S., AND BENDER, M. B.: Visual disturbances as the result of nystagmus on direct forward gaze. Effect of amobarbital (amytal®) sodium. *Arch. Neurol. & Psychiat., 69:*427, 1953.

761. NEIDING, AND FRANKFURTER: Cited by C. Frank. Ueber Lokalisation der Augenmuskelnervenkerne. *J. Psychol. u. Neurol., 26:*200, 1921.

762. NEIDLE, E. A.: Pilocarpine sensitization in the parasympathetically denervated pupil of the cat. *Am. J. Physiol., 160:*467, 1950.

763. NEUMANN: Konglomerattuberkel des Pons. *Deutsche med. Wchnschr., 44:*871, 1918.

764. NEUMANN, H.: *Der Otitische Kleinhirnabscess.* Leipzig, F. Deuticke, 1907, 118 pp.

765. NICKELL, R.: Das Centrum des reflectorischen Lidschlusses. *Arch. ges. Physiol., 42:*547, 1888.

766. NICOLAI, H.: Objective Sehschärfenbestimmung auf der Grundlage des optokinetischen Nystagmus mit eigenem Gerät. *Klin. Monatsbl. Augenh., 122:*402, 1953.

767. NIESSL VON MAYENDORF, [E.]: Die sogenannte Radiatio optica. *Arch. f. Ophth., 104:*293, 1921.

768. DE NIGRIS, G.: Sindrome oculocefalogira in sogetto neuroluetica. *Riv. oto-neuro-oftal., 10:*73, 1933.

769. NOEHTE: Ueber Nystagmus bei Verletzungen des Fusses der II. Stirnhirn-windung. *Deutsche med. Wchnschr., 41(2):*1217, 1915.

770. NOJI, R.: Ueber optisch erzwungene parallele Rollunger der Augen. *Arch. f. Ophth., 122:*562, 1929.

771. NORDMANN, J.: Le nystagmus optocinétique du nouveau-né. *Bull. Soc. opht. Paris,* No. *5:*273, 1928. Abs. *Zentralbl. ges. Ophth., 20:*685, 1929.

772. NORDMANN, J., AND LIEAU, Y. C.: Le nystagmus optocinétique. *Rev. d'oto-neuro-opht., 6:*81, 1928.

773. NORTHINGTON, P., AND PIKE, F. H.: Some observations on the occurrence of and modifications in the type of vestibular nystagmus after experimental lesion of the central nervous system. *Laryngoscope, 42:*237, 1933.

774. NORTON, E. W. D., AND COGAN, D. G.: Spasmus nutans. *Arch. Ophth., 52:*442, 1954.

775. NULSEN, F. E., BLACK, S. P. W., AND DRAKE, C. G.: Inhibition and facilitation of motor activity by the anterior cerebellum. *Federation Proc., 7:*86, 1948.

776. NYLÉN, C. O.: A nystagmus phenomenon. *Acta oto-larygn., 3:*502, 1922.

777. NYLÉN, C. O.: Clinical study on positional nystagmus in cases of brain tumor. *Acta oto-laryng.,* Supple. *15:*1, 1931.

778. NYLÉN, C. O.: To the diagnosis of brain tumours: Head-position nystagmus and brain tumours. I. *Congr. internat. d'oto-rhino-laryng., 76,* 1929. Abs. *Zentralbl. ges. Ophth., 24:*667, 1931.

779. NYLÉN, C. O.: Oto-neurological diagnosis of tumours of brain. *Acta oto-laryng.,* Supple., 33, p. 1, 1939.

780. NYLÉN, C. O.: Positional nystagmus. *J. Laryng. & Otol., 64:*295, 1950.

781. OBREGIA, A.: Ueber Augenbewegungen auf Sehsphaerenreizung. *Arch. Anat. u. Physiol.* (Physiol. Abt.), p. 260, 1890. Abs. *Jahresb. Ophth., 21:*60, 1890.

782. OHM, J.: Drehnystagmus bei Taubstummen. *Monatsschr. Ohrenh., 65:*805, 1931. Abs. *Zentralbl. ges. Ophth., 26:*555, 1932.

783. OHM, J.: Grundplan der Augenbewegung. I. Die gleichsinnigen waagerechten Augenbewegungen. *Arch. f. Ophth., 138:*1, 1938.

784. OHM, J.: Die Hebelnystagmographie. *Arch f. Ophth., 120:*235, 1928.

785. OHM, J.: Die klinische Bedeutung des optischen Drehnystagmus. *Klin. Monatsbl. Augenh., 68:*323, 1922(1).

786. OHM, J.: Der latente Nystagmus nach Verlust eines Auges. *Arch. f. Ophth., 144:*617, 1942.

787. OHM, J.: Objectivadaptationsprüfung mittels des optokinetischen Nystagmus in einem Falle von abgelaufener Neuritis retrobulbaris. *Arch. f. Ophth., 144:*453, 1942.

788. OHM, J.: Der optische Drehnystagmus bei Augen- und Allgemeinleiden. *Arch. f. Ophth., 114:*169, 1924.

789. OHM, J.: Der optokinetische Nystagmus bei hysterischer Blindheit. *Ztschr. Augenh., 85:*65, 1935.

790. OHM, J.: Optokinetischer Nystagmus und Nystagmographie im Dienste der Hirndiagnostik. *Arch. Augenh., 106:*185, 1932.

791. OHM, J.: Ueber die Beziehungen der Augenmuskeln zu den Ampullen der Bogengänge beim Menschen und Kaninchen. *Klin. Monatsbl. Augenh., 62:* 289, 1919(1).

792. OHM, J.: Ueber die Beziehungen zwischen motorische Sprachlähmung und optokinetischen Nystagmus. *Deutsche Ztschr. Nervenh., 154:* 237,1943.

793. OHM, J. Ueber optischen Drehnystagmus. *Klin. Monatsbl. Augenh., 68:*234, 1922(1).

794. OHM, J.: Ueber Registrierung des optischen Drehnystagmus. *München. med. Wchnschr., 68:*1451, 1921. Abs. *Zentralbl. ges. Ophth., 6:*547, 1922.

795. OHM, J.: Die Vestibulariskerne als Bestandteil der optokinetischen Reflexbahn. *Deutsche Ztschr. Nervenh., 154:*68, 1942.

796. OHM, J.: Zur Augenzitternkunde. 20 Mitteilung. Zum 2000. Fall von Augenzittern der Bergleute. Part I. *Arch. f. Ophth., 125:*245, 1930.

797. OHM, J.: Zur Augenzitternkunde. 23 Mitteilung. Zum 2000. Fall von Augenzittern der Bergleute. Part 2. *Arch. f. Ophth., 126:*221, 1931.

798. OHM, J.: Zur Augenzitternkunde. 38 Mitteilung. Ueber den Einfluss der gleichseitigen Halbblindheit auf den optokinetischen Nystagmus. *Arch. f. Ophth., 135:*200, 1936.

799. OHM, J.: Zur Augenzitternkunde. 40 Mitteilung. Ueber die Beziehungen zwischen der Halbblindheit und dem optokinetischen Nystagmus. *Arch. f. Ophth., 136:*341, 1936.

800. OHM, J.: "Zur Lehre vom Augenzittern." Erwiderung auf den Aufsatz von Raudnitz "Kritisches zur Lehre vom Spasmus nutans." *Jahrb. Kinderh., 88:*397, 1918.

801. OHM, J.: Ueber einseitige bzw. nicht assoziierte Innervationen der Augenmuskeln. *von Graefes Arch. Ophth., 149:*364, 1949.

802. OHM, J.: Die objektive Sehschärfenbestimmung mit Hilfe des optokinetischen Nystagmus bei einem einäugigen 'Kriegsblinden.' *Klin. Monatsbl. Augenh., 115:*193, 1949.

803. OHM, J.: Familiäres Vorkommen von Augenzittern der Bergleute, Dunkelzittern kleiner Kinder und ähnlichem Augenzittern. *von Graefes Arch. Ophth., 152:*121, 1951.

804. OHM, J.: Ueber die Anwendung bewegter Spiegelmarken in Verbindung mit dem optokinetischen Nystagmus zwecks objectiver Sehschärfenbestimmung. *Klin. Monatsbl. Augenh., 120:*144, 1952.

805. OLMSTED, J. M. D., MARGUTTI, M., AND YANAGISAWA, K.: Adaptation to transposition of eye muscles. *Am. J. Physiol., 116:*245, 1936.

806. OLMSTED, J. M. D., AND MORGAN, M. W., JR.: The influence of the cervical sympathetic nerve on the lens of the eye. *Am. J. Physiol., 133:*720, 1941.

807. OLOFF, [H.]: Ueber die hemianopische Pupillenreaktion. *München. med. Wchnschr., 69* (1):462, 1922.

808. OLOFF, H., AND KORBSCH, H.: Ueber das Hertwig-Magendiesche Phänomen (Vertikaldivergenz der Augen). *Klin. Monatsbl. Augenh., 77:*618, 1926 (2).

809. OLSEN, C. W., AND MILLITZER, M. M.: Parinaud's syndrome; case with autopsy. *Bull. Los Angeles Neurol. Soc., 5:*224, 1940.

810. OPPENHEIM, H.: Zur Symptomatologie der Pseudobulbärparalyse. *Fortschr. Med., 13:*1, 1895.

811. OPPENHEIM, H.: *Lehrbuch der Nervenkrankheiten für Ärzte und Studierende.* ed. 6. Berlin, S. Karger, 1913, vol. 2, 1926 pp.

812. ORZECHOWSKI, C.: De l'ataxie dysmétrique des yeux. Remarques sur l'ataxie des yeux dite myolconique (opsoclonie, opsochorie). *J. Psychol. u. Neurol., 35:*1, 1927. Abs. *Zentralbl. ges. Ophth., 19:*322, 1928.

813. OUGHTERSON, A. W.: Cited by J. F. Fulton. *Physiology of the Nervous System*. London, Oxfosd Univ. Press, 1938, 675 pp.

814. PALOMAR COLLARDE, F.: Characteristics de la dinamica ocular y so terminologia. *Arch. Soc. oftal. hispano-am., 10:922*, 1950.

815. PAPEZ, J. W.: Reticulo-spinal tracts in cat; Marchi method. *J. Comp. Neurol., 41:365*, 1926.

816. PARSONS, J. H.: On dilatation of the pupil from stimulation of the cortex cerebri. *J. Physiol., 26:366*, 1900/01.

817. PARSONS, J. H.: The fourth cranial nerve. *Brit. J. Ophth., 5:529*, 1921.

818. PATERSON, D., AND ELLIS, R. W. B.: Spasmus nutans (head-nodding) as associated with defective lighting in the home. *Lancet, 2:736*, 1931.

819. PATHOVEN, W. J.: Kontralaterale Abducenslähmung bei otogener Meningitis. *Arch. Ohren-, Nasen- u. Kehlkopfh., 147:348*, 1940.

820. PATON, L., AND MANN, I. C.: The development of the third nerve nucleus and its bearing on the Argyll-Robertson pupil. *Tr. Ophth. Soc. U. Kingdom, 45*, pt. 2:610, 1925.

821. PEARSON, A. A.: The trochlear nerve in human fetuses. *J. Comp. Neurol., 78:29*, 1943.

822. PENFIELD, W.: Focal epileptic discharge in a case of tumor of the posterior temporal region. *Canad. M. A. J., 33:32*, 1935.

823. PENFIELD, W., AND RASMUSSEN, T.: *The Cerebral Cortex of Man: A Clinical Study of Localization of Function*. New York, Macmillan, 1950.

824. PERLIA: Die Anatomie des Oculomotoriuscentrums beim Menschen. *Arch. f. Ophth., 35* (4):287, 1889.

825. PERLMAN, H. B., AND CASE, T. J.: Nystagmus: some observations based on electrical method for recording eye movements. *Laryngoscope, 49:217*, 1939.

826. PETERS, A.: Ueber Convergenzlähmungen. *Centralbl. Augenh., 13:225*, 1889.

827. PETERSON, E. W., AND HENNEMAN, E.: Corticocollicular connections in the macaque. *Tr. Am. Neurol. A., 73:119*, 1948.

828. PFLUGFELDER, M., AND HAUSER, F.: Komplette Blicklähmung in einem Falle von Heine-Medinscher Poliomyelitis acuta. *Ophthalmologica, 118:378*, 1949.

829. PHILIBERT, A., AND ROSE, F.: Un cas de syndrome de l'artère cérébelleuse postéroinférieure. *Progrès méd., 52:229*, 1924. Abs. *Zentralbl. ges. Ophth., 13:95*, 1925.

830. PHILLIPS, G. B., VICTOR, M., ADAMS, R. D., AND DAVIDSON, C. S.: A study of the nutritional defect in Wernicke's syndrome. *J. Clin. Investigation, 31:859*, 1952.

831. PIPER, H. F.: Der Einfluss des Adaptationszustandes auf den Ablauf unwillkürlicher Augenbewegungen. *Berl. deutsch. ophth. Gesellsch., 57:260*, 1951.

832. POCHIN, E. E.: Ocular effects of sympathetic stimulation in man. *Clin. Sc., 4:79*, 1939.

833. POLJAK, S.: An experimental study of the association callosal, and projection fibers of the cerebral cortex of the cat. *J. Comp. Neurol., 44:197*, 1927.

834. POLJAK, S.: *The Main Afferent Systems of the Cerebral Cortex in Primates*. Berkeley, Univ. California Press, 1932, 370 pp. (Univ. Calif. Publ. Anat. vol. 2).

835. POLJAK, S.: Die Verbindungen der Area Striata (intrahemisphaerale, kommissurale, palliodienzephalische, palliotektale Fasern) bei der Katze und

deren funktionelle Bedeutung. *Ztschr. ges. Neurol. u. Psychiat., 100:*545, 1926.

836. Poos, F.: Zur Frage der sympathischen Innervation des Ziliarmuskels und ihrer Bedeutung für die Akkommodation. *Klin. Monatsbl. Augenh., 80:*749, 1928 (1).

837. Popper, L.: Ueber die Pupillen in schweren zerebrallen Insulten. *Wien. med. Wchnschr., 83:*120, 1933.

838. Posner, M., and Horrax, G.: Eye signs in pineal tumors. *J. Neurosurg., 3:*15, 1946.

839. Post, L.: Unilateral nystagmus. *Am. J. Ophth., 8:*632, 1925.

840. Pötzl, O.: Lokaldiagnostische Bemerkungen zu der einseitigen Übererregbarkeit eines Labyrinths bei Kleinhirnerkrankungen. *Med. Klin., 24:*167, 1928.

841. Pötzl, O., and Sittig, O.: Klinische Befunde mit Hertwig-Magendie Augeneinstellung. *Ztschr. ges. Neurol. u. Psychiat., 95:*701, 1925.

842. Powell, W. H.: Ocular manifestations of alcohol and consideration of individual variations in seven cases studied. *J. Aviation Med., 9:*97, 1938.

843. Prevost, J. L.: Prevost, J. L.: *De la Déviation Conjugée des Yeux et de la Rotation de la Tête dans Certains Cas d'Hémiplégie.* Paris, Masson, 1868, 135 pp.

844. Preyer, W.: *The Mind of the Child. Part I. The Senses and the Will.* New York, D. Appleton, 1895, 353 pp.

845. Prezzolini, M.: Deviazione coniugata dei bulbi oculari, associata alla chiuslera delle palpebre, nell' emiplegia. *Bull. sc. med., 84:*285, 1913.

846. Pritchard, E .A. B.: Tumour of sphenoidal region with external ocular palsies. *Proc. Roy. Soc. Med., 31:*663, 1937-1938.

847. Probst, M.: Ueber den Verlauf der centralen Sehfasern (Rinden-Sehhügelfasern) und deren Endigung im Zwischen- und Mittelhirne und über die Associations- und Commissurenfasern der Sehsphäre. *Arch. Psychiat., 35:* 22, 1901.

848. Putnam, T. J.: Studies on the central visual system. IV. The details of the organization of the geniculostriate system in man. *Arch. Neurol. & Psychiat., 16:*683, 1926.

849. Quensel: Cited by M. Bartels. Auge und Ohr (Die Ohr-Augen-Bewegungen.), in *Kurzes Handbuch der Ophthalmologie,* edited by F. Schieck and A. Brückner. Berlin, J. Springer, 1930, vol. 3, p. 652.

850. Raeder, J. G.: Paratrigeminal paralysis of oculo-pupillary sympathetic. *Brain, 47:*149, 1924.

851. Raimondo, N.: Torcicollo oculare da nistagmo. *Ann. ottal. e clin. ocul., 78:* 949, 1952.

852. Ramón y Cajal: Cited by M. Bartels. Auge und Ohr (Die Ohr-Augen-Bewegungen.), in *Kurzes Handbuch der Ophthalmologie,* edited by F. Schieck and A. Brückner. Berlin, J. Springer, 1930, vol. 3, p. 652.

853. Rand, R. W.: An anatomical and experimental study of the cerebellar nuclei and their efferent pathways in the monkey. Thesis, University of Michigan, 1952.

854. Ranson, S. W.: *The Anatomy of the Nervous System: Its Development and Function,* 8th ed. Revised by Clark. Philadelphia, Saunders, 1947.

855. RANSON, S. W., AND MAGOUN, H. W.: The central path of pupilloconstrictor reflex in response to light. *Arch. Neurol. & Psychiat., 30:*1193, 1933.

856. RANSON, S. W., AND MAGOUN, H. W.: Respiratory and pupillary reactions induced by electrical stimulation of the hypothalamus. *Arch. Neurol. & Psychiat., 29:*1179, 1933.

857. RASMUSSEN, A. T.: *The Principal Nervous Pathways.* New York: Macmillan, 1945.

858. RASMUSSEN, T., AND PENFIELD, W.: Movement of head and eyes from stimulation of human frontal cortex. *Res. Publ. A. Nerv. & Ment. Dis., 27:*346, 1948.

859. RAUDNITZ, [R. W.]: Demonstration von experimentellen Nystagmus. *Klin. Monatsbl. Augenh., 40:*271, 1902 (2).

860. RAUDNITZ, R. W.: Versuche über experimentellen Spasmus nutans und über die Einwirkung von Harnzersetzungprodukten auf junge Hunde. *Jahrb. Kinderh., 73:*259, 1911.

861. RAUDNITZ, R. W.: Zur Lehre von Spasmus nutans. *Jahrb. Kinderh., 45:*145 and 416, 1897.

862. RAY, B. S., HINSEY, J. C., AND GEOHEGAN, W. A.: Observations on the distribution of the sympathetic nerves to the pupil and upper extremity as determined by stimulation of the anterior roots in man. *Ann. Surg., 118:*647, 1943.

863. REDSLOB, E.: Le nystagmus des aveugles. *Rev. oto-neuro-ocul., 5:*490, 1927.

864. REDSLOB, [E.], AND KELLER: Paralysie oculaire apres rachi-anesthésie. *Bull. Soc. opht. Paris, 4:*294, 1939.

865. REESE, W. S., AND YASKIN, J. C.: Preservation of convergence with paralysis of all lateral movements in a case of intra-medullary tumor of the pons. *Am. J. Ophth., 24:*544, 1941.

866. REICH: Ueber die Anatomie des peripheren und zentralen Bogengangapparates. *Verhandl. Gesellsch. deutsch. Naturforsch. u. Aertze, 85:*251, 1913. Abs. *Neurol. Centralbl., 32:*1395, 1913.

867. REID, G.: Rate of discharge of extraocular motoneurones. *J. Physiol., 110:* 217, 1949.

867a. REID, W. L., AND CONE, W. V.: Mechanism of fixed dilation of pupil resulting from ipsilateral cerebral concussion. *J.A.M.A., 112:*2030, 1939.

868. REISSER, O., AND NEUSCHLOSS, S. M.: Physiologische und kolloid-chemische Untersuchungen ueber den Mechanismus der durch Gifte bewirkten Kontraktur quergestreiften Muskeln. I. Ueber die durch Azetylcholin bewirkte Erregungskontraktur des Froschmuskels und ihre antagonistische Beeinflussung durch Atropin, Novakain und Kurare. *Arch. exper. Path. u. Pharmakol., 91:*342, 1921.

869. RENARD, G.: La synergie pupillaire a la convergence. *Rev. oto-neuro-opht., 19:*240, 1947.

870. RHESE, [H.]: Ueber die traumatische Läsion der Vestibularisbahn, insbesondere über den Sitz der Läsion. *Ztschr. Ohrenh., 70:*262, 1914.

871. RICHTER, H.: Anatomische Veränderungen nach Verschluss der Arteria cerebelli inf. post. mit retroovinärem Erweichungsherd. *Arch. f. Psychiat., 71:*272, 1924. Abs. *Zentralbl. ges. Ophth., 13:*470, 1925.

872. RIDDOCH, G.: On the relative perceptions of movement and a stationary ob-

ject in certain visual disturbances due to occipital injuries. *Proc. Roy. Soc. Med., 10* (Part 2):13 (Sect. of Neurol.), 1916-1917.

873. RIEGER, H.: Zur Pathologie des Ganglion Ciliare. *Klin. Monatsbl. Augenh., 120:*337, 1952.

874. RIEKEN, H.: Objektive Adaptometrie. *Klin. Monatsbl. Augenh., 107:*1, 1941.

875. VAN RIJNBERK, G.: Das Kleinhirn, in *Ergebnisse der Physiologie,* edited by L. Asher and K. Spiro. Munich, J. F. Bergmann, 1931, vol. 31, p. 592. Abs. *Zentralbl. ges. Ophth., 25:*194, 1931.

876. VAN RIJNBERK, G.: Weitere Beiträge zum Lokalisationproblem im Kleinhirn. *Folia neuro-biol., 6:*Suppl., p. 143, 1912.

877. RINALDI, F., AND FERRARI, E.: Contribution to the study of experimental nystagmus. II Action of pentothal in unilaterally and bilaterally labyrinthectomized rabbits. *Acta neurol., 6:*129, 1951. Abs., Ophthalmology Sect. XII, *Excerpta Medica, 5:*2138, 1951.

878. RINALDI, F., AND FERRARI, E.: Experimental nystagmus. I Pentothal nystagmus in rabbits. *Acta neurol., 6:*11, 1951. Abs. Ophthalmology Sect. XII, *Excerpta Medica, 6:*1276, 1952.

879. RIOCH, D. M., AND BRENNER, C.: Experiments on the corpus striatum and rhinencephalon. *J. Comp. Neurol., 68:*491, 1938.

880. RIZZO, A.: Sulla natura funzionale dei centri corticali pei movimenti degli occhi nel cane. *Riv. oto-neuro-oftal., 2:*127, 1925. Abs. *Zentralbl. ges. Ophth., 15:*711, 1926.

881. ROBBINS, A. R.: Divergence paralysis with autopsy report. *Am. J. Ophth., 24:*556, 1941.

882. ROELOFS, C. O., AND VAN DER BEND, J. H.: Betrachtungen und Untersuchungen über den optokinetischen Nystagmus. *Arch. Augenh., 102:*551, 1930.

883. ROSENBACH, P.: Zur Frage über die "epileptogene Eigenschaft" des hinteren Hirnrindengebietes. *Neurol. Centralbl., 8:*249, 1889.

884. ROSENFELD, M.: Der galvanische Nystagmus. (Ein Beitrag zu seiner Physiologie und Pathologie.) *Monatsschr. Psychiat. u. Neurol., 74:*257, 1930.

885. ROSENFELD, M.: Untersuchungen über den calorischen Nystagmus bei Gehirnkranken mit Störungen des Bewusstseins. *Ztschr. ges. Neurol. u. Psychiat., 3:*271, 1910.

886. ROTH, W.: Pseudobulbärparalyse. XVI internat. med. Kong., Budapest. *Neurol. Centralbl., 28:*1126, 1909.

887. ROTH, W. C.: Demonstration von Kranken mit Ophthalmoplegie. *Neurol. Centralbl., 20:*922, 1901.

888. Not used.

889. ROTHFELD, J.: Ueber den Einfluss akuter und der chronischer Alkoholverigiftung auf die vestibularen Reaktionen. *Arb. neurol. Inst. Wien. Univ., 20:*89, 1912-1913.

890. ROTHMANN: Cited by F. Best. Die Augenveränderungen bei den organischen nichtentzündlichen Erkrankungen des Zentralnervensystems, in *Kurzes Handbuch der Ophthalmologie,* edited by F. Schieck and A. Brückner. Berlin, J. Springer, 1931, vol. 6, p. 531.

891. ROTHMANN, M.: The symptoms of cerebellar disease and their significance. XVII internat. Congr. med., London, 1913, Sec. XI Neuropath. p. 59.

892. RUBINO, A., AND QUARTI, M.: Sindrome esoftalmoplegica da aneurisma della carotide interna nel seno cavernoso. *Riv. oto-neuro-oftal., 16:*214, 1939.

893. Rückert, W.: Ueber die tonischen Eigenschaften foetalle Muskeln. *Arch. exper. Path. u. Pharmakol., 150:*221, 1930.

894. Russel, R.: An experimental investigation of eye movements. *J. Physiol., 17:* 1, 1894.

895. Ruttin, E.: Bemerkungen zu der Arbeit "Ueber vertikalen Nystagmus" by S. H. Mygind. *Arch. Ohren-, Nasen- u. Kehlkopfh., 129:*60, 1931. Abs. *Zentralbl. ges. Ophth., 25:*796, 1931.

896. Ruttin, E.: *A Clinical Study of the Serous and Purulent Diseases of the Labyrinth.* New York, Rebman [1914], 232 pp.

897. Ruttin, E.: Ohrbefunde bei Tumoren der mittleren Schädelgrube. *Passow-Schaefer's Beitr. prakt. u. theoret. Hals-, Nasen- u. Ohrenh., 27:*461, 1929. Abs. *Zentralbl. ges. Ophth., 22:*188, 1930.

898. Ruttin, E.: Ueber Lage-Schwindel und Schwindel-Lage, Lage-Nystagmus und Nystagmos-Lage. *Monatsschr. Ohrenh., 70:*257, 455, and 523, 1936. Abs. *Zentralbl. ges. Ophth., 38:*48, 1937.

899. Ruttin, E.: Diagnose der Tumoren der mittleren Schädelgrube. *Monatsschr. Ohrenh., 49:*383, 1915.

900. Sachs, E.: On the structure and functional relations of the optic thalamus. *Brain, 32:*95, 1909.

901. Sager, O., and Voiculescu, V.: Experimental studies on tracts from the cortex to centers for vertical eye movements. Abs., Ophthalmology Sect. XII, *Ercerpta Medica, 5:*2316, 1951.

902. Sahlgren, E., and Hofman-Bang, E.: A case of internuclear ophthalmoplegia. *Acta psychiat., 25:*429, 1950.

903. Sala, G.: Su di un caso di paralisi dello sguardo in alto con rari sintomi associati. *Bull. ocul., 17:*841, 1938.

904. Sandifer, P. H.: Chronic progressive ophthalmoplegia of myopathic origin. *J. Neurol., Neurosurg. & Psychiat., 9:*81, 1946.

905. von Sántha, K.: Zur Symptomatologie der Ponstumoren. Klinisch-anato-mischer Beitrag zur Pathophysiologie der willkürlichen und der vestibular-reflektorischen Augenbewegungen. *Arch. Psychiat., 102:*249, 1934.

906. Sauvineau, C.: Nouvelle théorie pathogénique du nystagmus. *Arch. opht., 29:*416, 1909.

907. Savitsky, N., and Madonick, M. J.: Divergence paralysis and head trauma. *Arch. Neurol. & Psychiat., 53:*135, 1945.

908. Savitsky, N., and Madonick, M. J.: Divergence paralysis associated with tumor of the brain. *Arch. Neurol. & Psychiat., 55:*232, 1946.

909. Savitsky, N., and Rangell, L.: The ocular findings in multiple sclerosis. *Res. Publ. A. Nerv. & Ment. Dis., 28:*403, 1950.

910. Scala, N. P., and Spiegel, E. A.: The mechanism of optokinetic nystagmus. *Tr. Am. Acad. Ophth., 43:*277, 1938.

911. Scala, N. P., and Spiegel, E. A.: Subcortical (passive) optokinetic nystagmus in lesions of the midbrain of the vestibular nuclei. *Confinia neurol., 3:*53, 1940.

912. Schäfer, E. A.: Experiments on the electrical excitation of the visual area of the cerebral cortex in the monkey. *Brain, 11:*1, 1888.

913. Schäfer, E. A.: On electrical excitation of the occipital lobe and adjacent parts of the monkey's brain. *Proc. Roy. Soc., London, 43:*408, 1888.

914. Schäfer, E. A.: On the relative length of the period of latency of the ocular

muscles, when called into action by electrical excitation of the motor and of the sensory regions of the cerebral cortex. *Internat. Monatsschr. Anat. u. Physiol., 5:*149, 1888.

915. SCHALL, L. A.. AND REAGAN, D. J.: Malignant exophthalmos. *Ann. Otol. Rhin. & Laryng., 54:*37, 1945.

916. SCHEIE, H. G.: Site of disturbance of Adie's syndrome. *Arch. Ophth., 24:*225, 1940.

917. SCHENK, V. W. D.: Ein Hemicephalus. *Ztschr. ges. Neurol. u. Psychiat., 142:* 469, 1932.

918. SCHIEFFERDECKER, P.: Eine Eigentümlichkeit im Baue des Augenmuskels, 1904. Abs. *Ztschr. Augenh., 14:*186, 1905.

919. SCHIFF: Cited by H. Oloff and H. Korbsch. Ueber das Hertwig-Magendiesche Phänomenon (Vertikaldivergenz der Augen). *Klin. Monatsbl. Augenh., 77:*618, 1926 (2).

920. SCHILLING, R.: Ein Beitrag zur Funktion des Vestibularapparates. *Arch. Ohren-, Nasen- u. Kehlkopfh., 104:*120, 1919.

921. SCHMELZER, H.: Eine einfache Untersuchungsmethode auf hemianopische Pupillenstarre mittels der Spaltlampe. *Klin. Monatsbl. Augenh., 87:*200, 1931 (2).

922. SCHMERE, E., AND STEINBERG, B.: Separation of diencephalic centres concerned with pupillary motility and ocular tension. *Am. J. Ophth., 33:*1379, 1950.

923. SCHNEIDER, R. C., KAHN, E. A., AND CROSBY, E. C.: Extradural hematoma of posterior fossa. *Neurology, 1:*386, 1951.

924. SCHORCHER, F.: Ueber die Ursachen der einseitigen Pupillenerweiterung beim epi- und subduralen Hämatom. *Deutsche Ztschr. Chir., 248:*420, 1937.

925. SCHOTT, E.: Ueber die Registrierung des Nystagmus und andere Augenbewegungen vermittels des Saitengalvanometers. *Deutsches Arch. klin. Med., 140:*79, 1922.

926. SCHOTT, E.: Ueber die Verwendbarkeit des Sympotoms der Stereoagnosie in der topischen Diagnostik. *Deutsche Ztschr. Nervenh., 80:*357, 1923-1924.

927. SCHUBERT, G.: Notiz über das Rindenfeld für einseitige Augenbewegungen beim Hunde. *Arch. ges. Physiol., 222:*765, 1929.

928. SCHUBERT, G.: Die Leistungen der Augenmuskeln und ihre Steuerung. *Wien. klin. Wchnschr., 63:*632, 1951.

929. SCHUBERT, G., AND BRECHER, G. A.: Labyrinthäre Vertikalabweichungen der Augen beim erwachsenen Menschen. *Ztschr. Hals-, Nasen- u. Ohrenh., 43:* 451, 1938. Abs. *Zentralbl. ges. Ophth., 43:*117, 1939.

930. SCHUSTER, P.: Beiträge zur Pathologie des Thalamus opticus. IV Mitteilung. Motorische Störungen, Thalamushand, mimische und Affektbewegungen, dysarthrische Störungen, vegetative Funkitionen, Blicklähmung, Beziehungen zu den psychischen Funktionen. *Arch. Psychiat., 106:*201, 1937.

931. SCHWANN: Cited by H. Oloff and H. Korbsch. Ueber das Hertwig-Magendiesche Phänomen (Vertikaldivergenz der Augen). *Klin. Monatsbl. Augenh., 77:*618, 1926 (2).

932. SCHWARZ, G. A., AND CHAN-NAO LIU: Chronic progressive external ophthalmoplegia (a clinical and neuropathologic report). *Arch. Neurol. & Psychiat., 71:*31, 1954.

933. SCOBEE, R. G., AND GREEN, E. L.: A center for ocular divergence: does it exist? *Am. J. Ophth., 29:*422, 1946.

934. SECUNDA, L., AND TROWBRIDGE, E. H., JR.: The occurrence of polyneuritis and abnormal pupillary reactions in chronic alcoholism. *Quart. J. Stud. Alcohol,* 2:669, 1942.

935. SEEFELDER, R.: Die Aniridie als eine Entwicklungshemmung der Retina. *Arch. f. Ophth.,* 70:65, 1909.

936. SEIFERTH, L. B.: Commotio cerbri und Lagennystagmus unter Berücksichtigung der übrigen Vestibularis- und Cochlearissymptome. *Arch. Ohren-, Nasen- u. Kehlkopfh.,* 149:241, 1941.

937. SEIFERTH, L. B.: Ueber Lagennystagmus. *München. med. Wchnschr.,* p. 310, 1936 (1). Abs. *Zentralbl. f. d. ges. Ophth.,* 36:291, 1936.

938. SEIFERTH, L. B.: Die Bedeutung des Lagennystagmus für die otologische und neurologische Diagnostik. *Arch. Ohren-, Nasen- u. Kehlkopfh.,* 143:52, 1937.

939. SEMERIA, C.: Studio delle modificazioni del diametre e delle reflettivita pupillare dopo interventi sull'orecchio medio. *Minerva oto-rino-laring.,* 2:490, 1952.

940. SEYFFARTH, H.: The behavior of motor units in voluntary contractions. Cited by Bjork and Kugelberg, 1953.

941. SHARPLEY, F. W.: Vision and illumination in coal mines with reference to miners' nystagmus. *Brit. J. Ophth.,* 20:129, 1936.

942. SHERRINGTON, C. S.: Further experimental note on the correlation of action of antagonistic muscles. *Brit. M. J.,* 1:1218, 1893.

943. SHERRINGTON, C. S.: *The Integrative Action of the Nervous System* (Silliman Memorial Lectures). London, Constable and Co., 1906, 412 pp.

944. SHERRINGTON, C. S.: Observations on sensual role of proprioceptive nerve supply of extrinsic ocular muscles. *Brain, 41:*332, 1918.

945. SHERRINGTON, C. S.: On reciprocal innervation of antagonistic muscles. *Proc. Roy. Soc., London, 60:*414, 1896-1897.

946. SHERRINGTON, C. S.: Antagonistic muscles and reciprocal innervation. *Proc. Roy. Soc., 62:*183, 1897/98.

947. SHERRINGTON, C. S.: On the anatomical constitution of nerves of skeletal muscles; with remarks on recurrent fibres in the ventral spinal nerveroot. *J. Physiol., 17:*211, 1894-1895.

948. SHIGEMATSU, T.: Die Pupilleninnervation des Luysschen Körpers. *Fukuoka acta med., 23:*1751, 1930. Abs. *Zentralbl. ges. Ophth., 26:*150, 1932.

949. SHINOMIYA, M., KAWAHARA, D., AND SAWADA, S.: Upon the relationship of the cerebellum to spontaneous nystagmus. *J. Orient. Med., 15:*93, 1931. Abs. *Zentralbl. ges. Ophth., 26:*838, 1932.

950. SHINOSAKI, T.: Reizversuche zur zentralen Pupilleninnervation am Corpus Luysi. *Ztschr. ges. exper. Med., 66:*171, 1929. Abs. *Zentralbl. ges. Ophth., 22:*538, 1930.

951. SIEBECK, R.: Wahrnehmungsformen bei experimentellen Augenmuskellähmungen. *Deutsch. ophth. Gesell., 58:*24, 1953.

952. SIEBECK, R.: Wahrnehmungsstörung und Störungswahrnehmung bei Augenmuskellähmungen. *von Graefes Arch. Ophth., 155:*26, 1954.

953. SIEBECK, R., AND FREY, R.: Die Wirkungen muskelerschlaffender Mittel auf die Augenmuskeln. *Anaesthesist., 2:*138, 1953.

954. SIEBENS, A., AND WOOLSEY, C. N.: Cortical autonomic center of the eyes on the mesial surface of the frontal lobe in the cat. *Federation Proc., 5:*95, 1946.

955. Siemerling, E.: Ein Fall von gummöser Erkrankung der Hirnbasis mit Beteilung des Chiasma nervorum Opticorum. Ein Beitrag zur Lehre vom Faserverlauf im optischen Leitungsapparat. *Arch. Psychiat., 20:*401, 1888.

956. Silberpfennig, J.: Contributions to the problem of eye movements. III. Disturbances of ocular movements with pseudohemianopsia in frontal lobe tumors. *Confinia neurol., 4:*1, 1941.

957. Simonelli, G., and di Giorgio, A. M.: Il comportamento del nistagmo spontaneo provocato nelle lesioni asimmetriche del cerveletto. *Boll. Soc. ital. biol. sper., 6:*206, 1931. Abs. *Zentralbl. ges. Ophth., 25:*798, 1931.

958. Simmons, A.: Kopfhaltung und Muskeltonus. Klinische Beobachtungen. *Ztschr. ges. Neurol. u. Psychiat., 80:*499, 1923.

959. Sklodowski, J.: Die konjurgierte Augenoszillation im Verlaufe einer Herderkrankung des Gehirns. *Ztschr. ges. Neurol. u. Psych., 31:*166, 1916.

960. Smelser, G. K.: Experimental production of exophthalmos resembling that found in Graves' Disease. *Proc. Soc. Exper. Biol. & Med., 35:*128, 1936.

961. Smith, K. U.: The effect of partial and complete decortication upon the extinction of optic nystagmus. *J. Gen. Psychol., 25:*3, 1941.

962. Smith, K. U.: The neurologic centers concerned in optic nystagmus. *Am. J. Physiol., 126:*631, 1939

963. Smith, W. K.: Ocular responses elicited by electrical stimulation of the cerebral cortex. *Anat. Rec., 64* (Suppl.):45, 1936.

964. Smyth, G. E., and Stern, K.: Tumours of the thalamus. A clinico-pathological study. *Brain, 61:*339, 1938.

965. Snell, A. C.: The optokinetoscope. *Tr. Am. Acad. Ophth., 44:*396, 1939.

966. Snider, R. S.: Recent contributions to anatomy and physiology of cerebellum. *Arch. Neurol. & Psychiat., 64:*196, 1950.

967. Snider, R. S., and Stowell, A.: Receiving areas of tactile, auditory, and visual systems in cerebellum. *J. Neurophysiol., 7:*331, 1944.

968. Sommer, J.: Vertikaler Nystagmus als einziges Krankheitsymptom. *Monatsschr. Ohrenh., 62:*498, 1928.

969. Soriano, V., and Fulton, J. F.: Interrelation between anterior lobe of the cerebellum and the motor area. *Federation Proc., 6:*207, 1947.

970. Sorsby, A.: Latent nystagmus. *Brit. J. Ophth., 15:*1, 1931.

971. Souders, B. F.: Hysterical convergence spasm. *Arch. Ophth., 27:*361, 1942.

972. Spaeth, E. B.: A classification for congenital ptosis. *Arch. Ophth., 29:*164, 1943.

973. Spiegel, E. A.: Experimentalstudien am Nervensystem. V. Mitteilung. Ueber den Erregungszustand der medullären Zentren nach doppelseitiger Labyrinthauschaltung. (Vestibulare Ausfallerscheinungen nach einseitiger Verletzung der Vestibulariskerne trotz Labyrinthmangels by Ginichi Sato.) *Arch. ges. Physiol., 215:*106, 1927.

974. Spiegel, E. A.: Role of vestibular nuclei in cortical innervation of the eye muscles. *Arch. Neurol. & Psychiat., 29:*1084, 1933.

975. Spiegel, E. A., and Aronson, L.: Continuous stimulation of the labyrinth with sustained nystagmus. *Arch. Otolaryng., 17:*311, 1933.

976. Spiegel, E. A., and Démetriades, T. D.: Die Zentrali Kompensation des Labyrinthverlustes. *Arch. ges. Physiol., 210:*215, 1925.

977. Spiegel, E. A., and Hunsicker, W. C., Jr.: The conduction of cortical impulses to the autonomic system. *J. Nerv. & Ment. Dis., 83:*252, 1936.

978. Spiegel, E. A., and Nagasaka, G.: Experimentalstudien am Nervensystem;

über die Beziehung des Pupillenreflexbogens zum vorderen Vierhügel. *Arch. ges. Physiol., 215:*120, 1926.

979. SPIEGEL, E. A., AND PRICE, J. B.: Origin of quick component of labyrinthine nystagmus. *Arch. Otolaryng., 30:*576, 1939.

980. SPIEGEL, E. A., AND SCALA, N. P.: The cortical innervation of ocular movements. *Arch. Ophth., 16:*967, 1936.

981. SPIEGEL, E. A., AND SCALA, N. P.: Ocular disturbances associated with experimental lesions of the mesencephalic central gray matter, with special reference to vertical ocular movements. *Arch. Ophth., 18:*614, 1937.

982. SPIEGEL, E. A., AND SCALA, N. P.: Positional nystagmus in cerebellar lesions. *J. Neurophysiol., 5:*247, 1942.

983. SPIEGEL, E. A., AND SCALA, N. P.: Effects of quadrigeminal lesions upon labyrinthine nystagmus. *Confinia neurol., 7:*68, 1946.

984. SPIEGEL, E. A., AND SOMMER, I.: *Neurology of the Eye, Ear, Nose, and Throat.* New York, Grune & Stratton, 1944.

985. SPIEGEL, E. A., AND TAKANO, K.: Zur Analyse der vom Streifenhügel erhaltener Reizwirkung. *Ztschr. ges. Neurol. u. Psychiat., 118:*429, 1929.

986. SPIEGEL, E. A., AND TESCHLER, L.: Experimentalstudien am Nervensystem. XII. Mitt. Ueber die Beziehung der Blickbahn zu dem Vestibulariskernen. *Arch. ges. Physiol., 222:*359, 1929.

987. SPIEGEL, E. A., AND TOKAY, L.: Experimentalstudien am Nervensystem. XVI. Mitt. Der Einfluss labyrinthären und corticaler Reizung auf die Augenstellung nach Durchschneidung des hinteren Längsbündels. *Arb. neurol. Inst. Wien. Univ., 32:*138, 1930. Abs. *Zentralbl. ges. Ophth., 25:*406, 1931.

988. SPIELMEYER, W.: Veränderungen des Nervensystems nach Stovainanästhesie. *München. med. Wchnschr., 56:*1629, 1908.

989. SPILLER, W. G.: The importance in clinical diagnosis of paralysis of associated movements of the eyeballs, especially of upward and downward associated movements. *J. Nerv. & Ment. Dis., 32:*417, 1905.

990. SPILLER, W. G.: The oculopupillary fibers of the sympathetic system: Division of the first thoracic root in man. *Am. J. M. Sc., 159:*325, 1920.

991. SPILLER, W. G.: Ophthalmoplegia internuclearis anterior; a case with necropsy. *Brain, 47:*345, 1924.

992. SPILLER, W. G.: Subcortical epilepsy. *Brain, 50:*171, 1927.

993. SPITZER, A.: Anatomie und Physiologie der zentralen Bahnen des Vestibularis. *Arb. neurol. Inst. Wien. Univ., 25:*423, 1924.

994. STEINERT, [H.], AND BIELSCHOWSKY, [A.]: Ein Beitrag zur Physiologie und Pathologie der vertikalen Blickbewegungen. *München. med. Wchnschr., 53:* 1613, 1906.

995. DE STELLA, H.: Deux signes importants du syndrome cérébelleux pour le diagnostic de l'abcès cérébelleux: Les troubles du language et les paralysies oculaires. *Ann. oto-laryng., 6:*535, 1938. Abs. *Zentralbl. ges. Ophth., 42:*234, 1939.

996. STENGEL, E.: Zur Frage der Herdlokalisation bei spontanem Vertikalnystagmus. *Ztschr. ges. Neurol. u. Psychiat., 153:*417, 1935.

997. STENVERS, H. W.: On the optic (opto-kinetic, opto-motorial) nystagmus. *Acta oto-laryng., 4:*545, 1925.

998. STENVERS, [H. W.]: Sur le nystagmus opto-kinétique. *Rev. oto-neuro-opht., 5:*917, 1927.

999. STENVERS, H. W.: Ueber die klinische Bedeutung des optischen Nystagmus für die cerebrale Diagnostik. *Schweiz. Arch. Neurol. u. Psychiat.*, *14:*279, 1924. Abs. *Zentralbl. ges. Ophth.*, *13:*261, 1925.

1000. STERN, F:. Ueber psychische Zwangsvorgänge und ihre Entstehung bei encephalitischen Blickkrämpfen, mit Bemerkungen über die Genese der encaphalitischen Blickkrämpfe. *Arch. Psychiat.*, *81:*522, 1927.

1001. STIEREN, E.: Congenital absence of both inferior recti muscles. *Am. Med.*, *5:* 581, 1903; cited by G. Stevens, *A Treatise on the Motor Apparatus of the Eyes.* Philadelphia, F. A. Davis, 1906, p. 487.

1002. STILL, G. F.: Head-nodding with nystagmus in infancy. *Lancet*, *2:*207, 1906.

1003. STILL, G. F.: On head-rolling and other curious movements in children. *Clin. J.*, *29:*87, 1906.

1004. STRAUSS, H.: Ueber die hirnlokalisatoriche Bedeutung des einseitigen Ausfalls des optokinetischen Nystagmus und der hemianopischen Aufmerksamkeitsschwäche. *Ztschr. ges. Neurol. u. Psychiat.*, *143:*427, 1933.

1005. STRICKROOT, F. L., SCHAEFFER, R. L., AND BERGO, H. L.: Myasthenia gravis occurring in infant born of myasthenic mother. *J.A.M.A.*, *120:*1207, 1942.

1006. SUNDERLAND, S.: The projection of the cerebral cortex on the pons and cerebellum in the macaque monkey. *J. Anat.*, *74:*201, 1940.

1007. SUNDERLAND, S.: Mechanism responsible for changes in the pupil unaccompanied by disturbances of extraocular muscle function. *Brit. J. Ophth.*, *36:*638, 1952.

1008. SUNDERLAND, S., AND BRADLEY, K. G.: Disturbances of oculomotor function accompanying extradural haemorrhage. *J. Neurol., Neurosurg. & Psychiat.*, *16:* 35, 1953.

1009. SUNDERLAND, S., AND HUGHES, E. S. R.: The pupillo-constrictor pathway and the nerves to the ocular muscles in man. *Brain*, *69:*301, 1946.

1010. SZENTÁGOTHAI, J.: Die innere Gliederung des oculomotoriuskernes. *Arch. Psychiat.*, *115:*126, 1942.

1011. TAIT, J., AND MCNALLY, W. J.: An analysis of the limb responses to semicircular canal stimulation in the frog. *Tr. Am. Acad. Ophth.*, *34:*241, 1929.

1012. TEN CATE, J.: Akustische und optische Reaktionen der Katzen nach teilweisen und totalen Exstirpationen des Neopalliums. *Arch. néerl. physiol.*, *19:*191, 1934.

1013. TEN CATE, J., AND VAN HERK, H. W. H.: Beobachtungen an Kaninchen nach Exstirpationen im Neopallium. *Arch. néerl. physiol.*, *18:*337, 1933.

1014. TER BRAAK, J. W. G.: Untersuchungen über optokinetischen Nystagmus. *Arch. néerl. physiol.*, *21:*309, 1936.

1015. TEN DOESSCHATE, J.: Can amblyopia nystagmus be elicited in subjects without amblyopia. *Nederl. tijdschr. geneesk.*, *96:*1228, 1952. Abs., Ophthalmology Sect. XII, *Excerpta Medica*, *7:*817, 1953.

1016. TERGAST, P.: Ueber das Verhältniss von der Nerv und Muskel. *Arch. mikr. Anat.*, *9:*36, 1873.

1017. TERRIEN, F.: *Semeiologie Oculaire: Statique et Dynamique Occularies.* Paris, Masson, 1928, 224 pp.

1018. TICHOMIROFF, P. E.: Zur Frage der ophthalmoplegischen Migräne. Sbornik v osn. sorok. nauc. dejat. sals. dejat. nauki M. I. Averbach p. 481, 1935. Abs. *Zentralbl. ges. Ophth.*, *36:*598, 1936.

1019. TILING: Cited by C. Wernicke. I. Herderkrankung des unteren Scheitelläppchens. *Arch. Psychiat., 20:*243, 1889.

1020. TOPOLANSKI, A.: Das Verhalten der Augenmuskeln bei centraler Reizung. Das Coordinationscentrum und die Bahnen für coordinirte Augenbewegungen. *Arch. f. Ophth., 46:*452, 1898.

1021. TORDA, C., AND WOLFF, H. G.: Effect of blood serum from patients with myasthenia gravis on synthesis of acetylocholine in vitro. *J. Clin. Investigation, 23:*649, 1944.

1022. TORDA, C., AND WOLFF, H. G.: Effect of ether extract of thymus and pancreas on synthesis of acetylcholine. *Proc. Soc. Exper. Biol. & Med., 57:*69, 1944.

1023. TORDA, C., AND WOLFF, H. G.: Release of curare-like agent from healthy muscle and its bearing on myasthenia gravis. *Proc. Soc. Exper. Biol. & Med., 58:* 242, 1945.

1024. TOSELLI, C., AND MENZIO, P.: Fenomeni di eteroforia di origine vestibolare. *Bol. Soc. ital. biol. sper., 28:*349, 1952.

1025. TOURNIER, C.: Double hémiplégie, trismus persistant; syndrome de paralysie glosso-labio-faciale pseudobulbaire d'origine cérébrale; ophthalmoplégie ne portant que sur les mouvements voluntaires avec conservation des mouvements réflexes. *Rev. méd., Paris, 18:*671, 1898.

1026. TOZER, F. M., AND SHERRINGTON, C. S.: Receptors and afferents of the third, fourth, and sixth cranial nerves. *Proc. Roy. Soc., London,* s. B. *82:*450, 1910.

1027. TRETHEWIE, E. R., AND WRIGHT, R. D.: Acetylcholine synthesis and myasthenia gravis. *Australian & New Zealand J. Surg., 12:*244, 1944.

1028. TRONCELLITI, E. T.: Myasthenia gravis in a 9-year-old boy. *Arch. Neurol. & Psychiat., 59:*546, 1948.

1029. TSCHERMAK, A.: Augenbewegungen, in *Handbuch der Normalen und Pathologischen Physiologie,* edited by A. Bethe, G. v. Bergmann, G. Embden and A. Ellinger. Berlin, J. Springer, 1931, vol. 12, pt. 2, p. 1001.

1030. TSCHERMAK, A.: Cited by H. Oloff and H. Korbsch. Ueber das Hertwig-Magendiesche Phänomen (Vertikaldivergenz der Augen). *Klin. Monatsbl. Augenh., 77:*618, 1926 (2).

1031. TSCHIRREN, B., AND WIESINGER, K.: Untersuchungen über den zeitlichen Verlauf des konsensuellen. Pupillenreflexes beim Übergang in die Höhe. *Helvet. physiol. et pharmacol. acta, 6:*554, 1948.

1032. TSENG, H. C., AND KU, Y. C.: Paralysis of extraocular muscles following spinal anaesthesia. *Chinese M. J., 68:*81, 1950. Abs., Ophthalmology Sect. XII, *Excerpta Medica, 5:*886, 1951.

1033. TSUCHIDA, U.: Ueber die Ursprungskerne der Augenbewegungsnerven. Arb. a. d. hirnanat. Inst. in Zurich. Wiesbaden, J. F. Bermann, 1906, Part 2, p. 1. Abs. *Jahresb. Ophth., 37:*5, 1906.

1034. VAN DER TWEEL, L. H., AND BLEEKER, G. M.: Recording pupillograph of simple design. *Brit. J. Ophth., 35:*632, 1951.

1035. UFFENORDE, [W.]: Spontan auftretender Spätnystagmus bei Ohrnormalen. *Beitr. Anat., Physiol., Path. u. Therap. Ohres, 18:*37, 1922. Abs. *Zentralbl. ges. Ophth., 8:*326, 1923.

1036. UFFENORDE, W.: Zur Entstehungsweise des Nystagmus bei der thermischen Prüfung des Ohrlabyrinths. *Sitzungsb. Gesellsch. z. Beförd. ges. Naturw. Marburg, 62:*247, 1927.

1037. UNDRIC, V.: Zur Frage über die nystagmatischen Bewegungen isolierte Augen-muskeln. *Russk. oto-laring., 21:*5, 1928. Abs. *Zentralbl. Hals-, Nasen- u. Ohrenh., 12:*535, 1928.

1038. UNDRITZ, W.: Ueber den Einfluss verschiedener Versuchsbedingungen auf den Drehnystagmus und über die Bedeutung der kontralateralen Verbindungs-fasern des N. vestibularis. *Ztschr. Hals-, Nasen- u. Ohrenh., 19:*444, 1928. Abs. *Zentralbl. ges. Ophth., 20:*655, 1929.

1039. URBANEK: Zur Ätiologie der Abducensparese. *Ztschr. Augenh., 62:*399, 1927.

1040. URIST, M. J.: Simulated divergence paralysis. *Arch. Ophth., 48:*581, 1952.

1041. URY, B., AND GELLHORN, E.: Role of the sympathetic system in reflex dilatation of pupil. *J. Neurophysiol., 2:*268, 1939.

1042. VANDERGRIFT, G. W., AND LOSEY, R. R.: A case of paralysis of convergence and paresis of accommodation. *Arch. Ophth., 51:*405, 1922.

1043. VELHAGEN, K.: Heterophoria unter der Bedingungen des Hohenflüges. *Luftfahrt. med. Abhandl., 1:*344, 1937.

1044. VELZEBOER, C. M. J.: Bilateral cortical hemianopsia and optokinetic nystagmus. *Nederl. tijdschr. geneesk, 96:*59, 1952. Abs., Ophthalmology Sect XII, *Excerpta Medica, 6:*1259, 1952.

1045. VERHAGE, J. W. C.: Eine klinische Studie über den Nystagmus latens. *Ophthalmologica, 103:*209, 1942.

1046. VERHOEFF, F. H.: Cycloduction. *Tr. Am. Ophth. Soc., 32:*208, 1934.

1047. VERHOEFF, F. H.: Hyperphoria tests based on a new principle. *Arch. Ophth., 22:*743, 1939.

1048. VERHOEFF, F. H.: Letter to the Editor. *Am. J. Ophth., 25:*227, 1942.

1049. VERHOEFF, F. H.: A new theory of binocular vision. *Arch. Ophth., 13:*151, 1935.

1050. VERHOEFF, F. H.: Occlusion hypertropia. *Arch. Ophth., 25:*780, 1941.

1051. VERHOEFF, F. H.: Recurring attacks of concomitant exotropia, each followed by transient esotropia; migraine the probable cause. *Arch. Ophth., 30:*727, 1943.

1052. VERHOEFF, F. H.: Problems concerning convergence. *Tr. Am. Acad. Ophth., 52:*15, 1947.

1053. VERHOEFF, F. H.: Unpublished.

1054. VERSTEEGH, C.: Ergebnisse partieller Labyrinthexstirpation bei Kaninchen. *Acta oto-laryng., 11:*393, 1927.

1055. VILA-CORO, A.: Hinterer Ansatz der Muskeln der Augenhöhle. *Klin. Monatsbl. Augenh., 96:*466, 1936(1).

1056. VOGEL, H.: Der sogenannte Gradenigosche Symptomenkomplex. Kritisches Sammelreferat. *Internat. Zentralbl. Ohrenh. u. Rhino-Laryng., 18:*293 and *19:* 1, 1921. Abs. *Zentralbl. ges. Ophth., 6:*450, 1922.

1057. VOGT, A.: Zwei Fälle von Kupferkatarakt, der eine mit Chalkosis retinae (letztere Beobachtung gemeinsam mit Dr. Knüsel). *Klin. Monatsbl. Augenh., 69:*119, 1922(2).

1058. VOGT, C., AND VOGT, O.: Zur Kenntnis der elektrisch erregbaren Hirnrinden-gebiete bei den Säugetieren. *J. Psychol. u. Neurol., 8:*277, 1906-7.

1059. VORIS, H. C., ADSON, A. W., AND MOERSCH, F. P.: Tumors of the frontal lobe. Clinical observations in a series verified microscopically. *J.A.M.A., 104:*93, 1935.

1060. VOSS: Cited by W. Klestadt. Symptomatologie der Erkrankungen des N. VIII einschliesslich Leitung im Hirnstamm, in *Handbuch der Neurologie* edited by O. Bumke and O. Foerster. Berlin, J. Springer, 1936, vol. 4, p. 359.

1061. VULPIAN: Cited by H. Oloff and H. Korbsch. Ueber das Hertwig-Magendiesche Phänomen (Vertikaldivergenz der Augen). *Klin. Monatsbl. Augenh., 77:* 618, 1926(2).

1062. WAGGONER, R. W., AND BOYD, D. A.: Sex-linked hereditary nystagmus. *Am. J. Ophth., 25:*177, 1942.

1063. WALKER, C. B.: Topical diagnostic value of the hemiopic pupillary reaction and the Wilbrand hemianopic prism phenomenon; with a new method of performing the latter. *J.A.M.A., 61:*1152, 1913.

1064. WALKER, E. A., AND WEAVER, T. A., JR.: Ocular movements from the occipital lobe in the monkey. *J. Neurophysiol., 3:*353, 1940.

1065. WALKER, M. B.: Treatment of myasthenia gravis with physostigmine. *Lancet, 1:*1200, 1934.

1066. WALKER, M. B.: Case showing effect of prostigmine on myasthenia gravis. *Proc. Roy. Soc. Med., 28:*759, 1935.

1067. WALKER, M. B.: Myasthenia gravis: case in which fatigue of forearm muscles could induce paralysis of extraocular muscles. *Proc. Roy. Soc. Med., 31:* 722, 1938.

1069. WALLENBERG, [A.]: Beitrag zur Lehre vom Ursprung des Levator palpebrae superioris und seinen angeblichen Beziehungen zur Grosshirnrinde. *Neurol. Centralbl.,* No. 8, 1910. Abs. *Jahresb. Ophth., 41:*7, 1910.

1069. WALLENBERG, A.: Neuere Fortschritte in der topischen Diagnostik des Pons und der Oblongata. *Deutsche Ztschr. Nervenh., 41:*8, 1911.

1070. WALLER, W. H., AND BARRIS, R. W.: Pupillary inequality in the cat following experimental lesions of the occipital cortex. *Am. J. Physiol., 120:*144, 1937.

1071. WALSH, F. B.: Supranuclear lesions as they affect ocular movements. *Arch. Ophth., 27:*1026, 1942.

1072. WALSH, F. B.: Myasthenia gravis and its ocular signs: a review. *Am. J. Ophth., 28:*13, 1945.

1073. WALSH, F. B.: Ocular signs of thrombosis of the intracranial venous sinuses. *Arch. Ophth., 17:*46, 1937.

1074. WALSH, F. B.: *Clinical Neuro-Ophthalmology.* Baltimore, Williams & Wilkins, 1947.

1075. WALSH, F. B.: Ocular signs of intracranial saccular aneurisms. *Tr. Ophth. Soc. Australia, 8:*18, 1948.

1076. WALSH, F. B.: Myasthenia gravis. *Tr. Ophth. Soc. Australia, 8:*39, 1948.

1077. WALSH, F. B., AND KING, A. B.: Ocular signs of intracranial saccular aneurysms; experimental work on collateral circulation through ophthalmic artery. *Arch. Ophth., 27:*1, 1942.

1078. WALSH, F. B., AND SLOAN, L. L.: Results of cervical sympathectomy in pigmentary degeneration of the retina. *Arch. Ophth., 14:*699, 1933.

1079. WALSHE, F. M. R.: On the pathogenesis of diphtheritic paralysis. *Quart. J. Med., 11:*191, 1917-1918.

1080. WALSHE, F. M. R.: On the pathogenesis of diphtheritic paralysis. Part II. Clinical observations on the paralysis of faucial and extra-faucial diphtheria, with an analysis of thirty cases following skin and wound infections. *Quart. J. Med., 12:*14, 1918-1919.

1081. WANG, G., LU, T., AND LAU, T.: Pupillary constriction from cortical stimulation. *Chinese J. Physiol., 5:*205, 1931. Abs. *Zentralbl. ges. Ophth., 26:*739, 1932.

1082. WARD, A. A., JR., AND REED, H. L.: Mechanism of pupillary dilatation elicited by cortical stimulation. *J. Neurophysiol., 9:*329, 1946.

1083. WARTENBERG, R.: Associated movements in the oculomotor and facial muscles. *Arch. Neurol. & Psychiat., 55:*439, 1946.

1084. WARWICK, R.: A study of retrograde degeneration in the oculomotor nucleus of the rhesus monkey, with a note on a method of recording its distribution. *Brain, 73:*532, 1950.

1085. WEEKERS, R.: Pupille tonique provoquee par injection retrobulbaire d'alcohol. Contribution a la pathogenie du syndrome d'Adie. *Ann. ocul., 181:*193, 1948.

1086. WEHRLI, E.: Ueber sechs Fälle von latentem Rücknystagmus (Nystagmus saccadé Javal). *Klin. Monatsbl. Augenh., 56:*444, 1916(1).

1087. WEINSTEIN, E. A., AND BENDER, M. B.: Pupillodilator reactions to sciatic and diencephalic stimulation; comparative study in cat and monkey. *J. Neurophysiol., 4:*44, 1941.

1088. WEINSTEIN, E. A., AND DOLGER, H.: External ocular muscle palsies occurring in diabetes mellitus. *Arch. Neurol. & Psychiat., 60:*597, 1948.

1089. WEISINGER, K., AND PLÜSS, H. R.: Untersuchungen mit einer photographischen Methode. *Helvet. physiol. et pharmacol. acta, 6:*528, 1948.

1090. WEISINGER, K., AND WERNER, H.: Die Pupillenweite und ihre Schwankung beim Übergang ins Hochgebirge. II Teil Untersuchungen mit eimem Doppelbild-Pupillometer. *Helvet. physiol. et pharmacol. acta, 6:*540, 1948.

1091. WELLS, H. S.: The demonstration of tonic neck and labyrinthine reflexes and positive heliotropic responses in normal human subjects. *Science, 99:*36, 1944.

1092. WERNICKE, C.: Ein Fall von Ponserkrankung. *Arch. Psychiat., 7:*513, 1877.

1093. WERNICKE, C.: I. Herderkrankung des unteren Scheitelläppchens. *Arch. Psychiat., 20:*243, 1889.

1094. WERNICKE, C.: Ueber hemiopische Pupillenreaktion. *Fortschr. Med., 1:*49, 1883.

1095. WERNICKE, C.: *Lehrbuch der Gehirnkrankheiten.* Kassel and Berlin, T. Fischer, 1881-3.

1096. WERNICKE, O.: Ueber Lähmung der Seitwärtswender. *Arch. Augenh., 42:*183, 1901.

1097. WERNØE, T. B.: Eisenbahnnystagmus. *Bibliot. f. laeger, 114:*1, 1922.

1098. WERNØE, T. B.: Eisenbahnnystagmus. *Ugesk. laeger, 83:*1516, 1921. Abs. *Zentralbl. ges. Ophth., 7:*252, 1922.

1099. WERNØE, T. B.: Ueber die Bedeutung des Thalamus opticus als Zentraler sensorischer Einstellungsapparat sowie als Durchgangslied der Willensbahnen, besonders derjenigen Bahnen, deren Abbrechung die motorische Aphasie bedingt. *Bibliot. laeger, 114:*29, and 69, 1922. Abs. *Zentralbl. ges. Ophth., 8:* 248, 1923.

1100. WEST, L. C.: Coincident inheritance of strabismus and nystagmus. *J. Hered., 30:*496, 1939.

1101. WESTHEIMER, G.: Mechanism of saccadic eye movements. *Arch. Ophth., 52:* 710, 1954.

1102. WESTHEIMER, G.: A case of voluntary nystagmus. *Ophthalmologica, 128:*300, 1954.

1103. WESTPHAL, C.: Ueber einen Fall von chronischer progressiver Lähmung der Augensmuskeln (Ophthalmoplegia externa) nebst Beschreibung von Ganglienzellengruppen im Bereiche des Oculomotoriuskerns. *Arch. Psychiat., 18:*846, 1887. Abs. *Jahresb. Ophth., 18:*71, 1887.

1104. WHITE, J. W.: Paralysis of the superior rectus and inferior oblique muscles of the same eye. *Arch. Ophth., 27:*366, 1942.

1105. WHITNALL, S. E.: *The Anatomy of the Human Orbit, and Accessory Organs of Vision,* 2nd ed. London, Humphrey Milford, Oxford, 1932.

1106. WIEDERSHEIM, O.: Ueber Photonystagmographie. *Klin. Monatsbl. Augenh., 86:*32, 1931(1).

1107. VAN WIJHE, J. W.: Ueber die Mesodermsegmente und der Entwickelung der Nerven des Selachierkopfes. *Verhandl. Akad. Wetensch., 22:*1883 (50 pp.).

1108. WILBRAND, H.: Ueber die diagnostische Bedeutung des Prismenversuches zwischen der basalen und der supranucleären homonymen Hemianopsie. *Ztschr. Augenh., 1:*125, 1899.

1109. WILBRAND, H., AND SAENGER, A.: *Die Neurologie des Auges; ein Handbuch für Nerven- und Augenärzte.* Wiesbaden, J. F. Bermann, 1900, vol. 1, Parts 1 and 2, 696 pp.

1110. WILBRAND, H., AND SAENGER, A.: *Die Neurologie des Auges; ein Handbuch für Nerven- und Augenärzte.* Wiesbaden, J. F. Bergmann, 1904, vol. 3, Part 1, 474 pp.

1111. WILBRAND, H., AND SAENGER, A.: *Die Neurologie des Auges; ein Handbuch für Nerven- und Augenärzte.* Munich, J. F. Bergmann, 1921, vol. 8, 480 pp.

1112. WILBRAND, H., AND SAENGER, A.: *Die Neurologie des Auges in ihren heutigen Stande.* Munich, J. F. Bergmann, 1927, Part 1, 288 pp.

1113. WILKE, G.: Zur Frage des Nystagmus retractorius. Zugleich ein Beitrag zur Pathophysiologie der vestibulo-okulären Reflexe. *Arch. Psychiat., 113:*388, 1941.

1114. WILKINSON, H. J.: The innervation of striated muscle. *M. J. Australia, 2:*768, 1929.

1115. WILSON, A., MAW, G. A., AND GEOGHEGAN, H.: Cholinesterase activity of blood and muscle in myasthenia gravis. *Quart. J. Med., 20:*13, 1951.

1116. WILSON, A., AND STONER, H. B.: Myasthenia gravis: consideration of its causation in study of 14 cases. *Quart. J. Med., 13:*1, 1944.

1117. WILSON, J. G., AND PIKE, F. H.: The mechanism of labyrinthine-nystagmus and its modifications by lesions in the cerebellum and cerebrum. *Arch. Int. Med., 15:*31, 1915.
*J. Neurol. & Psychopath., 2:*1, 1921.

1118. WILSON, S. A. K.: Some problems in neurology. I. The Argyll-Robertson pupil.

1119. WILSON, S. A. K., AND GERSTLE, M., JR.: Argyll-Robertson sign in mesencephalic tumors. *Arch. Neurol. & Psychiat., 22:*9, 1929.

1120. WILSON, S. A. K., AND RUDOLF, G. DE M.: Case of mesencephalic tumor with double Argyll-Robertson pupil. *J. Neurol. & Psychopath., 3:*140, 1922.

1121. WINCKLER: Cited by P. van Gehuchten. Syndrome de Parinaud. Etude anatomique. *J. belge de neurol. et de psychiat., 40:*126, 1940.

1122. WINCKLER, G.: L'innervation sensitive et motrice des muscles extrinsèques de l'oeil chez quelques ongulés. *Arch. anat., histol. et embryol., 23:*219, 1937.

1123. WIRTHS, M.: Beitrag zum klinischen Bilde der assoziierten Blicklähmung mit besonderer Berücksichtigung des vestibulären und optischen Nystagmus. *Ztschr. Augenh., 26:*318, 1911.

1124. WISHART, D. E. S.: Neuro-otological examination in eleven verified cases of brain tumour. *J. Laryng. & Otol., 38:*109, 1923.

1125. WITTMAACK, K.: Ueber Veränderungen im inneren Ohre nach Rotationen. *Verhandl. deutsch. otol. Gesellsch., 18:*150, 1909.

1126. WOHLFAHRT, G.: Ueber das Vorkommen verschiedener Arten von Muskelfasern in der Skeletmuskulatur des Menschen und einiger Säugetiere. *Acta psychiat. et neurol.,* Suppl. 12:1, 1937.

1127. WOLF, E.: On the relation between measurements of intensity discrimination and of visual acuity in the honey bee. *J. Gen. Physiol., 16:*773, 1933.

1128. WÖLFFLIN, E.: Zur Frage der experimentellen Halssympathikusreizung. *Klin. Monatsbl. Augenh., 68:*460, 1922(2).

1129. WOLTER, J. R.: Die nervenendigungen in der äusseren augenmuskulatur. *Berl. deutsch. ophth. gesellsch., 57:*285, 1951.

1130. WOLTER, J. R.: Ueber Nervenendungen in der äusseren augenmuskulatur. *Acta neuroveg., 4:*342, 1952.

1131. WOLTER, J. R.: Die Gefässnerven in der äusseren, quergestreiften Augenmuskulatur des Menschen. *Acta neuroveg., 5:*257, 1953.

1132. WOOLLARD, H. H.: The innervation of the ocular muscles. *J. Anat., 65:*215, 1930-1931.

1133. WOOLLARD, H. H.: The innerveation of the ocular muscles and the mesencephalic root of the V nerve. *Tr. Ophth. Soc. U. Kingdom, 57:*84, 1937.

1134. WOOLLARD, H. H.: The innervation of voluntary muscle. *J. Anat., 61:*498, 1926-1927.

1135. WORMSER, P.: Die Reaktion der Pupille auf Mydriatica nach Unterbrechung der sympathischen Pupillenbahn. *Ophthalmologica,* Suppl. 33, 1948.

1136. WOTZILKA, G.: Ein neuer, klinisch verwendbarer Nystagmograph. *Ztschr. Hals-, Nasen- u. Ohrenh., 8:*93, 1924. Abs. *Zentralbl. ges. Ophth., 13:*237, 1925.

1137. WRIGHT, E. S.: Bilateral ophthalmoplegia in acute anterior poliomyelitis. *Am. J. Ophth., 30:*1294, 1947.

1138. WRIGHT, E. S.: Extraocular muscle paralysis from spinal injection of pantopaque. *California Med., 71:*214, 1949.

1139. YASUDA, H.: Ueber den Einfluss der Analeptica und Narkotica auf den experimentellen Nystagmus. *Fukuoka acta med., 31:*191, 1938. Abs. *Zentralbl. ges. Ophth., 42:*69, 1939.

1140. ZAVALIA, A. U.: Paralisis bilateral congenita del musculo oblique inferior. *Arch. oftal. Buenos Aires, 23:*1, 1948.

1141. ZIBA, S.: Ueber die Beziehungen des dorsalen Längsbündels zur Labyrinthären Ophthalmostatik. *Arch. Ohrenh., 86:*189, 1911.

INDEX

This Book

Neurology of the
Ocular Muscles

(Second Edition)

By

DAVID G. COGAN, M.D.

was set, printed and bound by George Banta Company, Inc. of Menasha, Wisconsin. The engravings were made by Northwestern Engraving Company of Menasha, Wisconsin. The page trim size is 6 × 9 inches. The type page is 26 × 43 picas. The type face is Linotype Baskerville, set 11 point on 13 point. The text paper is 70 lb. White Woodbine Folding Enamel. The cover is Holliston Sturdite, Q 18, Color 78249, Grain T. Roller, Finish A.

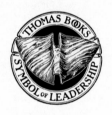

With **THOMAS BOOKS** *careful attention is given to all details of manufacturing and design. It is the Publisher's desire to present books that are satisfactory as to their physical qualities and artistic possibilities and appropriate for their particular use.* **THOMAS BOOKS** *will be true to those laws of quality that assure a good name and good will.*